PRAISE FOR

The 4-Hour Workweek

"This is a whole new ball game. Highly recommended." —Dr. Stewart D. Friedman, adviser to Jack Welch and former director of the Work/Life Integration Program at the Wharton School, University of Pennsylvania

"It's about time this book was written. It is a long-overdue manifesto for the mobile lifestyle, and Tim Ferriss is the ideal ambassador. This will be huge." —Jack Canfield, co-creator of *Chicken Soup for the Soul*®, 100+ million copies sold

"Stunning and amazing. From mini-retirements to outsourcing your life, it's all here. Whether you're a wage slave or a Fortune 500 CEO, this book will change your life!" —Phil Town, *New York Times* bestselling author of *Rule #1*

"*The 4-Hour Workweek* is a new way of solving a very old problem: just how can we work to live and prevent our lives from being all about work? A world of infinite options awaits those who would read this book and be inspired by it!" —Michael E. Gerber, founder and chairman of E-Myth Worldwide and the world's #1 small business guru

"Timothy has packed more lives into his 29 years than Steve Jobs has in his 51." —Tom Foremski, journalist and publisher of SiliconValleyWatcher.com

"If you want to live life on your own terms, this is your blueprint." —Mike Maples, co-founder of Motive Communications (IPO to $260M/£162M market cap) and founding executive of Tivoli (sold to IBM for $750M/£468M)

"Thanks to Tim Ferriss, I have more time in my life to travel, spend time with family, and write book blurbs. This is a dazzling and highly useful work." —A. J. Jacobs, editor-at-large of *Esquire* magazine and author of *The Know-It-All*

"Tim is Indiana Jones for the digital age. I've already used his advice to go spearfishing on remote islands and ski the best hidden slopes of Argentina. Simply put, do what he says and you can live like a millionaire." —Albert Pope, derivatives specialist at UBS World Headquarters

"Reading this book is like putting a few zeros on your income. Tim brings lifestyle to a new level—listen to him!" —Michael D. Kerlin, McKinsey & Company consultant to Bush-Clinton Katrina Fund and a J. William Fulbright Scholar

"Part scientist and part adventure hunter, Tim Ferriss has created a road map for an entirely new world. I devoured this book in one sitting—I have seen nothing like it." —Charles L. Brock, chairman and CEO of Brock Capital Group; former CFO, COO, and general counsel of Scholastic, Inc.; and former president of the Harvard Law School Association

"Outsourcing is no longer just for Fortune 500 companies. Small and mid-sized firms, as well as busy professionals, can outsource their work to increase their productivity and free time for more important commitments. It's time for the world to take advantage of this revolution." —Vivek Kulkarni, CEO of Brickwork India and former IT secretary of Bangalore; credited as the "techno-bureaucrat" who helped make Bangalore an IT destination in India

"Tim is the master! I should know. I followed his rags to riches path and watched him transform himself from competitive fighter to entrepreneur. He tears apart conventional assumptions until he finds a better way." —Dan Partland, Emmy Award-winning producer of *American High* and *Welcome to the Dollhouse*

"*The 4-Hour Workweek* is an absolute necessity for those adventurous souls who want to live life to its fullest. Buy it and read it before you sacrifice any more!" —John Lusk, group product manager at Microsoft World Headquarters

"If you want to live your dreams now, and not in 20 or 30 years, buy this book!" —Laura Roden, chairman of the Silicon Valley Association of Startup Entrepreneurs and a lecturer in Corporate Finance at San Jose State University

"With this kind of time management and focus on the important things in life, people should be able to get 15 times as much done in a normal workweek." —Tim Draper, founder of Draper Fisher Jurvetson, financiers to innovators including Hotmail, Skype and Overture.com

"Tim has done what most people only dream of doing. I can't believe he is going to let his secrets out of the bag. This book is a must read!" —Stephen Key, top inventor and team designer of Teddy Ruxpin and Lazer Tag and a consultant to the television show *American Inventor*

The 4-Hour Body

Also by Timothy Ferriss

The 4-Hour Work Week

The 4-Hour Body

AN UNCOMMON GUIDE TO
RAPID FAT-LOSS, INCREDIBLE SEX
AND BECOMING SUPERHUMAN

Timothy Ferriss

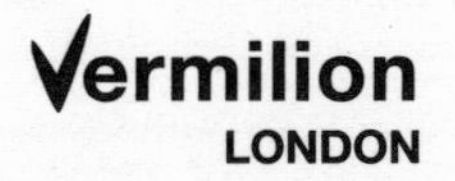
Vermilion
LONDON

14

Published in 2011 by Vermilion, an imprint of Ebury Publishing

First published in the United States by Crown Archetype, an imprint of the Crown Publishing Group, a division of Random House, Inc., New York, in 2010

Ebury Publishing is a Random House Group company

The Random House Group Limited Reg. No. 954009

Addresses for companies within The Random House Group can be found at: www.randomhouse.co.uk

A CIP catalogue record for this book is available from the British Library

The Random House Group Limited supports The Forest Stewardship Council® (FSC®), the leading international forest-certification organisation. Our books carrying the FSC label are printed on FSC®-certified paper. FSC is the only forest-certification scheme supported by the leading environmental organisations, including Greenpeace. Our paper procurement policy can be found at www.randomhouse.co.uk/environment

Printed and bound in Great Britain by Clays Ltd, St Ives plc

ISBN 9780091939526

Copies are available at special rates for bulk orders. Conact the sales development team on 020 7840 8487 for more information.

To buy books by your favourite authors and register for offers, visit www.randomhouse.co.uk

For my parents, who taught a little troublemaker that marching to a different drummer was a good thing. I love you both and owe you everything. Mum, sorry about all the crazy experiments.

Support good science—
10% of all author royalties are donated to cure-driven research, including the excellent work of St. Jude Children's Research Hospital.

CONTENTS

START HERE

FUNDAMENTALS—FIRST AND FOREMOST

GROUND ZERO—GETTING STARTED AND SWARAJ

SUBTRACTING FAT

BASICS

GETTING STRONGER

FROM SWIMMING TO SWINGING

ON LONGER AND BETTER LIFE

CLOSING THOUGHTS

APPENDICES AND EXTRAS

The 4-Hour Body

TIM'S DISCLAIMER

Please don't be stupid and kill yourself. It would make us both quite unhappy. Consult a doctor before doing anything in this book.

PUBLISHER'S DISCLAIMER

ON THE SHOULDERS OF GIANTS

I am not the expert. I'm the guide and explorer.

If you find anything amazing in this book, it's thanks to the brilliant minds who helped as resources, critics, contributors, proofreaders and references. If you find anything ridiculous in this book, it's because I didn't heed their advice.

Though indebted to hundreds of people, I wish to thank a few of them upfront, here listed in alphabetical order (still more in the acknowledgements):

Alexandra Carmichael
Andrew Hyde
Ann Miura-ko PhD
Barry Ross
Ben Goldacre MD
Brian MacKenzie
Casey Viator
Chad Fowler
Charles Poliquin
Charlie Hoehn
Chris Masterjohn
Chris Sacca
Club H Fitness
Craig Buhler
Daniel Reda
Dave Palumbo
David Blaine
Dean Karnazes
Dorian Yates
Doug McGuff MD
Dr. John Berardi
Dr. Justin Mager
Dr. Lee Wolfer
Dr. Mary Dan Eades
Dr. Michael Eades
Dr. Ross Tucker
Dr. Seth Roberts
Dr. Stuart McGill
Dr. Tertius Kohn
Dr. Timothy Noakes
Dustin Curtis
Ellington Darden PhD
Eric Foster
Gary Taubes
Gray Cook
Jaime Cevallos
JB Benna
Jeffrey B. Madoff
Joe DeFranco
Joe Polish
John Romano
Kelly Starrett
Marie Forleo
Mark Bell
Mark Cheng
Marque Boseman
Marty Gallagher
Matt Brzycki
Matt Mullenweg
Michael Ellsberg
Michael Levin
Mike Mahler
Mike Maples
Nate Green
Neil Strauss
Nicole Daedone
Nina Hartley
Pavel Tsatsouline
Pete Egoscue
Phil Libin
Ramit Sethi
Ray Cronise
Scott Jurek
Sean Bonner
Tallulah Sulis
Terry Laughlin
The Dexcom Team
(especially Keri Weindel)
The OneTaste Team
The Kiwi
Thomas Billings
Tracy Reifkind
Trevor Claiborne
Violet Blue
William Llewellyn
Yuri V. Griko PhD
Zack Even-Esh

START HERE

THINNER, BIGGER, FASTER, STRONGER?

How to Use This Book

Does history record any case in which the majority was right?

—Robert Heinlein

I love fools' experiments. I'm always making them.

—Charles Darwin

MOUNTAIN VIEW, CALIFORNIA, 10 P.M., FRIDAY

Shoreline Amphitheatre was rocking.

More than 20,000 people had turned out at northern California's largest music venue to hear Nine Inch Nails, loud and in charge, on what was expected to be their last tour.

Backstage, there was more unusual entertainment.

"Dude, I go into the stall to take care of business, and I look over and see the top of Tim's head popping above the divider. He was doing f*cking air squats in the men's room in complete silence."

Glenn, a videographer and friend, burst out laughing as he re-enacted my technique. To be honest, he needed to get his thighs closer to parallel.

"Forty air squats, to be exact," I offered.

Kevin Rose, founder of Digg, one of the top-500 most popular websites in the world, joined in the laughter and raised a beer to toast the incident. I, on the other hand, was eager to move on to the main event.

In the next 45 minutes, I consumed almost two full-size barbecue chicken pizzas and three handfuls of mixed nuts, for a cumulative total of about 4,400 calories. It was my fourth meal of the day, breakfast having consisted of two glasses of grapefruit juice, a large cup of coffee with cinnamon, two chocolate croissants and two doughnuts.

The more interesting portion of the story started well after Trent Reznor left the stage.

Roughly 72 hours later, I tested my body fat percentage with an ultrasound analyser designed by a physicist out of Lawrence Livermore National Laboratory.

Charting the progress on my latest experiment, I'd dropped from 11.9% to 10.2% body fat, a 14% reduction of the total fat on my body, in 14 days.

How? Timed doses of garlic, sugar cane and tea extracts, among other things.

The process wasn't punishing. It wasn't hard. Tiny changes were all it took. Tiny changes that, while small in isolation, produced enormous changes when used in combination.

Want to extend the fat-burning half-life of caffeine? Naringenin, a useful little molecule in grapefruit juice, does just the trick.

Need to increase insulin sensitivity before bingeing once per week? Just add some cinnamon to your pastries on Saturday morning, and you can get the job done.

Want to blunt your blood glucose for 60 minutes while you eat a high-carb meal guilt-free? There are a half-dozen options.

But 2% body fat in two weeks? How can that be possible if many general practitioners claim that it's *impossible* to lose more than 2lb (900g) of fat per week? Here's the sad truth: most of the one-size-fits-all rules, this being one example, haven't been field-tested for exceptions.

You can't change your muscle fibre type? Sure you can. Genetics be damned.

Calories in and calories out? It's incomplete at best. I've lost fat while grossly overfeeding. Cheesecake be praised.

The list goes on and on.

It's obvious that the rules require some rewriting.

That's what this book is for.

Diary of a Madman

The spring of 2007 was an exciting time for me.

My first book, after being turned down by 26 out of 27 publishers, had just hit the *New York Times* bestseller list and seemed headed for Number 1 on the business list, where it landed several months later. No one was more dumbfounded than me.

One particularly beautiful morning in San Jose, I had my first major media phone interview with Clive Thompson of *Wired* magazine. During our pre-interview small chat, I apologized if I sounded buzzed. I was. I had just finished a 10-minute workout following a double espresso on an empty stomach. It was a new experiment that would take me to single-digit body fat with two such sessions per week.

Clive wanted to talk to me about e-mail and websites like Twitter. Before we got started, and as a segue from the workout comment, I joked that the major fears of modern man could be boiled down to two things: too much e-mail and getting fat. Clive laughed and agreed. Then we moved on.

The interview went well, but it was this offhand joke that stuck with me. I retold it to dozens of people over the subsequent month, and the response was always the same: agreement and nodding.

This book, it seemed, had to be written.

The wider world thinks I'm obsessed with time management, but they haven't seen the other—much more legitimate, much more ridiculous—obsession.

I've recorded almost every workout I've done since age 18. I've had more than 1,000 blood tests[1] performed since 2004, sometimes as often as every two weeks, tracking everything from complete lipid panels, insulin and haemoglobin A1c, to IGF-1 and free testosterone. I've had stem cell growth factors imported from Israel to reverse "permanent" injuries, and I've flown to rural tea farmers in China to discuss Pu-Erh tea's effects on fat loss. All said and done, I've spent more than $250,000 (£156,000) on testing and tweaking over the last decade.

Just as some people have avant-garde furniture or artwork to decorate their homes, I have pulse oximeters, ultrasound machines and medical de-

1. Multiple tests are often performed from single blood draws of 10–12 vials.

vices for measuring everything from galvanic skin response to REM sleep. The kitchen and bathroom look like an A&E department.

If you think that's craziness, you're right. Fortunately, you don't need to be a guinea pig to benefit from one.

Hundreds of men and women have tested the techniques in *The 4-Hour Body* (4HB) over the last two years, and I've tracked and graphed hundreds of their results (194 people in this book). Many have lost more than 20lb (9kg) of fat in the first month of experimentation, and for the vast majority, it's the first time they've ever been able to do so.

Why do 4HB approaches work where others fail?

Because the changes are either small or simple, and often both. There is zero room for misunderstanding, and visible results compel you to continue. If results are fast and measurable,[2] self-discipline isn't needed.

I can give you every popular diet in four lines. Ready?

- Eat more greens.
- Eat less saturated fat.
- Exercise more and burn more calories.
- Eat more omega-3 fatty acids.

We won't be covering any of this. Not because it doesn't work—it does. . . up to a point. But it's not the type of advice that will make friends greet you with "What the #$%& have you been doing?!", whether in the dressing room or on the playing field.

That requires an altogether different approach.

The Unintentional Dark Horse

Let's be clear: I'm neither a doctor nor a PhD. I am a meticulous data cruncher with access to many of the world's best athletes and scientists.

This puts me in a rather unusual position.

I'm able to pull from disciplines and subcultures that rarely touch one another, and I'm able to test hypotheses using the kind of self-

2. Not just noticeable.

experimentation mainstream practitioners can't condone (though their help behind the scenes is critical). By challenging basic assumptions, it's possible to stumble upon simple and unusual solutions to long-standing problems.

Over-fat? Try timed protein and pre-meal lemon juice.

Under-muscled? Try ginger and sauerkraut.

Can't sleep? Try upping your saturated fat or using cold exposure.

This book includes the findings of more than 100 PhDs, NASA scientists, medical doctors, Olympic athletes, professional sports trainers (from the NFL to MLB), world-record holders, Super Bowl rehabilitation specialists, and even former Eastern Bloc coaches. You'll meet some of the most incredible specimens, including before-and-after transformations, you've ever seen.

I don't have a publish-or-perish academic career to preserve, and this is a good thing. As one MD from a well-known American Ivy League university said to me over lunch:

> *We're trained for 20 years to be risk-averse. I'd like to do the experimentation, but I'd risk everything I've built over two decades of schooling and training by doing so. I'd need an immunity necklace. The university would never tolerate it.*

He then added: "You can be the dark horse."

It's a strange label, but he was right. Not just because I have no prestige to lose. I'm also a former industry insider.

From 2001 to 2009, I was CEO of a sports nutrition company with distribution in more than a dozen countries, and while we followed the rules, it became clear that many others didn't. It wasn't the most profitable option. I have witnessed blatant lies on nutritional fact panels, marketing executives budgeting for FTC fines in anticipation of lawsuits, and much worse from some of the best-known brands in the business.[3] I understand how and where consumers are deceived. The darker tricks of the trade in supplements and sports nutrition—clouding results of "clinical trials" and creative labelling as just two examples—are nearly the same as in biotech and Big Pharma.

3. There are, of course, some outstanding companies with solid R&D and uncompromising ethics, but they are few and far between.

I will teach you to spot bad science, and therefore bad advice and bad products.[4]

Late one evening in the autumn of 2009, I sat eating cassoulet and duck legs with Dr. Lee Wolfer in the clouds of fog known as San Francisco. The wine was flowing, and I told her of my fantasies to return to a Berkeley or Stanford and pursue a doctorate in the biological sciences. I was briefly a neuroscience major at Princeton University and dreamed of a PhD at the end of my name. Lee is regularly published in peer-reviewed journals and has been trained at some of the finest programmes in the world, including the University of California at San Francisco (UCSF) (MD), Berkeley (MS), Harvard Medical School (residency), the Rehabilitation Institute of Chicago (fellowship) and Spinal Diagnostics in Daly City, California (fellowship).

She just smiled and raised a glass of wine before responding:

"You—Tim Ferriss—can do more outside the system than inside it."

A Laboratory of One

> Many of these theories have been killed off only when some decisive experiment exposed their incorrectness . . . thus the yeoman work in any science . . . is done by the experimentalist, who must keep the theoreticians honest.
>
> *—Michio Kaku (Hyperspace), theoretical physicist and co-creator of string field theory*

Most breakthroughs in performance (and appearance) enhancement start with animals and go through the following adoption curve:

> *Racehorses → AIDS patients (because of muscle wasting) and body builders → elite athletes → rich people → the rest of us*

The last jump from the rich to the general public can take 10–20 years, if it happens at all. It often doesn't.

I'm *not* suggesting that you start injecting yourself with odd substances never before tested on humans. I *am* suggesting, however, that government agencies (the U.S. Department of Agriculture, the Food and Drug Admin-

4. I have absolutely no financial interest in any of the supplements I recommend in this book. If you purchase any supplement from a link in this book, an affiliate commission is sent directly to the non-profit DonorsChoose.org, which helps public schools in the United States.

istration) are at least 10 years behind current research, and at least 20 years behind compelling evidence in the field.

More than a decade ago, a close friend named Paul was in a car accident and suffered brain damage that lowered his testosterone production. Even with supplemental testosterone treatments (creams, gels, short-acting injectables) and after visiting scores of top endocrinologists, he still suffered from the symptoms of low testosterone. Everything changed—literally overnight—once he switched to testosterone enanthate, a variation seldom seen in the medical profession in the United States. Who made the suggestion? An advanced body builder who knew his biochemistry. It shouldn't have made a difference, yet it did.

Do doctors normally take advantage of the 50+ years of experience that professional body builders have testing, even synthesizing, esters of testosterone? No. Most doctors view body builders as cavalier amateurs, and body builders view doctors as too risk-averse to do anything innovative.

This separation of the expertise means both sides suffer suboptimal results.

Handing your medical care over to the biggest man-gorilla in your gym is a bad idea, but it's important to look for discoveries outside of the usual suspects. Those closest to a problem are often the least capable of seeing it with fresh eyes.

Despite the incredible progress in some areas of medicine in the last 100 years, a 60-year-old in 2009 can expect to live an average of only 6 years longer than a 60-year-old in 1900.

Me? I plan on living to 120 while eating the best rib-eye steaks I can find. More on that later.

Suffice to say: for uncommon solutions, you have to look in uncommon places.

The Future's Already Here

In our current world, even if proper trials are funded for obesity studies as just one example, it might take 10–20 years for the results. Are you prepared to wait?

I hope not.

"Kaiser can't talk to UCSF, who can't talk to Blue Shield. *You* are the arbiter of your health information." Those are the words of a leading surgeon at UCSF, who encouraged me to take my papers with me before hospital records claimed them as their property.

Now the good news: with a little help, it's never been easier to collect a few data points (at little cost), track them (without training), and make small changes that produce incredible results.

Type 2 diabetics going off medication 48 hours after starting a dietary intervention? Wheelchair-bound seniors walking again after 14 weeks of training? This is not science fiction. It's being done today. As William Gibson, who coined the term "cyberspace", has said:

"The future is already here—it is just unevenly distributed."

The 80/20 Principle: From Wall Street to the Human Machine

This book is designed to give you the most important 2.5% of the tools you need for body recomposition and increased performance. Some short history can explain this odd 2.5%.

Vilfredo Pareto was a controversial economist-cum-sociologist who lived from 1848 to 1923. His seminal work, *Cours d'économie politique*, included a then little explored "law" of income distribution that would later bear his name: "Pareto's Law", or "the Pareto Distribution". It is more popularly known as "the 80/20 Principle".

Pareto demonstrated a grossly uneven but predictable distribution of wealth in society—80 per cent of the wealth and income is produced and possessed by 20 per cent of the population. He also showed that this 80/20 principle could be found almost everywhere, not just in economics. Eighty per cent of Pareto's garden peas were produced by 20% of the pea pods he had planted, for example.

In practice, the 80/20 principle is often much more disproportionate.

To be perceived as fluent in conversational Spanish, for example, you need an active vocabulary of approximately 2,500 high-frequency words. This will allow you to comprehend more than 95% of all conversation. To get to 98% comprehension would require at least five years of practice instead of five months. Doing the maths, 2,500 words is a mere 2.5% of the estimated 100,000 words in the Spanish language.

This means:

1. 2.5% of the total subject matter provides 95% of the desired results.
2. This same 2.5% provides just 3% less benefit than putting in 12 times as much effort.

This incredibly valuable 2.5% is the key, the Archimedes lever, for those who want the best results in the least time. The trick is finding that 2.5%.[5]

This book is not intended as a comprehensive treatise on all things related to the human body. My goal is to share what I have found to be the 2.5% that delivers 95% of the results in rapid body redesign and performance enhancement. If you are already at 5% body fat or bench-pressing 181kg (400lb), you are in the top 1% of humans and now in the world of incremental gains. This book is for the other 99% who can experience near-unbelievable gains in short periods of time.

How to Use This Book—Five Rules

It is important that you follow five rules with this book. Ignore them at your peril.

RULE #1. THINK OF THIS BOOK AS A BUFFET.

Do *not* read this book from start to finish.

Most people won't need more than 150 pages to reinvent themselves. Browse the table of contents, pick the chapters that are most relevant and discard the rest . . . for now. Pick one appearance goal and one performance goal to start.

The only mandatory sections are "Fundamentals" and "Ground Zero". Here are some popular goals, along with the corresponding chapters to read in the order listed:

5. Philosopher Nassim N. Taleb noted an important difference between language and biology that I'd like to underscore: the former is largely known and the latter is largely unknown. Thus, our 2.5% is not 2.5% of a perfect finite body of knowledge, but the most empirically valuable 2.5% of what we know now.

RAPID FAT LOSS

All chapters in "Fundamentals"
All chapters in "Ground Zero"
"The Slow-Carb Diet I and II"
"Building the Perfect Posterior"
Total page count: 98

RAPID MUSCLE GAIN

All chapters in "Fundamentals"
All chapters in "Ground Zero"
"From Geek to Freak"
"Occam's Protocol I and II"
Total page count: 97

RAPID STRENGTH GAIN

All chapters in "Fundamentals"
All chapters in "Ground Zero"
"Effortless Superhuman" (pure strength, little mass gain)
"Pre-hab: Injury-Proofing the Body"
Total page count: 92

RAPID SENSE OF TOTAL WELL BEING

All chapters in "Fundamentals"
All chapters in "Ground Zero"
All chapters in "Improving Sex"
All chapters in "Perfecting Sleep"
"Reversing 'Permanent' Injuries"
Total page count: 143

Once you've selected the bare minimum to get started, get started.

Then, once you've committed to a plan of action, dip back into the book at your leisure and explore. Immediately practical advice is contained in every chapter, so don't discount something based on the title. Even if you are a meat-eater (as I am), for example, you will benefit from "The Meatless Machine".

Just don't read it all at once.

RULE #2. SKIP THE SCIENCE IF IT'S TOO DENSE.

You do not need to be a scientist to read this book.

For the geeks and the curious, however, I've included a lot of cool details. These details can often enhance your results but are not required reading. Such sections are boxed and labelled "Geek's Advantage" with a "GA" symbol.

Even if you've been intimidated by science in the past, I encourage you to browse some of these GA sections—at least a few will offer some fun "holy sh*t!" moments and improve results 10% or so.

If you ever feel overwhelmed, though, skip them, as they're not mandatory for the results you're after.

RULE #3. PLEASE BE SCEPTICAL.

Don't assume something is true because I say it is.

As the legendary Timothy Noakes PhD, author or co-author of more than 400 published research papers, is fond of saying: "Fifty per cent of what we know is wrong. The problem is that we do not know which 50% it is." Everything in this book works, but I have surely got some of the mechanisms completely wrong. In other words, I believe the how-to is 100% reliable, but some of the why-to will end up on the chopping block as we learn more.

RULE #4. DON'T USE SCEPTICISM AS AN EXCUSE FOR INACTION.

As the good Dr. Noakes also said to me about one Olympic training regimen: "This [approach] could be totally wrong, but it's a hypothesis worth disproving."

It's important to look for hypotheses worth disproving.

Science starts with educated (read: wild-ass) guesses. Then it's all trial and error. Sometimes you predict correctly from the outset. More often, you make mistakes and stumble across unexpected findings, which lead to new questions. If you want to sit on the sidelines and play full-time sceptic, suspending action until a scientific consensus is reached, that's your choice. Just realize that science is, alas, often as political as a dinner party with die-hard Democrats and Republicans. Consensus comes late at best.

Don't use scepticism as a thinly veiled excuse for inaction or remaining in your comfort zone. Be sceptical, but for the right reason: because you're looking for the most promising option to test in real life.

Be *proactively* sceptical, not defensively sceptical.

Let me know if you make a cool discovery or prove me wrong. This book will evolve through your feedback and help.

RULE #5. ENJOY IT.

I've included a lot of odd experiences and screw-ups just for simple entertainment value. All fact and no play makes Jack a dull boy.

Much of the content is intended to be read as the diary of a madman. Enjoy it. More than anything, I'd like to impart the joy of exploration and discovery. Remember: this isn't a homework assignment. Take it at your own pace.

The Billionaire Productivity Secret and the Experimental Lifestyle

"How do you become more productive?"

Richard Branson leant back and thought for a second. The tropical sounds of his private oasis, Necker Island, murmured in the background. Twenty people sat around him at rapt attention, wondering what a billionaire's answer would be to one of the big questions—perhaps *the* biggest question—of business. The group had been assembled by marketing impresario Joe Polish to brainstorm growth options for Richard's philanthropic Virgin Unite. It was one of his many new ambitious projects. Virgin Group already had more than 300 companies, more than 50,000 employees, and $25 billion (£16 billion) per year in revenue. In other words, Branson had personally built an empire larger than the GDP of some developing countries. Then he broke the silence:

"Work out."

He was serious and elaborated: working out gave him at least four additional hours of productive time every day.

The cool breeze punctuated his answer like an exclamation point.

4HB is intended to be much more than a book.

I view 4HB as a manifesto, a call to arms for a new mental model of living: the experimental lifestyle. It's up to you—not your doctor, not the newspaper—to learn what you best respond to. The benefits go far beyond the physical.

If you understand politics well enough to vote for a president, or if you have ever filed taxes, you can learn the few most important scientific rules for redesigning your body. These rules will become your friends, 100% reliable and trusted.

This changes everything.

It is my sincere hope, if you've suffered from dissatisfaction with your body, or confusion regarding diet and exercise, that your life will be divided into before-4HB and after-4HB. It can help you do what most people would consider superhuman, whether losing 100lb (45kg) of fat or running 100 miles. It all works.

There is no high priesthood—there is cause and effect.

Welcome to the director's chair.

Alles mit Maß und Ziel,

Timothy Ferriss
San Francisco, California
10 June, 2010

FOR YOUR READING PLEASURE

Getting Tested

There are dozens of tests mentioned throughout this book. If you ever ask yourself "How do I get that tested?" or wonder where to start, the "Getting Tested" list on page 472 is your step-by-step guide.

Quick Reference

Not sure how much a gram is, or what the hell 4 ounces is? Just flip to the common measurements on page 470 and unleash your inner Julia Child.

Endnotes and Citations

This book is very well researched.

It's also big enough to club a baby seal. If you really want to make your eyes glaze over, more than 30 scientific citations can be found at www.fourhourbody.com/endnotes, divided by chapter and with relevant sentences included.

Resources

To spare you the headache of typing out paragraph-long URLs, all long website addresses have been replaced with a short www.fourhourbody.com address that will send you to the right place.

Got it? Good. Let's move on to the mischief.

FUNDAMENTALS—FIRST AND FOREMOST

THE MINIMUM EFFECTIVE DOSE

From Microwaves to Fat-Loss

Perfection is achieved, not when there is nothing more to add, but when there is nothing left to take away.

—Antoine de Saint-Exupéry

Arthur Jones was a precocious young child and particularly fond of crocodiles.

He read his father's entire medical library before he was 12. The home environment might have had something to do with it, seeing as his parents, grandfather, great-grandfather, half-brother and half-sister were all doctors.

From humble beginnings in Oklahoma, he would mature into one of the most influential figures in the exercise science world. He would also become, in the words of more than a few, a particularly "angry genius".

One of Jones's protégés, Ellington Darden PhD, shares a prototypical Jones anecdote:

> *In 1970, Arthur invited Arnold [Schwarzenegger] and Franco Colombu to visit him in Lake Helen, Florida, right after the 1970 Mr. Olympia. Arthur picked them up at the airport in his Cadillac, with Arnold in the passenger seat and Franco in the back. There are probably 12 stoplights in between the airport and the Interstate, so it was a lot of stop-and-go driving.*
>
> *Now, you have to know that Arthur was a*

man who talked loud and dominated every conversation. But he couldn't get Arnold to shut up. He was just blabbing in his German or whatever and Arthur was having a hard time understanding what he was saying. So Arthur was getting annoyed and told him to quiet down, but Arnold just kept talking and talking.

By the time they got onto the Interstate, Arthur had had enough. So he pulled over to the side of the road, got out, walked around, opened Arnold's door, grabbed him by the shirt collar, yanked him out, and said something to the effect of, "Listen here, you son of a bitch. If you don't shut the hell up, a man twice your age is going to whip your ass right out here in front of I-4 traffic. Just dare me."

Within five seconds Arnold had apologized, got back in the car, and was a perfect gentlemen for the next three or four days.

Jones was more frequently pissed off than anything else.

He was infuriated by what he considered stupidity in every corner of the exercise science world, and he channelled this anger into defying the odds. This included putting 4.5st (28.67kg) on champion body builder Casey Viator in 28 days and putting himself on the Forbes 400 list by founding and selling exercise equipment manufacturer Nautilus, which was estimated to have grossed $300 million (£187 million) per year at its zenith.

He had no patience for fuzzy thinking in fields that depended on scientific clarity. In response to researchers who drew conclusions about muscular function using electromyography (EMG), Arthur attached their machines to a cadaver and moved its limbs to record similar "activity". Internal friction, that is.

Jones lamented his fleeting time: "My age being what it is, universal acceptance of what we are now doing may not come within my lifetime; but it will come, because what we are doing is clearly established by simple laws of basic physics that cannot be denied forever." He passed away on 28 August 2007, of natural causes, 80 years old and as ornery as ever.

Jones left a number of important legacies, one of which will be the cornerstone of everything we'll discuss: the minimum effective dose.

The Minimum Effective Dose

The minimum effective dose (MED) is defined simply: the smallest dose that will produce a desired outcome.

Jones referred to this critical point as the "minimum effective load", as he was concerned exclusively with weight-bearing exercise, but we will look at precise "dosing" of both exercise and anything you ingest.[1]

Anything beyond the MED is wasteful.

To boil water, the MED is 100°C (212°F) at standard air pressure. Boiled is boiled. Higher temperatures will not make it "more boiled". Higher temperatures just consume more resources that could be used for something else more productive.

If you need 15 minutes in the sun to trigger a melanin response, 15 minutes is your MED for tanning. More than 15 minutes is redundant and will just result in burning and a forced break from the beach. During this forced break from the beach, let's assume one week, someone else who heeded his natural 15-minute MED will be able to fit in four more tanning sessions. He is four shades darker, whereas you have returned to your pale pre-beach self. Sad little manatee. In biological systems, exceeding your MED can freeze progress for weeks, even months.

In the context of body redesign, there are two fundamental MEDs to keep in mind:

To remove stored fat → do the least necessary to trigger a fat loss cascade of specific hormones.

To add muscle in small or large quantities → do the least necessary to trigger local (specific muscles) and systemic (hormonal[2]) growth mechanisms.

Knocking over the dominos that trigger both of these events takes surprisingly little. Don't complicate them.

For a given muscle group like the shoulders, activating the local growth mechanism might require just 80 seconds of tension using 23kg (50lb) once every seven days, for example. That stimulus, just like the 100°C (212°F)

1. Credit is due to Dr. Doug McGuff, who's written extensively on this and who will reappear later.
2. In fancier and more accurate terms, *neuroendocrine*.

for boiling water, is enough to trigger certain prostaglandins, transcription factors and all manner of complicated biological reactions. What are "transcription factors"? You don't need to know. In fact, you don't need to understand any of the biology, just as you don't need to understand radiation to use a microwave oven. Press a few buttons in the right order and it's done.

In our context: 80 seconds as a target is all you need to understand. That is the button.

If, instead of 80 seconds, you mimic a glossy magazine routine—say, an arbitrary 5 sets of 10 repetitions—it is the muscular equivalent of sitting in the sun for an hour with a 15-minute MED. Not only is this wasteful, it is a predictable path for preventing and reversing gains. The organs and glands that help repair damaged tissue have more limitations than your enthusiasm. The kidneys, as one example, can clear the blood of a finite maximum waste concentration each day (approximately 450 mmol, or millimoles per litre). If you do a marathon three-hour workout and make your bloodstream look like an LA traffic jam, you stand the real chance of hitting a biochemical bottleneck.

Again: the good news is that you don't need to know anything about your kidneys to use this information. All you need to know is:

80 seconds is the dose prescription.

More is not better. Indeed, your greatest challenge will be resisting the temptation to do more.

The MED not only delivers the most dramatic results, but it does so in the least time possible. Jones's words should echo in your head: "REMEMBER: it is impossible to evaluate, or even understand, anything that you cannot measure."

80 secs of 9kg (20lb)
10:00 mins of 12.2°C (54°F) water
200 mg of allicin extract before bed

These are the types of prescriptions you should seek, and these are the types of prescriptions I will offer.

RULES THAT CHANGE THE RULES

Everything Popular Is Wrong

Everything popular is wrong.

—Oscar Wilde, *The Importance of Being Earnest*

Know the rules well, so you can break them effectively.

—Dalai Lama XIV

"This is clearly a lie. Gaining 44.5 kg (98 lb) in 28 days requires a caloric surplus of 4,300 calories per day, so for a guy his size, he must have eaten 7,000 calories a day. He expects me to believe that he dropped 4% in body fat as a result of eating 7,000 calories? . . ."

I took a big swig of Malbec and read the blog comment again. Ah, the Internet. How far we haven't come.

It was amusing, and one of hundreds of similar comments on this particular blog post, but the fact remained: I had gained 15.4kg (34lb) of muscle, lost 1.8kg (4lb) of fat, and decreased my total cholesterol from 222 to 147, all in 28 days, without anabolics or statins like artovestin.

The entire experiment had been recorded by Dr. Peggy Plato, director of the Sport and Fitness Evaluation Program at San Jose State University, who used hydrostatic weighing tanks, medical scales and a tape measure to track everything from waist circumference to body fat percentage. My total time in the gym over four weeks?

Four hours.[3] Eight 30-minute workouts.

The data didn't lie.

But isn't weight loss or gain as simple as calories in and calories out?

It's attractive in its simplicity, yes, but so is cold fusion. It doesn't work quite as advertised.

German poet Johann Wolfgang Goethe had the right perspective: "Mysteries are not necessarily miracles." To do the impossible (sail around the world, break the four-minute mile, reach the moon), you need to ignore the popular.

Charles Munger, right-hand adviser to Warren Buffett, the richest man on the planet, is known for his unparalleled clear thinking and near-failure-proof track record. How did he refine his thinking to help build a $3 trillion (£2 trillion) business in Berkshire Hathaway?

The answer is "mental models", or analytical rules-of-thumb[4] pulled from disciplines outside of investing, ranging from physics to evolutionary biology.

Eighty to 90 models have helped Charles Munger develop, in Warren Buffett's words, "the best 30-second mind in the world. He goes from A to Z in one move. He sees the essence of everything before you even finish the sentence."

Charles Munger likes to quote Charles Darwin:

Even people who aren't geniuses can outthink the rest of mankind if they develop certain thinking habits.

In the 4HB, the following mental models, pulled from a variety of disciplines, are what will separate your results from the rest of mankind.

New Rules for Rapid Redesign

NO EXERCISE BURNS MANY CALORIES.

Did you eat half an Oreo cookie? No problem. If you're a 16st (98kg) male, you just need to climb 27 flights of stairs to burn it off.

3. In this case, the "4-Hour Body" is quite literal.
4. These "mental models" are often referred to as *heuristics* or *analytical frameworks*.

Put another way, moving 16st (98kg) 100 metres (about 27 flights of stairs) requires 100 kilojoules of energy, or 23.9 calories (known to scientists as kilocalories [kcal]). 450g (1lb) of fat contains 4,082 calories. How many calories might running a marathon burn? 2,600 or so.

The caloric argument for exercise gets even more depressing. Remember those 107 calories you burnt during that kick-ass hour-long Stairmaster™ session? Don't forget to subtract your basal metabolic rate (BMR), what you would have burnt had you been sitting on the sofa watching *The Simpsons* instead. For most people, that's about 100 calories per hour given off as heat (BTU).

That hour on the Stairmaster was worth seven calories.

As luck would have it, three small sticks of celery are six calories, so you have one calorie left to spare. But wait a minute: how many calories did that sports drink and big post-workout meal have? Don't forget that you have to burn more calories than you later ingest in larger meals due to increased appetite.

F*cking hell, right? It's enough to make a lumberjack cry. Confused and angry? You should be.

As usual, the focus is on the least important piece of the puzzle.

But why do scientists harp on the calorie? Simple. It's cheap to estimate, and it is a popular variable for publication in journals. This, dear friends, is referred to as "car park" science, so-called after a joke about a poor drunk man who loses his keys during a night on the town.

His friends find him on his hands and knees looking for his keys under a streetlight, even though he knows he lost them somewhere else. "Why are you looking for your keys under the streetlight?" they ask. He responds confidently, "Because there's more light over here. I can see better."

For the researcher seeking tenure, grant money or lucrative corporate consulting contracts, the maxim "publish or perish" applies. If you need to include 100 or 1,000 test subjects and can only afford to measure a few simple things, you need to paint those measurements as tremendously important.

Alas, mentally on your hands and knees is no way to spend life, nor is chafing your arse on a stationary bike.

Instead of focusing on calories-out as exercise-dependent, we will look at two underexploited paths: heat and hormones.

So relax. You'll be able to eat as much as you want, and then some. New exhaust pipes will solve the problem.

A DRUG IS A DRUG IS A DRUG

Calling something a "drug", a "dietary supplement", "over-the-counter" or a "nutriceutical" is a legal distinction, not a biochemical one.

None of these labels means that something is safe or effective. Legal herbs can kill you just as dead as illegal narcotics. Supplements, often unpatentable molecules and therefore unappealing for drug development, can decrease cholesterol from 222 to 147 in four weeks, as I have done, or they can be inert and do absolutely nothing.

Think "all-natural" is safer than synthetic? Split peas are all-natural, but so is arsenic. Human growth hormone (HGH) can be extracted from the brains of all-natural cadavers, but unfortunately it often brings Creutzfeldt-Jakob disease with it, which is why HGH is now manufactured using recombinant DNA.

Besides whole foods (which we'll treat separately as "food"), anything you put in your mouth or your bloodstream that has an effect—whether it's a cream, injection, pill or powder—is a *drug*. Treat them all as such. Don't distract yourself with labels that are meaningless to us.

THE 20lb (9kg) RECOMP GOAL

For the vast majority of you reading this book who weigh more than 8.5st (54kg), 1.4st (9kg) of *recomposition* (which I'll define below) will make you look and feel like a new person, so I suggest this as a goal. If you weigh less than 8.5st (54kg), aim for 10lb (4.5kg); otherwise, 20lb (9kg) is your new, specific goal.

Even if you have 7st (45kg) to lose, start with 20lb.

On a 1–10 attractiveness scale, 20lb (9kg) appears to be the critical threshold for going from a 6 to a 9 or 10, at least as tested with male perception of females.

The term "recomposition" is important. It does *not* mean a 1.4st (9kg) reduction in weight. It's a 1.4st (9kg) change in appearance. A 1.4st (9kg) "recomp" could entail losing 1.4st (9kg) of fat or gaining 1.4st (9kg) of muscle, but it most often involves losing 15lb (6.8kg) of fat and gaining 5lb (2.3kg) of muscle, or some blend in between.

Designing the best physique includes both subtraction and addition.

THE 100-UNIT SLIDER: DIET, DRUGS AND EXERCISE

How, then, do we get to 1.4st (9kg)?

Imagine a ruler with 100 lines on it, representing 100 total units, and two sliders. This allows us to split the 100 units into three areas that total 100. These three areas represent diet, drugs and exercise.

An equal split would look like this:

__________/__________/__________ (33% diet, 33% drugs, 33% exercise)

It is possible to reach your 1.4st (9kg) recomp goal with any combination of the three, but some combinations are better than others. One hundred per cent drugs can get you there, for example, but it will produce the most long-term side effects. One hundred per cent exercise can get you there, but if injuries or circumstances interfere, the return to baseline is fast.

/____________/ (100% drugs) = side effects
//____________ (100% exercise) = easy to derail

Here is the ratio of most of the fat-loss case studies in this book:

________/_/___ (60% diet, 10% drugs, 30% exercise)

If you're unable to follow a prescribed diet, as is sometimes the case with travel or vegetarianism, you'll need to move the sliders to increase the % attention paid to exercise and drugs. For example:

_/_____/______ (10% diet, 45% drugs, 45% exercise)

The numbers need not be measured, but this concept is critical to keep in mind as the world interferes with plans. Learning diet and exercise principles is priority #1, as these are the bedrock elements. Relying too much on drugs makes your liver and kidneys unhappy.

The percentages will also depend on your personal preferences and "adherence", which we cover next.

THE DUCT TAPE TEST: WILL IT STICK?

Eating at least one head of lettuce per day works well for losing fat and controlling insulin levels.

That is, if you're a critical intervention patient, such as a morbidly obese type 2 diabetic. The options for such people, as explained by their doctors, are (1) change your diet with this prescription, or (2) die. Not surprisingly, adherence is often incredible. For someone who would like to lose 1.4st (9kg) but is more interested in how their bum looks in a pair of jeans, the adherence will be abysmal. Chopping vegetables and cleaning the blender three times per day will lead to one place: abandonment of the method. Does that mean it won't work for some people? No. It just means that it will fail for *most* people. We want to avoid all methods with a high failure rate, even if you believe you are in the diligent minority. In the beginning, everyone who starts a programme believes they're in this minority.

Take adherence seriously: will you actually stick with this change until you hit your goal?

If not, find another method, even if it's less effective and less efficient. The decent method you follow is better than the perfect method you quit.

DON'T CONFUSE PHYSICAL RECREATION WITH EXERCISE

Physical recreation can be many things: football, swimming, yoga, rock-climbing, tipping cows . . . the list is endless. Exercise, on the other hand, means performing an MED of precise movements that will produce a target change. That's it. It's next to impossible to draw cause-and-effect relationships with recreation. There are too many variables. Effective exercise is simple and trackable.

Physical recreation is great. I love chasing dogs in the park as much as the next person. Exercise in our context, however, is the application of measurable stimuli to decrease fat, increase muscle or increase performance.

Recreation is for fun. Exercise is for producing changes. Don't confuse the two.

DON'T CONFUSE CORRELATION WITH CAUSE AND EFFECT

Want to look like a marathon runner, thin and sleek? Train like a marathoner.

Want to look like a sprinter, ripped and muscular? Train like a sprinter.

Want to look like a basketball player, 203cm (6ft 8in)? Train like a basketball player.

Hold on now. That last one doesn't work. Nor does it work for the first two examples. It's flawed logic, once again appealing and tempting in its simplicity. Here are three simple questions we can ask to avoid similar mistakes:

1. Is it possible that the arrow of causality is reversed? Example: do people who are naturally ripped and muscular often choose to be sprinters? Yep.
2. Are we mixing up absence and presence? Example: if the claim is that a no-meat diet extends average lifespan 5–15%, is it possible that it is the presence of more vegetables, not the absence of meat, that extends lifespan? It most certainly is.
3. Is it possible that you tested a specific demographic and that other variables are responsible for the difference? Example: if the claim is that yoga improves cardiac health, and the experimental group comprises upper-class folk, is it possible that they are therefore more likely than a control group to eat better food? You bet.

The point isn't to speculate about hundreds of possible explanations.

The point is to be sceptical, especially of sensationalist headlines. Most "new studies" in the media are observational studies that can, at best, establish correlation (A happens while B happens), but not causality (A causes B to happen).

If I pick my nose when the football cuts to a commercial, did I cause that? This isn't a haiku. It's a summary: correlation doesn't prove causation. Be sceptical when people tell you that A causes B.

They're wrong much more than 50% of the time.

USE THE YO-YO: EMBRACE CYCLING

Yo-yo dieting gets a bad press.

Instead of beating yourself up, going to the shrink, or eating an entire cheesecake because you ruined your diet with one biscuit, allow me to deliver a message: it's normal.

Eating more, then less, then more, and so on in a continuous sine wave is an impulse we can leverage to reach goals faster. Trying to prevent it—attempting to sustain a reduced-calorie diet, for example—is when yo-yoing becomes pathological and uncontrollable. Scheduling overeating at specific times, on the other hand, fixes problems instead of creating them.

The top body-builders in the world understand this and, even when in a pre-contest dieting phase, will cycle calories to prevent hormonal downregulation.[5] The daily average might be 4,000 calories per day, but it would be cycled as follows: Monday, 4,000; Tuesday, 4,500; Wednesday, 3,500, etc.

Ed Coan, described as the Michael Jordan of powerlifting, set more than 70 world records in his sport. Among other things, he deadlifted an unbelievable 409kg (901lb) at 99.7kg (220lb) bodyweight, beating even super-heavyweights. His trainer at the time, Marty Gallagher, has stated matter-of-factly that "maintaining peak condition year-round is a ticket to the mental ward".

You can have your cheesecake and eat it too, as long as you get the timing right. The best part is that these planned ups and downs accelerate, rather than reverse, progress.

Forget balance and embrace cycling. It's a key ingredient in rapid body redesign.

PREDISPOSITION V. PREDESTINATION: DON'T BLAME YOUR GENES

The marathoners of Kenya are legendary.

Kenyan men have won all but one of the last 12 Boston Marathons. In the 1988 Olympics, Kenyan men won gold in the 800-metre, 1,500-metre and 5,000-metre races, as well as the 3,000-metre steeplechase. Factoring in their population of approximately 30 million, the statistical likelihood of this happening at an international competition with the scope of the Olympics is about one in 1.6 billion.

If you've been in the world of exercise science for any period of time, you can guess their muscle fibre composition, which is an inherited trait: slow-twitch. Slow-twitch muscle fibres are suited to endurance work. Lucky bastards!

But here's the problem: it doesn't appear to be totally true. To the surprise of researchers who conducted muscle biopsies on Kenyan runners, there was a high proportion of fast-twitch muscle fibres, the type you'd expect to find in shot-putters and sprinters. Why? Because, as it turns out, they often train using low mileage and high intensity.

5. For example, proper conversion of T4 thyroid hormone to the more thermogenically active T3.

If you are overweight and your parents are overweight, the inclination is to blame genetics, but this is only one possible explanation.

Did fatness genes get passed on, or was it overeating behaviour? After all, fat people tend to have fat pets.

Even if you are *predisposed* to being overweight, you're not *predestined* to be fat.

Eric Lander, leader of the Human Genome Project, has emphasized repeatedly the folly of learned helplessness through genetic determinism:

> *People will think that because genes play a role in something, they determine everything. We see, again and again, people saying, "It's all genetic. I can't do anything about it." That's nonsense. To say that something has a genetic component does not make it unchangeable.*

Don't accept predisposition. You don't have to, and we can feed and train you towards a different physical future.[6] Nearly all of my personal experiments involve improving something that should be genetically fixed.

It is possible to redirect your natural-born genetic profile. From now on, "bad genetics" can't be your go-to excuse.

ELIMINATE PROPAGANDA AND NEBULOUS TERMS

> The word ***aerobics*** came about when the gym instructors got together and said, "If we're going to charge $10 (£6.24) an hour, we can't call it jumping up and down."
> —*Rita Rudner*

One question you must learn to ask when faced with advice or sales pitches is: "If this [method/product/diet/etc.] didn't work as advertised, what might their other incentives be for selling it?"

Aerobics classes? The reason you're sold: aerobics is more effective than alternative X. The real reason it's promoted: there's no equipment investment and the gym can maximize students per square metre per class. Many "new and improved" recommendations are based on calculating profit first and then working backwards to justify the method.

6. Genes alone cannot account for the diversity of characteristics we see around us. Messenger RNA (mRNA) is now thought to be responsible for much of the diversity, and there is good news: just as you can turn genes on and off, you can influence mRNA dramatically with environment—even shut down certain processes entirely through interference.

Marketer speak and ambiguous words have no place in 4HB or your efforts. Both will surface in conversations with friends who, in their best effort to help, will do more harm than good. If unprepared, one such conversation can single-handedly derail an entire programme.

These are two categories of words that you should neither use nor listen to. The first, **marketer-speak,** includes all terms used to scare or sell that have no physiological basis:

Toning
Cellulite
Firming
Shaping
Aerobics

The word *cellulite*, for example, first appeared in the 15 April 1968 issue of *Vogue* magazine, and this invented disease soon had a believer base worldwide:

> Vogue *began to focus on the body as much as on the clothes, in part because there was little they could dictate with the anarchic styles.... In a stunning move, an entire replacement culture was developed by naming a "problem" where it had scarcely existed before, centering it on the women's natural state, and elevating it to the existential female dilemma.... The number of diet-related articles rose 70 percent from 1968 to 1972.*

Cellulite is fat. Nothing special, neither a disease nor a unique female problem without solutions. It can be removed.

Less obvious, but often more damaging than marketer-speak, are **scientific-*sounding* words** that are so overused as to have no agreed-upon meaning:

Health
Fitness
Optimal

To eliminate words you shouldn't use in body redesign, the question to ask is: **can I measure it?**

"I just want to be healthy" is not actionable. "I want to increase my HDL cholesterol and improve my time for a one-mile jog (or walk)" is actionable. "Healthy" is subject to the fads and *regime du jour*. Useless.

The word *optimal* is also bandied about with much fanfare. "Your progesterone might fall within the normal range, but it's not optimal." The question here, seldom asked, should be: optimal for what? Triathlon training? Extending lifespan 40%? Increasing bone density 20%? Having sex three times a day?

"Optimal" depends entirely on what your goal is, and that goal should be numerically precise. "Optimal" is usable, but only when the "for what" is clear.

If it isn't, treat *optimal* as Wikipedia would: a weasel word.

WHY A CALORIE ISN'T A CALORIE

Calories are all alike, whether they come from beef or bourbon, from sugar or starch, or from cheese and crackers. Too many calories are just too many calories.

—Fred Stare, founder and former chair of the Harvard University Nutrition Department

The above statement is so ridiculous as to defy belief, but let's take a look at the issue through a more rational lens: hypothetical scenarios.

Scenario #1: Two male identical twins eat the exact same meals for 30 days. The only difference: one of the subjects just finished a strong course of antibiotics and now lacks sufficient good bacteria for full digestion.

Will the body composition outcomes be the same?

Of course not. **Rule #1: It's not what you put in your mouth that matters, it's what makes it to your bloodstream. If it passes through, it doesn't count.**

The creator of the "calorie" as we know it, 19th-century chemist Wilbur Olin Atwater, did not have the technology that we have today. He incinerated foods. Incineration does not equal human digestion; eating a fireplace log will not store the same number of calories as burning one will produce. Tummies have trouble with bark, as they do with many things.

Scenario #2: Three females of the same race, age and body composition each consume 2,000 calories daily for 30 days. Subject 1 consumes nothing but table sugar, subject 2 consumes nothing but lean chicken breast and subject 3 consumes nothing but mayonnaise (2,000 calories is just 19.4 tablespoons, if you'd care to indulge).

Will the body composition outcomes be the same?

Of course not. **Rule #2: The hormonal responses to carbohydrates (CHO), protein and fat are different.**

There is no shortage of clinical studies to prove that beef calories[7] do not equal bourbon calories.

One such study, conducted by Kekwick and Pawan, compared three groups put on calorically equal (isocaloric) semi-starvation diets of 90% fat, 90% protein or 90% carbohydrate. Though ensuring compliance was a challenge, the outcomes were clearly not at all the same:

1,000 cals. at 90% fat = weight loss of 408g (0.9lb) per day
1,000 cals. at 90% protein = weight loss of 272g (0.6lb) per day
1,000 cals. at 90% carbohydrate = weight *gain* of 108g (0.24lb) per day

7. Protein, for one, provokes a greater thermic effect of food (TEF) than either carbohydrate or fat—in simple terms, in digestion a higher percentage of protein calories are "lost" as heat v. carbohydrates or fat. This has led some scientists to suggest that the 4 calories per gram assumed for protein should be downgraded 20% to 3.2 calories per gram.

Different sources of calories = different results.

Things that affect calorie allocation—and that can be modified for fat loss and muscle gain—include digestion, the ratio of protein-to-carbohydrates-to-fat, and timing.

We'll address all three.

MARKETING 101: SEXISM SELLS

More than 50% of the examples in this book are of women.

Marketers have conditioned women to believe that they need specific programmes and diets "for women". This is an example of capitalism at its worst: creating false need and confusion.

Does this mean I'm going to recommend that a woman do exactly the same thing as an 18st (113kg) meathead who wants 51cm (20in) arms? Of course not. The two have different goals. But 99% of the time both genders want exactly the same thing: less fat and a bit more muscle in the right places. Guess what? In these 99 cases out of 100, men and women should therefore do *exactly* the same thing.

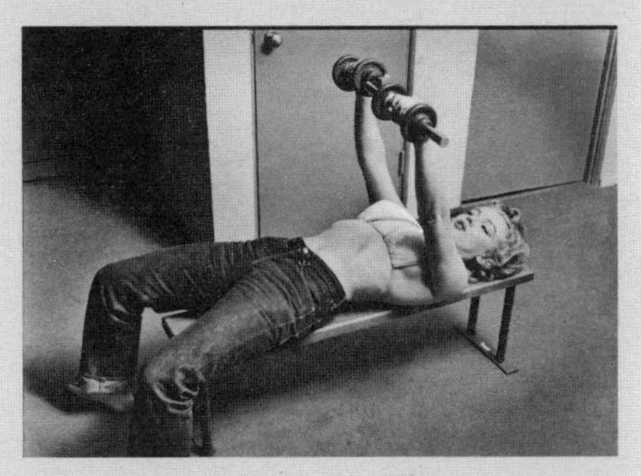

Marilyn Monroe building her world-famous sex appeal.

On average, women have less than one-tenth (often less than one-fortieth) the testosterone of men. This biochemical recipe just doesn't support rapid muscular growth unless you're an outlier, so, for the duration of this book, please suspend any fear of "getting bulky".

Even if you are a fast-responder, as you observe changes, you can omit pieces or reduce frequency. Don't worry about waking up looking like the Hulk the morning after a single workout. It won't happen, as much as men wish it did. There will be plenty of time to tweak and fine-tune, to cut back or shift gears, as you go.

One potential objection from the scientists in the group: *But don't women have more slow-twitch muscle fibres? Doesn't that mean women should train differently?* I propose not, and I'm not the first. Based on the data in this book and in the literature, you'll see that (1) muscle fibre composition can be changed, and (2) you should eat and train for your desired outcome, not to accommodate your current condition.

Don't fall victim to sexism in exercise. It's almost always a fraud or a sales pitch.

TOOLS AND TRICKS

***Seeking Wisdom: From Darwin to Munger* (www.fourhourbody.com/wisdom)** This is one of the best books on mental models, how to use them, and how not to make a fool of yourself. I was introduced to this manual for critical thinking by Derek Sivers, who sold his company CD Baby for $22 million (£14 million).

***Poor Charlie's Almanack: The Wit and Wisdom of Charles T. Munger* (www.fourhourbody.com/almanac)** This book contains most of the talks and lectures of Charlie Munger, the vice chairman of Berkshire Hathaway. It has sold nearly 50,000 copies without any advertising or bookshop placement.

Munger's Worldly Wisdom (www.fourhourbody.com/munger) This transcribed speech, given by Charlie Munger at USC Business School, discusses the 80–90 important mental models that cover 90% of the decisions he makes.

GROUND ZERO—

Getting Started and Swaraj

At the individual level Swaraj is vitally connected with the capacity for dispassionate self-assessment, ceaseless self-purification and growing self-reliance. . . . It is Swaraj when we learn to rule ourselves.

—Mahatma Gandhi, *Young India*, 28 June 1928, p. 772

I must not fear. Fear is the mind-killer. Fear is the little-death that brings total obliteration. I will face my fear. I will permit it to pass over me and through me. And when it has gone past I will turn the inner eye to see its path. Where the fear has gone there will be nothing. Only I will remain.

—Bene Gesserit "Litany Against Fear", from Frank Herbert's *Dune*

THE HARAJUKU MOMENT

The Decision to Become a Complete Human

For most of us, the how-to books on our shelves represent a growing to-do list, not advice we've followed.

Several of the better-known tech CEOs in San Francisco have asked me at different times for an identical favour: an index card with bullet-point instructions for losing abdominal fat. Each of them made it clear: "Just tell me exactly what to do and I'll do it."

I gave them all of the necessary tactical advice on one 76x127mm (3x5in) card, knowing in advance what the outcome would be. The success rate was impressive . . . 0%.

People suck at following advice. Even the most effective people in the world are terrible at it. There are two reasons:

1. Most people have an insufficient reason for action. The pain isn't painful enough. It's a *nice-to-have*, not a *must-have*. There has been no "Harajuku Moment".
2. There are no reminders. No consistent tracking = no awareness = no behavioural change. Consistent tracking, even if you

have no knowledge of fat loss or exercise, will often beat advice from world-class trainers.

But what is this all-important "Harajuku Moment"?

It's an epiphany that turns a nice-to-have into a must-have. There is no point in getting started until it happens. It applies to fat loss as much as strength gain, to endurance as much as sex. No matter how many bullet points and recipes I provide, you will need a Harajuku Moment to fuel the change itself.

Chad Fowler knows this.

Chad, CTO of InfoEther, Inc., spends much of his time solving hard problems for customers in the Ruby computer language. He is also co-organizer of the annual RubyConf and RailsConf conferences, where I first met him. Our second meeting was in Boulder, Colorado, where he used his natural language experience with Hindi to teach a knuckle-dragger (me) the primitive basics of Ruby.

Chad is an incredible teacher, gifted with analogies, but I was distracted in our session by something he mentioned in passing. He'd recently lost 5+st (32+kg) in less than 12 months.

It wasn't the amount of weight that I found fascinating. It was the timing. He'd been obese for more than a decade, and the change seemed to come out of nowhere. Upon landing back in San Francisco, I sent him one question via e-mail:

> What were the tipping points, the moments and insights that led you to lose the 5st?

I wanted to know what the defining moment was, the conversation or realization that made him pull the trigger after 10 years of business as usual.

His answer is contained in this chapter.

Even if you have no interest in fat loss, the key insights (partial completeness, data and oversimplification among them) will help you lift 227kg (500lb), run 31 miles (50km), gain 4st (23kg), or do anything else in this book.

But let's talk about one oddity upfront: calorie counting. I've just been thrashing calorie counting, and I'm including Chad's calorie-based approach to prove a point.

This book didn't exist when Chad lost his weight, and there are far better things to track than calories. But . . . would I recommend tracking calories as an alternative to tracking nothing? You bet. Tracking anything is better than tracking nothing.

If you are very overweight, very weak, very inflexible, or *very* anything negative, tracking even a mediocre variable will help you develop awareness that leads to the right behavioural changes.

This underscores an encouraging lesson: you don't have to get it all right. You just have to be crystal clear on a few concepts.

Results will follow.

Enter Chad Fowler.

The Harajuku Moment

"Why had I gone 10 years getting more and more out of shape (starting off pretty unhealthy in the first place) only to finally fix it now?

"I actually remember the exact moment I decided to do something.

"I was in Tokyo with a group of friends. We all went down to Harajuku to see if we could see some artistically dressed youngsters and also to shop for fabulous clothing, which the area is famous for. A couple of the people with us were pretty fashionable dressers and had some specific things in mind they wanted to buy. After walking into shops several times and leaving without seriously considering buying anything, one of my friends and I gave up and just waited outside while the others continued shopping.

"We both lamented how unfashionable we were.

"I then found myself saying the following to him: 'For me, it doesn't even matter what I wear; I'm not going to look good anyway.'

"I think he agreed with me. I can't remember, but that's not the point. The point was that, as I said those words, they hung in the air like when you say something super-embarrassing in a loud room but happen to catch the one randomly occurring slice of silence that happens all night long. Everyone looks at you like you're an idiot. But this time, it was me looking at myself critically. I heard myself say those words and I recognized them not for their content, but for their tone of helplessness. I am, in most of my endeavours, a solidly successful person. I decide I want things to be a certain way, and I make it happen. I've done it with my career, my learning of music, understanding of foreign languages and basically everything I've tried to do.

"For a long time, I've known that the key to getting started down the path of being remarkable in anything is to simply act with the intention of being remarkable.

"If I want a better-than-average career, I can't simply 'go with the flow' and get it. Most people do just that: they wish for an outcome but make no intention-driven actions towards that outcome. If they would just do *something* most people would find that they get some version of the outcome they're looking for. That's been my secret. Stop wishing and start doing.

"Yet here I was, talking about arguably the most important part of my life—my health—as if it was something I had no control over. I had been going with the flow for years. Wishing for an outcome and waiting to see if it would come. I was the limp, powerless ego I detest in other people.

"But somehow, as the school nerd who always got picked last for everything, I had allowed 'not being good at sports' or 'not being fit' to enter what I considered to be inherent attributes of myself. The net result is that I was left with an understanding of myself as an *incomplete* person. And though I had (perhaps) overcompensated for that incompleteness by kicking ass in every other way I could, I was still carrying this powerlessness around with me and it was very slowly and subtly gnawing away at me from the inside.

"So, while it's true that I wouldn't have looked great in the fancy clothes, the seemingly superficial catalyst that drove me to finally do something wasn't at all superficial. It actually pulled out a deep root that had been, I think, driving an important part of me for basically my entire life.

"And now I recognize that this is a pattern. In the culture I run in (computer programmers and tech people), this partial-completeness is not just common but maybe even the norm. My life lately has taken on a new focus: digging up those bad roots; the holes I don't notice in myself. And now I'm filling them one at a time.

"Once I started the weight loss, the entire process was not only easy but enjoyable.

"I started out easy. Just paying attention to food and doing relaxed cardio three to four times a week. This is when I started thinking in terms of making every day just slightly better than the day before. On day 1 it was easy. Any exercise was better than what I'd been doing.

"If you ask the average obese person: 'If you could work out for ONE year and be considered "in shape", would you do it?' I'd guess that just about every single one would emphatically say, 'Hell, yes!' The problem is that for most normal people there is no clear path from fat to okay in a year. For almost everyone, the path is there and obvious if you know what you're doing, but it's almost impossible to imagine an outcome like that so far in the distance.

"The number-one realization that led me to be able to keep doing it and make the right decisions was to **use data**.

"I learnt about the basal metabolic rate (BMR), also called resting metabolic rate, and was amazed at how many calories I would have to eat in order to stay the same weight. It was huge. As I started looking at calorie content for food that wasn't obviously bad, I felt like I'd have to just gluttonously eat all day long if I wanted to stay fat. The BMR showed me that (1) it wasn't going to be hard to cut calories, and (2) I must have been making BIG mistakes before in order to consume those calories—not small ones. That's good news. Big mistakes mean lots of low-hanging fruit.[1]

"Next was learning that 4,000 calories equals about 1lb (450g) of fat. I know that's an oversimplification, but that's okay. **Oversimplifying is one of the next things I'll mention as a tool.** But if 4,000 is roughly 1lb (450g) of fat, and my BMR makes it pretty easy to shave off some huge number of calories per day, it suddenly becomes very clear how to lose lots of weight without even doing any exercise. Add in some calculations on how many calories you burn doing, say, 30 minutes of exercise and you can pretty quickly come up with a formula that looks something like:

BMR = 2,900
Actual intake = 1,800
Deficit from diet = BMR – actual intake = 1,100
Burnt from 30 minutes cardio = 500
Total deficit = deficit from diet + burnt from 30 minutes cardio = 1,600

"So that's 1,600 calories saved in a day, or almost ½lb (225g) of bad weight I could lose in a single day. So for a big round number, I can

1. Tim: This type of low-hanging fruit is also commonly found by would-be weight gainers when they record protein intake for the first time. Many are only consuming 40–50 grams of protein per day.

lose 5lb (2.3kg) in a week and a half without even working too hard. When you're 4st (27kg) overweight, getting to 10% of your goal that fast is **real**.

"**An important thing I alluded to earlier is that all of these numbers are in some ways bullshit.** That's okay, and realizing that it was okay was one of the biggest shifts I had to make. When you're 4–5st (27–32kg) overweight (or I'd say whenever you have a BIG change to make), worrying about counting calories consumed or burnt slightly inaccurately is going to kill you. The fact of the matter is, there are no tools available to normal people which will tell us exactly how much energy we're burning or consuming. But if you're just *kinda* right and, more important, the numbers are *directionally* right, you can make a big difference with them.

"Here's another helpful pseudo-science number: apparently, 10lb (4.5kg) of weight loss is roughly a clothing size [XL → L → M]. That was a HUGE motivator. I loved donating clothes all year and doing guilt-free shopping.

"As a nerd, I find myself too easily discouraged by data collection projects where it's difficult or impossible to collect accurate data. Training myself to forget that made all the difference.

"Added to this knowledge was a basic understanding of how metabolism works. Here are the main things I changed: breakfast within 30 minutes of waking and five to six meals a day of roughly 200 calories each. How did I measure the calories? I didn't. I put together an exact meal plan for just ONE week, bought all the ingredients, stuck to it religiously. From that point on, I didn't have to do the hard work any more. I became aware after just one week of *roughly* how many calories were in a portion of different types of food and just guessed. Again, trying to literally *count* calories sucks and is demotivating. Setting up a rigid template for a week and then using it as a basic guide is sustainable and fun.

"Just a few more disconnected tips:

"I set up a workstation where I could pedal on a recumbent bike while working. I did real work, wrote parts of *The Passionate Programmer*, played video games, chatted with friends and watched ridiculous television shows I'd normally be ashamed to be wasting my time on all while staying in my aerobic zone. I know a lot of creative people who hate exercise because it's boring. I was in that camp too (I'm not any more. . . it changes once you get into it). The bike/desk was my saviour. That mixed with a measurement system:

"I got a heart rate monitor (HRM) and started using it for EVERYTHING. I used it while pedalling to make sure that even when I was having fun playing a game I was doing myself some good. If you know your heart rate zones (easy to find on the Internet), the ambiguity non-fitness-experts feel with respect to exercise is removed. Thirty minutes in your aerobic zone is good exercise and burns fat. Calculate how many calories you burn (a good HRM will do it for you), and the experience is fun and motivating. I started wearing my HRM when I was doing things like annoying chores around the house. You can clean house fast and burn serious fat. That's not some Montel Williams BS. It's real. Because of the constant use of an HRM I was able to combine fun and exercise or annoying chores and exercise, making all of it more rewarding and way less likely I'd get lazy and decide not to do it.

"Building muscle is, as you know, one of the best ways to burn fat. But geeks don't know how to build muscle. And as I've mentioned, geeks don't like to do things they don't *know* are going to work. We like data. We value expertise. So I hired a trainer to teach me what to do. I think I could have let go of the trainer after a few sessions, since I had learnt the 'right' exercises, but I've stayed with her for the past year.

"Finally, as a friend said of my difficulty in writing about my insights for weight loss, a key insight is my lack of specific insights.

"To some extent, the answer is just 'diet and exercise.' There were no gimmicks. **I used data we all have access to** and just trusted biology to work its magic. I gave it a trial of 20 days or so and lost a significant amount of weight. Even better, I started waking up thinking about exercising because I felt good.

"It was easy."

It was easy for Chad because of his Harajuku Moment. It worked because he used numbers.

In the next chapter, you'll get your numbers.

That's when the fun begins.

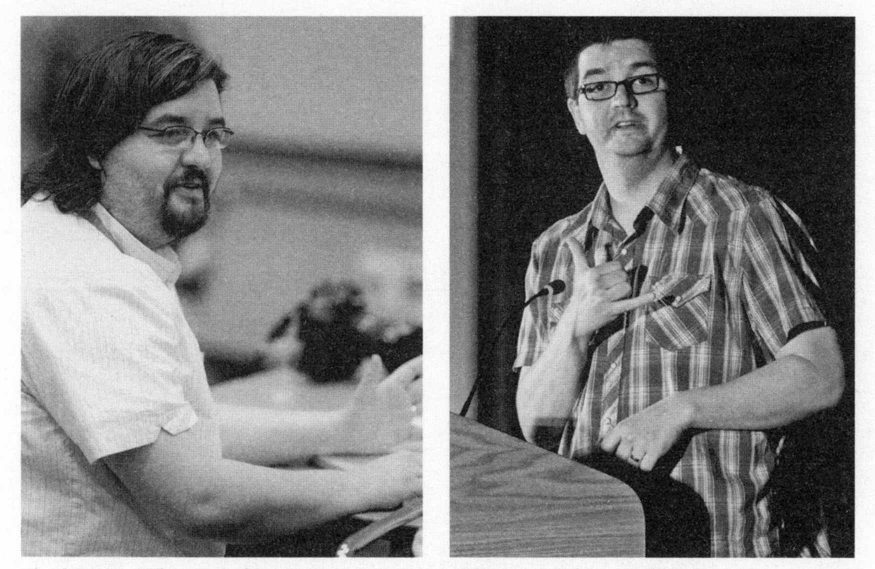

Chad Fowler, before and after his Harajuku Moment. (Photos: James Duncan Davidson)

TOOLS AND TRICKS

"Practical Pessimism: Stoicism as Productivity System", Google Ignite (www.fourhourbody.com/stoicism) This is a five-minute presentation I gave in 2009 on my personal Harajuku Moment. This video will show you how to inoculate your fears while leveraging them to accomplish what you want.

Clive Thompson, "Are Your Friends Making You Fat?" ***New York Times,*** **10 September 2009 (www.fourhourbody.com/friends)** Reaching your physical goals is a product, in part, of sheer proximity to people who exhibit what you're targeting. This article explains the importance and implications of choosing your peer group.

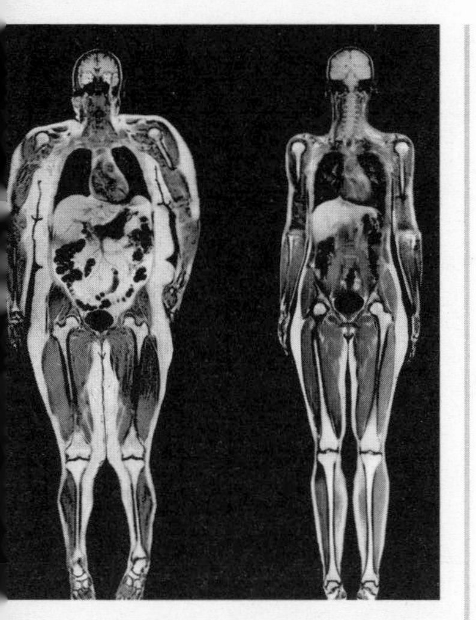

Think fat is just under the skin? Think again. The above MRI of an 18st (113kg) woman, compared to a 8.5st (54kg) woman, shows the large fat deposits around internal organs. The undigested food is a reader-gagging bonus.

The first principle is that you must not fool yourself, and you are the easiest person to fool.

—Richard P. Feynman, Nobel Prize-winning physicist

γνωθι σεαυτόυ
["Know Thyself"]

—Inscription at Temple of Apollo at Delphi

ELUSIVE BODY FAT

Where Are You Really?

Update E-Mail from Subject X, Male:

27/12/08
Beginning weight 17.5st (111kg).

30/1/09
End of month #1 16.3st (103kg).

1/3/09
End of month #2 15.9st (101kg).
[Too little protein in the morning for the past 4 weeks; added 30 grams within 30 minutes of waking to restart fat loss]

2/4/09
End of month #3 14.5st (92kg).
[90 day weight loss = 2.9st (19kg).]

1/5/09
End of month #4 14.3st (91kg).

1/6/09
End of month #5 13.8st (87.5kg).

1/7/09
End of month #6 13.3st (85kg).

31/7/09

End of month #7 13.2st (84kg).

It's somewhat demoralizing to only lose 3.5kg in the last two months. As far as my lifting exercises are concerned, there are five basic lifts.[2] The two weights I am giving you are kilograms and pounds when I started and my present kilograms and pounds.

1. Shoulder Press—10 slow reps[3]
Starting weight—6.8kg (15lb). Present weight—34kg (75lb).
2. Pulldown—8 slow reps
Starting weight—23kg (50lb). Present weight—61kg (135lb).
3. Bench Press—8 slow reps
Starting weight—13.6kg (30lb). Present weight—41kg (90lb).
4. Row—8 slow reps
Starting weight—23kg (50lb). Present weight—54kg (120lb).
5. Curl—12 slow reps
Starting weight—7kg (15lb). Present weight—23kg (50lb).

Subject X, aged 65, was depressed by his slowing rate of weight loss. The real question was: should he have been?

The Deceptive Scale

Looking at his exercise logs, he showed massive strength gains in the three months where he showed the least *weight* loss.

I didn't think this was a coincidence. He had almost tripled his strength in all movements, and to estimate 4.5kg (10lb) of lean muscle gain over those three months would be conservative. This would make his actual fat loss closer to 8kg (18lb), not the scale's 3.5kg (8lb).

His muscle gains slowed after this update e-mail, and the fat loss once again began to show on the scale. He dropped from 185 to 173lb. Total *weight* lost: 32kg (72lb).

But total *fat* lost? It's impossible to tell. In a rush to get started, I hadn't insisted on getting his body fat percentage measured.

2. This subject had more than 10 fractures in his knees and could not perform lower-body exercises.
3. For those unfamiliar with lifting parlance, "reps" are repetitions of a movement. If you do 20 push-ups, you've done 20 reps of the push-up.

Not that I cared much. For the first time in my life, I saw my father weighing less than me. During his annual check-up four months later, his doctor remarked: "You realize you're younger now than you were a year ago. You may just live forever." It was a stark contrast to his 17.5st (111kg) at 168cm (5ft 6in) just a year earlier. My dad had gone from risk of sudden heart attack to looking and feeling 10 years younger in 12 months.

Regardless, he had become depressed about his results precisely when he should have been giving people high-fives. It takes just one such incident to ruin an entire programme and months of progress.

How can *you* prevent unnecessary moments of doubt?

It just takes a few simple numbers to steer the ship—to know, without fail, when something is working and when it is not.

Until you finish this chapter, do not pass go.

If you want to skip directly to the actions, jump to "Starting Your Physical GPS" on page 51. In fact, I suggest this for the first read through.

Choosing the Right Tools

I used to have a signature move while driving.

About 0.4km (¼ mile) or so before arriving at my hard-fought destination, often within 60m (200ft), I would come to the unwavering conclusion that I'd gone too far. Then I would U-turn and drive in the opposite direction, only to repeat the drill like a dog tethered to a clothesline. Best-case scenario, this shuttle run doubled my travel time. Worst-case scenario, I got so frustrated that I abandoned the trip altogether.

This is exactly what most people do with fat loss and exercise.

Using a blunt instrument like a scale (the equivalent of the odometer in my example) people often conclude they're not making progress when, in fact, they are making tremendous progress. This leads to a musical chairs of fad diets and demoralizing last-ditch efforts that do more harm than good. To hit your target 1.4st (9kg) recomposition, you'll need to track the right numbers.

The scale is one tool, and you should use it, but it is not king. It can mislead. Take this unedited feedback from Angel, who was two weeks into the Slow-carb Diet at the time (see "The Slow-carb Diet I and II" chapters):

After my cheat day on Saturday, I gained 1 pound which is normal for me . . . week two, I lost that 1 pound. I didn't lose any [additional] weight on week two, but I'm not discouraged. I did manage to lose in inches. I lost ½ an inch off my hips which is absolutely great. I lost a total of 1 inch off my thighs. Not so shabby either. So that's a total of 1.5 inches for the week. I'll take the inches. The grand total of inches lost from Day One: 5 inches . . . Yippee! No exercise either.

My driving issues ended when I bought a GPS device.

The GPS fixed my problem because it could answer the simple question: was I getting *closer* to my destination?

In body redesign, our "destination" is a better ratio of body *composition*, not weight.

How much of you is useful muscle and how much of you is useless fat? Our constant companions will be circumference and body fat measurements. By the end of this chapter, you will have a starting point for your own physical GPS. This will guide you to your 1.4st (9kg) recomposition goal.

Circumference is easy enough: use a tape measure. We'll cover the details at the end of this chapter.

But how do we actually measure body fat percentage?

It turns out, there are a lot of options, and the most common are the worst.

Skinning the Cat

In one 24-hour period,[4] I took more than a dozen body fat measurements using the easiest-to-find, as well as the most sophisticated, equipment available.

Here are some of the results, from lowest to highest:

7%—3-point with SlimGuide calipers
7.1–9.4%—Accu-measure
9.5%—BodyMetrix ultrasound
11.3%—DEXA

4. From noon on 3 October 2009 to noon on 4 October 2009.

13.3%—BodPod
14.7–15.4%—Omron hand-held bio-impedance (second value after drinking two litres of water in five minutes)
15.46–16.51%—4-site SlimGuide calipers

The range is 7% to 16.51%. So then, which of these bad boys is accurate?

The truth is, none of them are accurate. Moreover, this doesn't matter. We just need to make sure that the method we choose is consistent.

This table shows the various techniques I considered, ordered from most to least error-prone.[5]

COMPARISON OF METHODS FOR ESTIMATING % BODY FAT

METHOD	Cost of Procedure	Time (minutes)	Technician Skill	Subject Comfort	Error in %BF	Comments
Circumference	Low	~5	Low to moderate	High	~3.0% ~ 3.6%	
Bio Electrical Impedance	Low	~5	Low	High	~2.5% ~ 4.0%	Sensitive to subject hydration
Skinfold	Low	~5	High	Low	~2.0% ~ 3.5%	Dependent on formula
Ultrasound	Low	~5	Moderate	High	~2.3% ~ 3.0%	Only low-cost method that can also measure muscle thickness
BodPod	High	~30	High	Moderate	~2.3% ~ 2.8%	
Underwater Weighing	High	~30 ~ 60	High	Low	~2.3% ~ 2.8%	Needs careful measurement and can be affected by subject
DEXA	High	~15 ~ 30	High	High	~1.2% ~ 2.5%	Can measure lean mass and bone
X-ray CT	High	~10 ~ 15	High	High	~1.0% ~ 2.0%	Significant radiation
MRI	High	~30 ~ 45	High	High	~1.0% ~ 2.0%	

Provided by Luiz Da Silva, PhD., scientific advisory board, UC Davis National Science Foundation Center for Biophotonics Science and Technology.

After dozens of trials with multiple subjects, and taking into account both constancy and convenience (including cost), there were three clear winners:[6]

5. These error ranges assume trained professionals and optimum conditions for measurements (e.g., good hydration for body-impedance). The order was determined using the median of their lower and upper error percentages.
6. In an ideal world, X-ray CT and MRI would be used, but I omitted them due to radiation and cost, respectively.

1. DEXA
2. BodPod
3. Ultrasound (BodyMetrix)

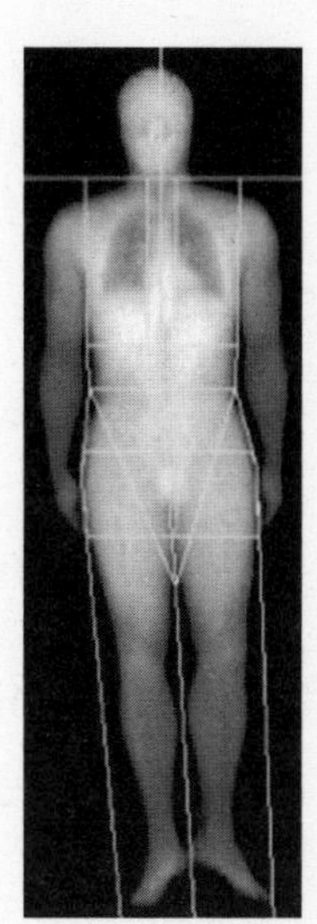
My DEXA scan image.

The Top 3

DEXA

Dual energy X-ray absorptiometry (DEXA), which costs $50–100 (£31–62) per session, ended up my favourite, as it is repeatable and offers valuable information besides body fat percentage. The GE Lunar Prodigy, the machine I used, is designed for bone density testing and splits the body into different zones.

If you're not concerned about osteoporosis, why is this interesting?

Because it highlights muscular imbalances between the left and right sides. In my case:

Left arm—4.6 kg
Right arm—4.7 kg (I'm right-handed, so not surprising)
Left leg—12.4 kg
Right leg—12.8 kg
Left trunk—18.9 kg
Right trunk—17.9 kg

As we'll see in "Pre-hab", making yourself injury-proof requires, above all, correcting left–right imbalances. In five to ten minutes, DEXA gives a crystal-clear picture of mass imbalances that even outstanding physical therapists can miss after hours of observation.

BODPOD

Costing just $25–50 (£15.50–31), BodPod uses air displacement and is comparable to the clinical "gold standard" of hydrostatic underwater weighing. The subject (you) sits inside a sealed capsule, and alternating air pressures determine body composition. Infinitely faster and more comfortable than underwater weighing, the BodPod is the official body fat measurement device of the NFL Combine, where the 330 best college football players are analysed by NFL coaches and scouts to determine their worth.

Unlike calipers and some other methods, BodPod can accommodate obese subjects of 35.7+st (227+kg).

BODYMETRIX

BodyMetrix is a hand-held ultrasound device that tells you the exact thickness of fat (in millimetres) wherever you place it. It ended up being the tool I used most often and still use most often.

Ultrasound has been used for more than a decade to determine the fat and muscular characteristics of livestock. Want to see how that intramuscular marbling is coming along on your living Kobe beef? Pull out the pregnancy cam!

It's amazing that it took so long to reach athletics. The next-generation BodyMetrix wand, small enough to fit in a jacket pocket, connects to any PC with a USB cable and is now used by world-famous teams like the New York Yankees and AC Milan football club. It is the picture of simplicity: I was able to take frequent readings in less than two minutes, and both data and images were automatically uploaded to my Mac. (The PC software actually runs faster on a Mac using Parallels®, a program that allows you to use PC software on Macs.)

Rather than attempt to find a gym that offered this for per-session fees, I decided to own a unit. At $2,000 (£1,250) for the professional unit, it was worth the convenience. There is a personal version in development that will cost less than $500 (£310).

Can't Find the Fancy Stuff?

If you choose to use calipers or bio-impedance (any tool you hold or stand on) out of convenience, or if you use them for more frequent measurement alongside one of the Top Three, here are critical points to consider:

1. NEVER COMPARE BEFORE-AND-AFTER RESULTS FROM DIFFERENT TOOLS.[7]

Results from different tools cannot be compared. In my 24-hour measurement marathon, I tested 13.3% with BodPod and 11.3% with DEXA. Let's say I had tested using only DEXA at 11.3% and then tested on BodPod for my follow-up, which resulted in 12.3%. I would wrongly conclude that I'd

7. Nor should you compare different algorithms on the same equipment. This most frequently causes confusion when you get caliper readings from different trainers. Use the same person and same algorithm (e.g., 3-point Jackson-Pollock).

gained 1% body fat, whereas I would have seen a more accurate 1% loss had I used BodPod for both.

2. IF YOU CHOOSE TO USE BIO-ELECTRICAL IMPEDANCE (BEI),[8] YOU NEED CONSISTENT HYDRATION.

Using bio-impedance devices, I have been able to make my body fat percentage jump almost 1% in five minutes by drinking 2 litres (64 fl oz) of water in between measurements. Here's a simple approach that largely fixes hydration issues:

Immediately upon waking, drink 1.5 litres (48 fl oz) of cold water[9]—ensure that water temperature is the same day to day—and wait 30 minutes. Urinate and then test body fat using bio-impedance. Do not eat or drink anything else before testing. I use two empty Bulleit bourbon bottles (750 millilitres × 2 = 1.5 litres) because I love the old-school bottles, but Nalgene bottles are generally 1 litre (32 fl oz) each and have line measurements on the side. Wine and most liquor is also standardized for a 750-millilitre bottle size.

3. IF YOU CHOOSE TO USE CALIPERS, YOU NEED A CONSISTENT ALGORITHM.

Even with the same calipers, using different maths = different results. I suggest asking the gym or trainer to use a 3-point or 7-point Jackson-Pollock algorithm, which I have found gives the most consistent results compared to the Top Three.[10] This should be as simple as selecting from a drop-down menu in their software.

Starting Your Physical GPS—The Steps

Starting a body recomposition programme without measurements is like planning a trip without a start address. I *guarantee* you will regret it later. Don't fly blind.

My father, who lost more than 5st (31.7kg) and more than tripled his strength, is still kicking himself for not having body fat numbers.

8. Also referred to as bio-impedance, or BI.

9. The coldness of the water will also help fat loss.

10. There are population-specific formulas that give better numbers, but they are not commonly used since most fitness clubs and personal trainers deal with the broad population.

Spend a pound or two and get your data. If need be, skip a few lattes and a dinner out.

Next steps:

1. Take your "before" circumference measurements. Get a simple tape measure and measure four locations: both upper arms (mid-bicep), waist (horizontal at navel), hips (at widest point below waist) and both legs (mid-thigh). Total these numbers to arrive at your **Total Inches (TI)**. Changes in this total will be meaningful enough to track.
2. Estimate your body fat (BF%) based on the "Eyeballing It" sidebar on page 54.
3. Choose the best tool and schedule a session.

If you're over 30% body fat, avoid calipers and use DEXA, BodPod or ultrasound, in that order. If you cannot find these, opt for bio-impedance and follow the hydration rules mentioned earlier.

If you are under 25%, still aim for DEXA, BodPod or ultrasound. If you cannot find these, opt for calipers with a qualified professional (use the same person for all follow-up visits) and request the 3-point or 7-point Jackson-Pollock algorithm. If neither is available, use another algorithm that includes a leg measurement and at least three points total. Leg fat is tricky and needs to be included. Record the name of the algorithm used for future reference.

TOOLS AND TRICKS

OrbiTape One-handed Tape Measure (www.fourhourbody.com/orbitape) Measure any body part with military precision using this tape measure, the armed services' choice for physical examinations.

Finding DEXA DEXA must be administered by licensed medical staff and so eliminates most gyms and health clubs. First, Google your city, plus "DEXA body fat". If that fails, search "DEXA", "osteoporosis testing" or "bone density testing" for your postcode or city. Add "facility" if the search returns too many results. I spent $49 (£31) on the test in Redwood City, California, at the Body Composition Center (www.bodycompositioncenter.com).

BodPod Locators (www.bodpod.com/clients/europeClients) The BodPod is used to test athletes at the NFL Combine for fat and fat-free mass, as well as respiratory volume. Use this site to find BodPod assessment centres which are located in the UK and Europe.

BodyMetrix (www.fourhourbody.com/bodymetrix) The hand-held BodyMetrix device uses ultrasound to measure body composition down to the millimetre. For those with the means, it is an outstanding option and my default choice.

Escali Bio-impedance Scale (www.fourhourbody.com/escalibio) Escali's bio-impedance scale measures weight and percentage of body fat for up to 10 users.

Slim Guide Skinfold Calipers (www.fourhourbody.com/slimguide) These are the most widely used calipers in the world. They're low-cost, but accurate enough for professional use. Be sure to include at least one leg measurement in all calculations.

Cosmetic Fat v. Evil Fat—How to Measure Visceral Fat (www.fourhourbody.com/evil) Ever wonder how some people, especially older men, can have beer bellies that seem as tight as a drum? Distended abdomens that seem like muscle if you poke them? The answer is unpleasant: rather than fat under the skin, it's fat around internal organs that presses the abdominal wall out.

One weakness of calipers and ultrasound is that they can only directly measure subcutaneous fat (under the skin) and not what's called visceral fat (around the organs).

This article, authored by Michael Eades MD and Mary Dan Eades MD, explains a low-tech method for estimating the latter, which is particularly important for those over 25% body fat or of middle age and older.

EYEBALLING IT: A VISUAL GUIDE TO BODY FAT

What should your body fat goals be? For most people, I suggest the following as a starting point:

For men:
If obese, aim for 20%.
If you have just a bit of extra padding, aim for 12%.

For women:
If obese, aim for 25%.
If you have just a bit of extra padding, aim for 18%.

If you (male or female) want to get to 5%, we'll help you later.

Use the pictures on pages 56–57 and descriptions (whatever is most helpful) to estimate your current body fat percentage. Where are you really? Look at the pics before reading the rest, as you might be able to skip the text.

The following percentages and descriptions are intended to reflect high-end caliper readings on males, but the guidelines are still helpful for women. Keep in mind that since calipers measure a skinfold, both subcutaneous fat and subcutaneous water are reflected in the numbers. Special credit to Surferph34 for the guidelines and photo links:[11]

20% Body fat

There is *no* visible muscle definition and only a hint of separation between major muscle groups if those groups are large and well developed. For examples, see:

www.fourhourbody.com/20a
www.fourhourbody.com/20b
www.fourhourbody.com/20c

15% Body fat

Some muscle separation appears between the shoulders (deltoids) and upper arms. Abs are not visible. For an example, see:

www.fourhourbody.com/15a

11. www.fourhourbody.com/bodyfat-examples

12% Body fat

More muscle separation appears, particularly in the chest and back, and an outline of the abs begins to appear. Standing under a ceiling light with favourable shadows, a pending four-pack might be visible. For examples, see:

www.fourhourbody.com/12a
www.fourhourbody.com/12b

10% Body fat

Muscle separations get deeper in the arms, chest, legs, and back, and six-pack abs are visible when flexed. For an example, see:

www.fourhourbody.com/10a

7–9% Body fat

Abs are clearly visible all the time, vascularity in arms is prominent, chest and back separation is obvious, and the face starts to appear more angular. For examples, see:

www.fourhourbody.com/7a
www.fourhourbody.com/7b

5–7% Body fat

Striations appear in large muscle groups when they are flexed. Vascularity appears in lower abdomen and in the legs. Competitive bodybuilders often aim for this state for competition day. For an example, see:

www.fourhourbody.com/5a

MALE EXAMPLES

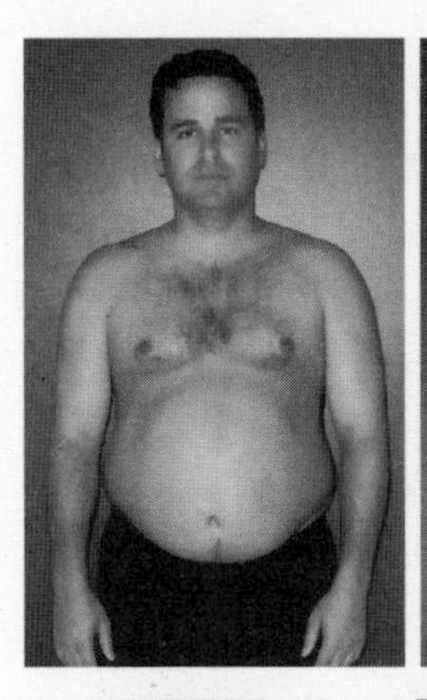
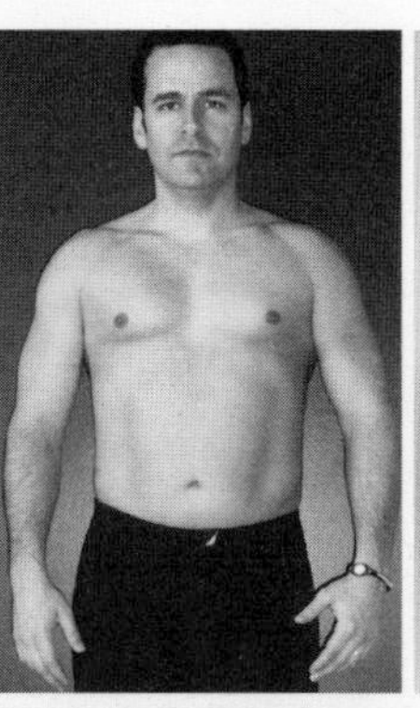
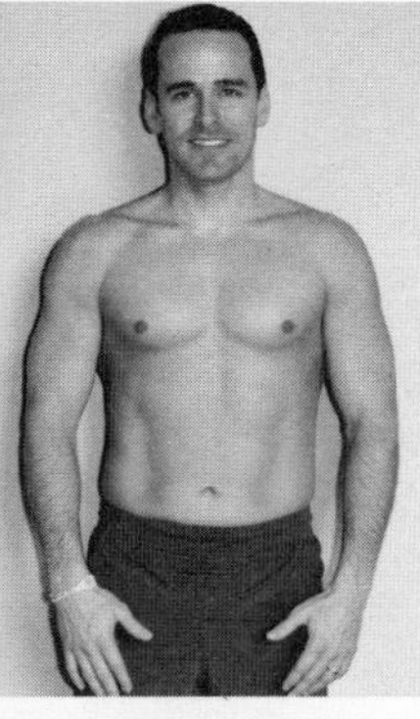

Trevor Newell
33% body fat,
19% body fat,
9% body fat

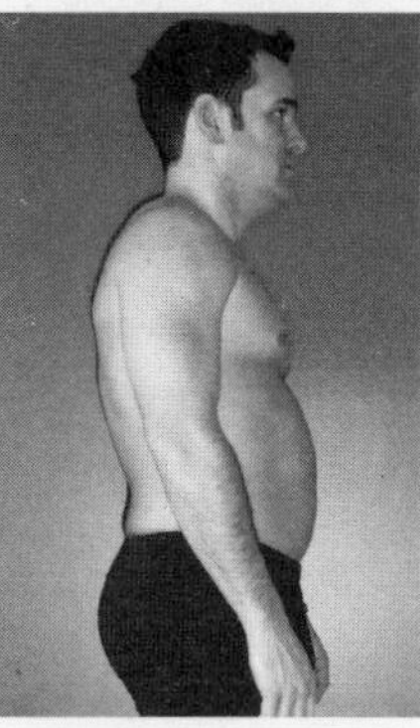
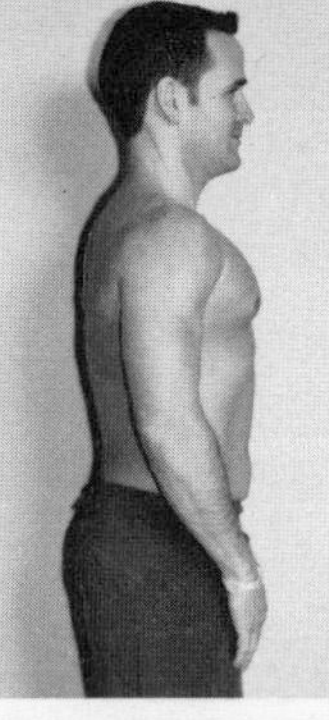

Trevor Newell
33% body fat,
19% body fat,
9% body fat

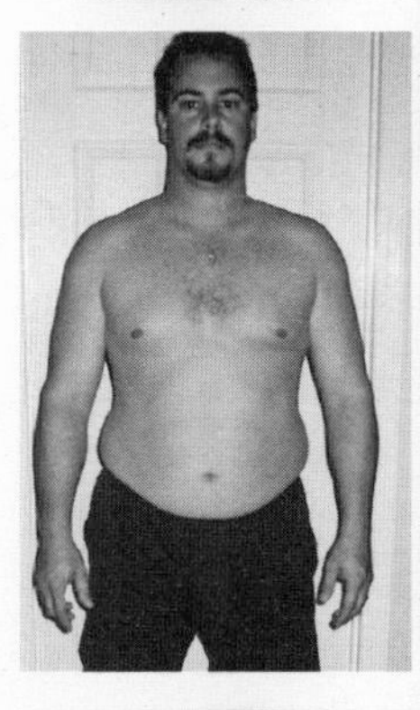
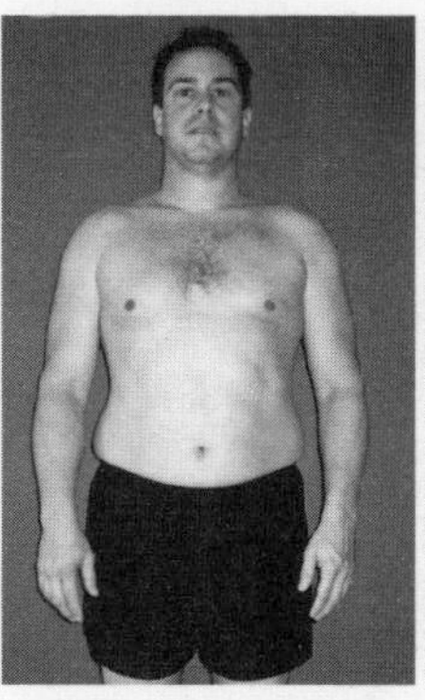
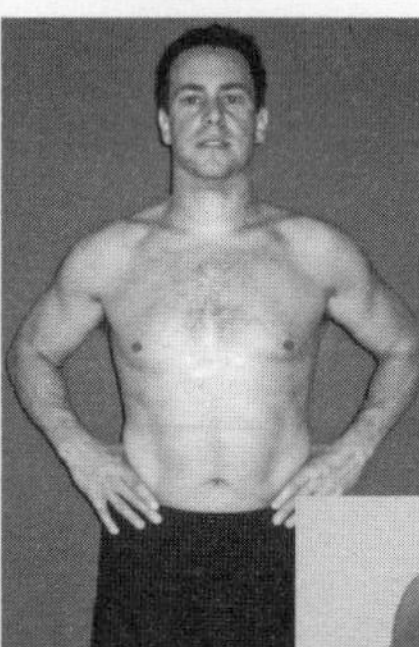

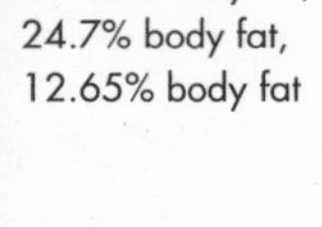

Ray Cronise
31.56% body fat,
24.7% body fat,
12.65% body fat

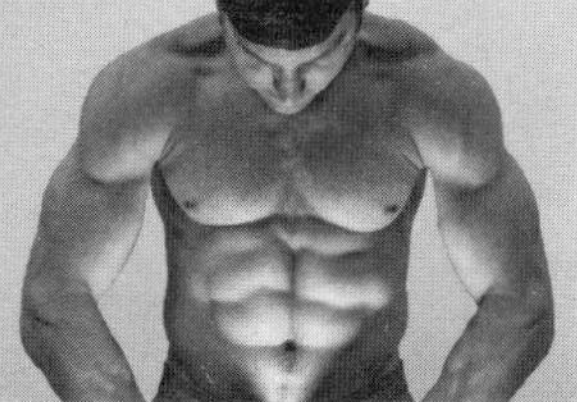

Nathan Zaru: 8% body fat. Despite the Incredible Hulk lighting, I believe this to be (among these photos) the best representative picture of what 8% body fat looks like for males with decent muscle tone. People dramatically underestimate body fat percentage. If you have a bit of muscle and are sub-10%, you should have definition similar to this.

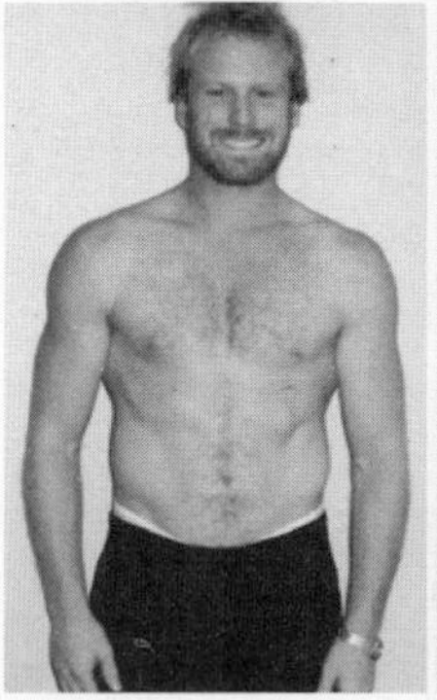
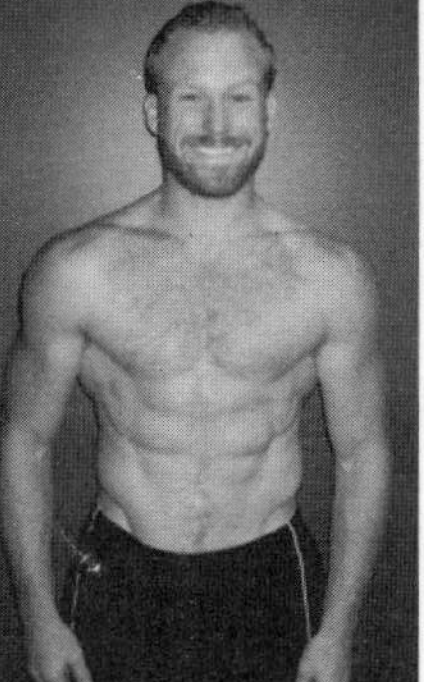

Nic Irwin
22% body fat, 5% body fat

FEMALE EXAMPLES

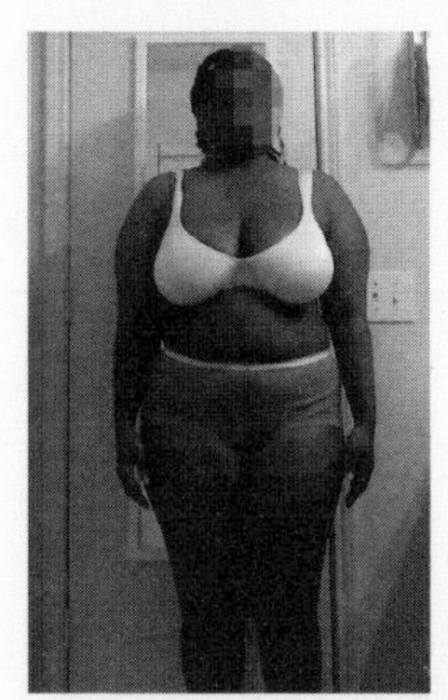

16.2st (103kg), 39.8% body fat

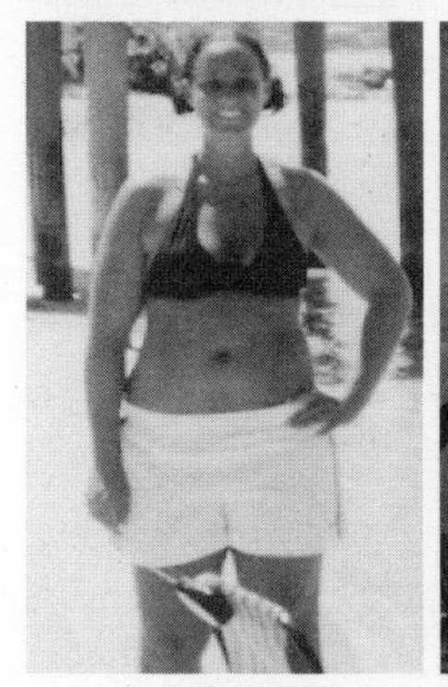

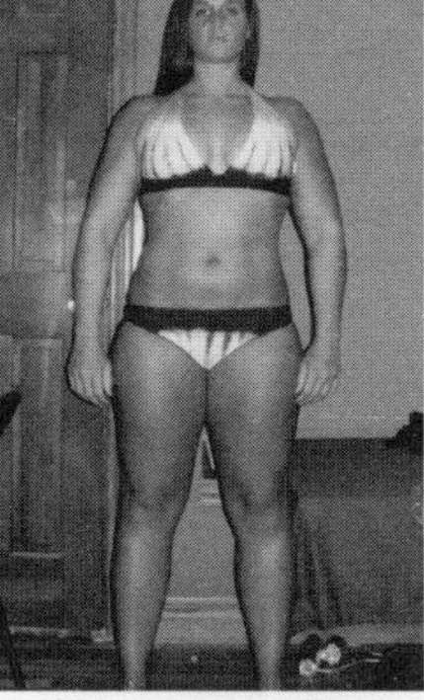

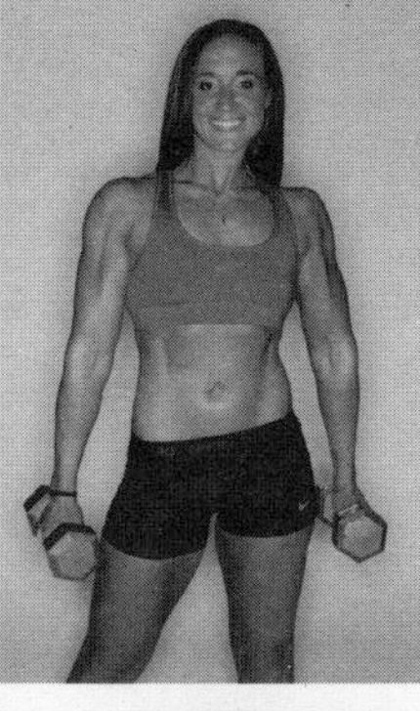

Erin Rhoades
30% body fat,
25% body fat,
12% body fat

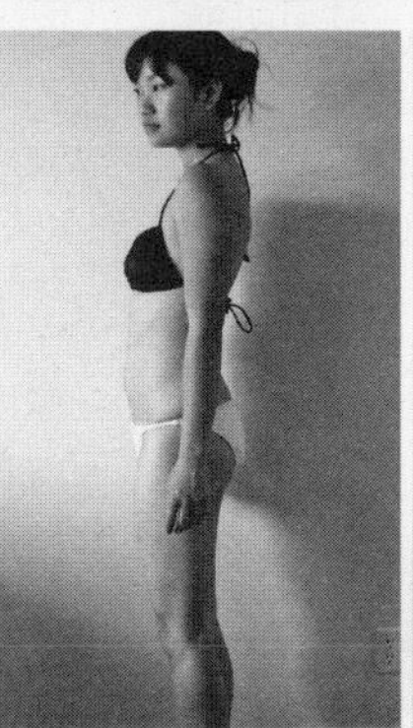

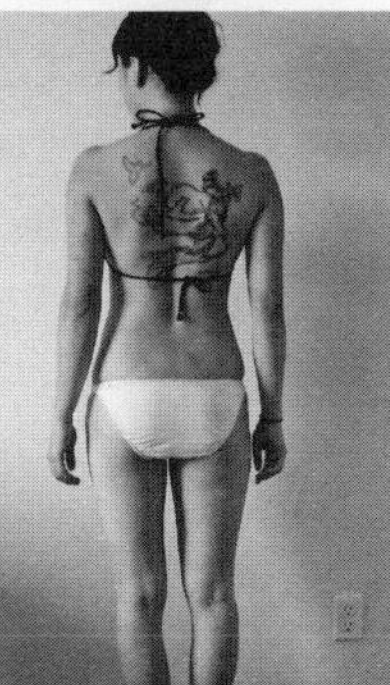

Julee
22% body fat (compare to Trevor or Nic in their 19–22% pics—the smooth appearance is similar)

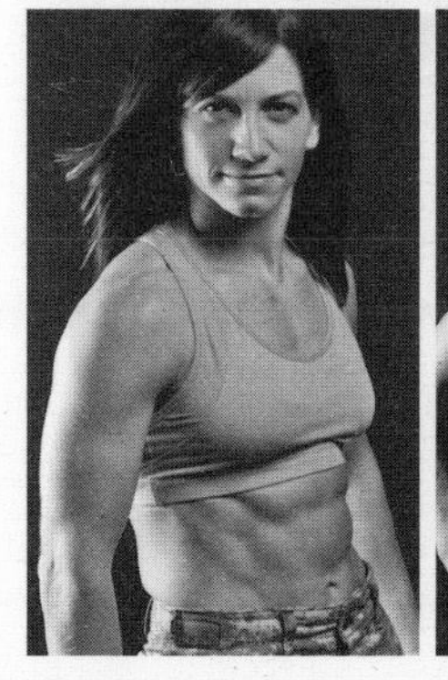

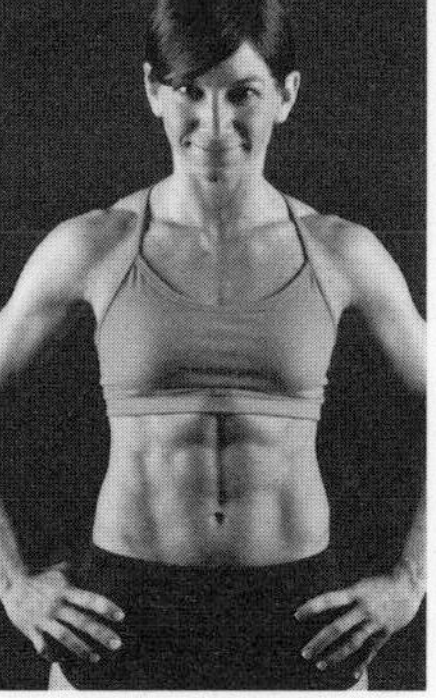

Andrea Bell
13.4% body fat

FROM PHOTOS TO FEAR

Making Failure Impossible

I have a great diet. You're allowed to eat anything you want, but you must eat it with naked fat people.

—Ed Bluestone

What gets measured gets managed.

—Peter Drucker, recipient of Presidential Medal of Freedom

199.2 . . .

Trevor stared at the LCD as it delivered the news. He blinked a few times. 199.2lb. Then he blinked a few more times.

"Holy crap!"

He'd put on about 10lb (4.5kg) a year after sophomore year in high school, tipping the scales at 17.1st (109kg) at college graduation. Now, for the first time since his teens, Trevor weighed less than 14.3st (91kg).

That had been the goal since stepping on a treadmill almost two years earlier, but a distant goal. Breaking the 14.3st (91kg) barrier had seemed unattainable. Now he'd done it. The question wasn't so much how he did it. The real question was: *why* did it work?

Simple. He'd made an agreement with a co-worker: they would go to the gym together three times per week, and if either of them missed a session, that person had to pay the other $1 (60p).

In his first gym visit, Trevor walked for four minutes on the treadmill.

Not long thereafter, he ran a mile for the first time since he was nine.

Now he has run two half-marathons.

It's not the $1 (60p) that matters (Trevor does quite well), it's the underlying psychology.

Whether it's 60 pence or 2.5cm (1in), there are ways to ensure that the first step takes you to where you want to go.

Cheap Insurance—
Four Principles of Failure-proofing

I love aeroplane magazines. But one fateful Tuesday, despite my best efforts to read about poolside hammocks and wall-sized maps, I couldn't concentrate. There was a battle being waged across the aisle on Frontier Airlines, and I had a front-row seat.

In stunned silence, I watched a man, so obese that he needed a belt extension to buckle himself in, eat a full bag of strawberry-flavoured liquorice sticks prior to take-off. He then proceeded to eat a full bag of Oreos, which he polished off before we had reached cruising altitude. It was an impressive display.

I recall asking myself: *How can he rationalize eating so much?* He had a cane, for God's sake. The answer was, of course, that he couldn't. I doubt he'd even tried. There was no logical justification for his behaviour, but then again, there is no logical justification for how I hit the snooze button every 10 minutes for an hour or two every Saturday.

We break commitments to ourselves with embarrassing regularity. How can someone trying to lose weight binge on an entire 600ml (20 fl oz) of ice cream before bed? How can even the most disciplined of executives fail to make 30 minutes of time per week for exercise? How can someone whose marriage depends on quitting smoking pick up a cigarette?

Simple: logic fails. If you were to summarize the last 100 years of behavioural psychology in two words, that would be the takeaway.

Fortunately, knowing this, it is possible to engineer compliance. Pulling from both new and often-neglected data, including photographic research and auctions, there are four principles of failure-proofing behaviour.

Think of them as insurance against the weaknesses of human nature—your weaknesses, my weaknesses, *our* weaknesses:

1. Make it conscious.
2. Make it a game.

3. Make it competitive.
4. Make it small and temporary.

1. MAKE IT CONSCIOUS: FLASHING AND "BEFORE" PHOTOS

The fastest way to correct a behaviour is to be aware of it in real time, not after-the-fact.

The curious case of the so-called "flash diet" is a prime example of the difference. Dr. Lydia Zepeda and David Deal of the University of Wisconsin–Madison enlisted 43 subjects to photograph all of their meals or snacks prior to eating. Unlike food diaries, which require time-consuming entries often written long after eating, the photographs acted as an instantaneous intervention and forced people to consider their choices *before* the damage was done. In the words of one participant: "I was less likely to have a jumbo bag of M&Ms. It curbed my choices. It didn't alter them completely, but who wants to take a photo of a jumbo bag of M&Ms?"

The researchers concluded that photographs are more effective than written food diaries. This is saying something, as prior studies had confirmed that subjects who use food diaries lose *three times* as much weight as those who don't. The upshot: use your camera phone to take a snapshot before opening your mouth. Even without a prescribed diet, this awareness alone will result in fat loss.

The camera can also be used to accentuate your flaws . . . to your benefit.

If we analyse the post-contest submissions of the winners of the Body-for-Life Challenge, the largest physique transformation contest in the last 50 years of publishing, we can isolate one common understated element: "before" photographs. The training methods and diet varied, but those who experienced the most dramatic changes credited the "before" photographs with adherence to the programme. The pictures were placed in an unavoidable spot, often on the refrigerator, and served as inoculation against self-sabotage.

Get an accurate picture of your baseline. It will look worse than you expect. This need not be bad news. Ignoring it won't fix it, so capture it and use it.

2. MAKE IT A GAME: JACK STACK AND THE STICKINESS OF FIVE SESSIONS

Jack Stack was nervous. It was 1983, and he had just joined his employees to purchase SRC, a near-bankrupt engine remanufacturer, from their parent company, International Harvester. It was done in remarkable fashion, with

$100,000 (£62,000) applied to a loan of $9 million (£5.6 million), for a debt ratio of 89-to-1. The bank officer who handled the loan was fired within hours of approving it.

The 13 managers who contributed their life savings to make it possible were also nervous, but they needn't have been. That $100,000 (£62,000) would be worth $23 million (£14 million) in 1993, just 10 years later. By 2008, sales had increased from $16 million (£10 million) to more than $400 million (£250 million), and stock value had risen from 10¢ (6p) per share to $234 (£146) per share.

What was to thank?

Games. Frequent games.

Jack Stack taught all of his employees how to read the financial statements, opened the books, and put numerical goals alongside individual performance numbers on grease boards around the plant. Daily goals and public accountability were combined with daily rewards and public recognition.

The Hawthorne plant of the Western Electric Company in Cicero, Illinois, also figured this out, albeit accidentally. The year was 1955, and their finding was significant: increasing lighting in the plant made workers more productive. Then someone pointed out (I have to imagine a sweaty-palmed intern) a confusing detail. Productivity also improved when they dimmed the lighting! In fact, making any change at all seemed to result in increased productivity.

It turned out that, with each change, the workers suspected they were being observed and therefore worked harder. This phenomenon—also called the "observer effect"—came to be known as "the Hawthorne Effect".

Reinforced by research in game design, Jack Stack and Western Electric's results can be condensed into a simple equation: **measurement = motivation**.

Seeing progress in changing numbers makes the repetitive fascinating and creates a positive feedback loop. Once again, the act of measuring is often more important than what you measure. To quote the industrial statistician George Box: "Every model is wrong, but some are useful."

It's critical that you measure something. But that begets the question: to replace self-discipline, how often do you need to record things?

That is, how many times do you need to log data to get hooked and never stop? In the experience of the brilliant Nike+ team, and in the experience of their users, more than 1.2 million runners who have tracked more than 209 million km (130 million miles), that magic number is five:

If someone uploads only a couple of runs to the site, they might just be trying it out. But once they hit five runs, they're massively more likely to keep running and uploading data. At five runs, they've gotten hooked on what their data tells them about themselves.

Aristotle had it right, but he was missing a number: "We are what we do repeatedly". A mere five times (five workouts, five meals, five of whatever we want) will be our goal.

When in doubt, "take five" is the rule.

3. MAKE IT COMPETITIVE: FEAR OF LOSS AND THE BENEFITS OF COMPARISON

Would you work harder to earn $100 (£62) or to avoid losing $100? If research from the Center for Experimental Social Science at New York University is any indication, fear of loss is the winner.

Their three-group experiment looked like this: the first group received $15 (£9.36) and was told the $15 would be taken back if they lost a subsequent auction; the second group was told they'd be given $15 if they won the auction; and the third group was a control with no incentive. The first group routinely overbid the most.

Participating economist Eric Schotter explained the results:

Economists typically attribute excessive bidding to risk aversion, or the joy of winning. What we found is that the actual cause of overbidding is a fear of losing, a completely new theory from past investigations.

This is not a depressing realization. It's a useful one. Knowing that potential loss is a greater motivator than potential reward, we can set you up for success by including a tangible risk of public failure. Real weight-loss numbers support this. Examining random 500-person samples from the 500,000+ users of DailyBurn, a diet and exercise tracking website, those who compete against their peers in "challenges" lose an average of 2.7kg (5.9lb) more than those who do not compete.

There is another phenomenon that makes groups an ideal environment for change: social comparison theory. In plain English, it means that, in a group, some people will do worse than you ("Sarah lost only 450g/1lb—good for me!") and others will do better ("Mike's nothing special. If he can do it, so can I."). Seeing inferior performers makes you proud of even minor progress, and superior performers in your peer group make greater results seem achievable.

Looking at DailyBurn's data set, those who have three or more "motivators" in their peer group lose an average of 2.6kg (5.8lb) more than those with fewer.

Embrace peer pressure. It's not just for kids.

4. MAKE IT SMALL AND TEMPORARY

That brings us to your most important next steps, detailed below.

Questions and Actions

Before you move on to another chapter, take (or in the case of #2, *start*) at least two of the following four actions. Your choice:

1. **Do I really look like that in underwear?** Take digital photos of yourself from the front, back and side. Wear either underwear or a bathing suit. Not eager to ask a neighbour for a favour? Use a camera with a timer or a computer webcam like the Mac iSight. Put the least flattering "before" photo somewhere you will see it often: the refrigerator, bathroom mirror, dog's forehead, etc.
2. **Do I really eat that?** Use a digital camera or camera phone to take photographs of everything you eat for 3–5 days, preferably including at least one weekend day. For sizing, put your hand next to each item or plate in the photographs. For maximum effect, put these photos online for others to see.
3. **Who can I get to do this with me?** Find at least one person to engage in a friendly competition using either total inches (TI) or body fat percentage. Weight is a poor substitute but another option. Use competitive drive, guilt and fear of humiliation to your advantage. Embrace the stick. The carrot is overrated.
4. **How do I measure up?** Get a simple tape measure and measure five locations: both upper arms (mid-bicep), waist (horizontal at navel), hips (widest point between navel and legs) and both legs (mid-thigh). Total these numbers to arrive at your **total inches (TI)**. I'm telling you again because I know you didn't do it after the last chapter. Get off your ass and get 'er done. It takes five minutes.

5. **What is the smallest meaningful change I can make?** Make it small. Small is achievable. For now, this means getting started on at least two of the above four steps before moving on. The rest and best is yet to come.

TOOLS AND TRICKS

Grossly Dramatic and Realistic Fat Replicas (www.fourhourbody.com/fatreplica) These are disgusting but effective motivators. I keep a 450g (1lb) fat replica in the drawer of my refrigerator. The 2.3kg (5lb) replica is the most effective visual aid I've ever seen for getting otherwise resistant people to lose fat. One biotech CEO I know goes so far as to carry one in his briefcase to show people who might benefit. If you want to thank yourself, be thanked, or perhaps be punched in the face, order one of these.

Services for Posting "Before" (and "After") Pictures
Posterous (www.posterous.com), **Evernote (www.evernote.com)**[12], **Flickr (www.flickr.com)**

PBworks Personal Wiki Pages (www.fourhourbody.com/pbworks) Ramit Sethi (in the next sidebar) set up a free PBworks page (a simple wiki page like those found on Wikipedia) and invited all his bettors to be notified when he updated his weight. He also used his PBworks page to talk a ridiculous amount of trash.

Eat.ly (http://eat.ly) Eat.ly is one of the easiest ways to start a photo-food journal. This site lets you track and keep a visual record of meals you've eaten.

Habit Forge (www.habitforge.com) Habit Forge is an e-mail check-in tool for instilling new habits into your daily routine. Decide on the habit you want to form, and Habit Forge will e-mail you for 21 days straight. If you don't follow through, the e-mail cycle will start all over again.

stickK (www.stickk.com) stickK was founded on the principle that creating incentives and assigning accountability are the two most important keys to achieving a goal. Co-founder Dean Karlan, an economics professor at Yale, came up with the idea of opening an online "Commitment Store", which eventually became stickK. If you don't fulfil your commitment with stickK, it automatically tells your friends and opens you up to endless mockery and derision.

BodySpace (www.bodybuilding.com/superhuman) or DailyBurn (www.dailyburn.com/superhuman) Need to find someone to keep you accountable? To encourage or harass you when needed? Join more than 600,000 members on BodySpace, or 500,000 on DailyBurn who are tracking the results of their diet and exercise regimens. The URLs above will link you to 4HB communities on these sites.

12. Full disclosure: I am now an adviser to both Posterous and Evernote because I believe in the services.

RAMIT THE GREAT TRASH-TALKER—HOW TO GAIN 2.3KG (5LB) A WEEK

Ramit Sethi has always joked about his "Indian frailty".

He had wanted to add muscle to his 9st (57.6kg) frame for years, but it didn't happen until he made one simple addition to his life: another bet. Ramit has an entire folder in his Gmail dedicated to bets against friends, all adding up to about $8,000 (£5,000) in prize money.

This time, he bet them all that he could gain 6.8kg (15lb) of muscle in three months.

In the first seven days alone, he gained 2.6kg (5lb) and was the heaviest he'd ever been. In the end, he added 20% to his bodyweight—surpassing 6.8kg (15lb)—while keeping his body fat low. Now, three years later, he's maintained his new muscular weight almost to the exact pound.

There were three reasons it worked after years of failing to gain weight.

1. He used a bet and tracked results publicly

Ramit set up a free PBworks wiki page (like the pages found on Wikipedia) and invited all the bettors to receive notifications when he updated his weight. He then proceeded to talk an ungodly amount of trash.

Needless to say, smack-talking would make him look doubly stupid if he didn't win the bet. Ramit elaborates on the accountability:

"Use psychology to help; don't just 'try harder'. If you've repeatedly tried (or committed to do) something and it hasn't worked, consider public compliance or a bet."

CHANGE	COMMENT (FEEL FREE TO ADD YOUR OWN)
STARTING WEIGHT	• The beginning of the end for my bettors. –Ramit
+3.2	• Be afraid. –Ramit
+2.2	• Almost near my highest weight ever. Women and children are beginning to be frightened of me. –Ramit
+2.2	• A new weight record for me, and more to come. I have not felt hunger since 9/29. –Ramit
–1.4	• A pall is cast over this challenger as i encounter my first–ever week of losing weight. I will recover. –Ramit
+1.4	• Back on the right track. –Ramit
–2.0	• Have i plateaued? –Ramit
+3.8	• I AM A HUGE MAN, THE LARGEST I HAVE EVER BEEN. I WON'T WALK ON BRIDGES BECAUSE I'M AFRAID THEY WILL TOPPLE OVER. I AM ALSO AVOIDING PICKING UP BABIES BECAUSE I AM AFRAID OF ACCIDENTALLY THROWING THEM INTO THE STRATOSPHERE. IT'S ON!!!!!!!!!!!!!!! –Ramit

2. He ignored almost everyone

From Ramit:

"Everyone has a damn opinion. Some people told me I would get fat, as if I would let that happen for a few hundred bucks. And of course, everyone had theories about what to eat, drink, and even what combination of weights to lift.

"More than a few people shrieked upon finding out my strategy (working out, running, and eating more): 'What!? You can't run! You'll lose too much weight!' All I could do was point out that it seemed to be working: I'd already completed one-third of the bet in the first seven days. There wasn't much they could say to that.

"Everyone's got an opinion about what you 'should' do. But the truth is, most of them are full of hot air and you can get it done using a few simple steps.

"I ignored every one of them."

3. He focused on the method, not the mechanism

"People warned me that I had to understand how lipids and carbs and fatty acids worked before I started. That's such nonsense. What if I just started working out and ate more? Could I learn all that fancy stuff later? You don't have to be a genius to gain or lose weight."

4. Make it small and temporary: the immense practicality of baby steps

"Take the pressure off."

Michael Levin has made a career of taking the pressure off, and it has worked. Sixty literary works later, from national non-fiction bestsellers to screenplays, he was suggesting that I (Tim) do the same: set a meagre goal of two pages of writing per day. I had made a mental monster of the book in your hands, and setting the bar low allowed me to do what mattered most: get started each morning.

Dr. B. J. Fogg, founder of the Persuasive Technology Lab at Stanford University, wrote his graduate dissertation with a far less aggressive commitment. Even if he came home from a party at 3:00 A.G., he had to write one sentence per day. He finished in record time while classmates languished for years, overwhelmed by the enormity of the task.

Understanding this principle, IBM led the computing world in sales for decades. The quotas for its salespeople were the lowest in the industry because management wanted the reps to be unintimidated to do one thing: pick up the phone. Momentum took care of the rest, and quotas were exceeded quarter after quarter.

Taking off the pressure in 4HB means doing experiments that are short in duration and not overly inconvenient.

Don't look at a diet change or a new exercise as something you need to commit to for six months, much less the rest of your life. Look at it as a test drive of one to two weeks.

If you want to walk an hour a day, don't start with one hour. Choosing one hour is automatically building in the excuse of not having enough time. Commit to a fail-proof five minutes instead. This is exactly what Dr. Fogg suggested to his sister, and that one change (the smallest meaningful change that created momentum) led her to buy running shoes and stop eating dessert, neither of which he suggested. These subsequent decisions are referred to in the literature as "consonant decisions", decisions we make to be aligned with a prior decision.

Take the pressure off and do something small.

Remember our target to log five sessions of new behaviours? It's the five sessions that are important, not the duration of those sessions. Rig the game so you can win. Do what's needed to make those first five sessions as painless as possible. Five snowflakes are all you need to start the snowball effect of consonant decisions.

Take the pressure off and put in your five easy sessions, whether meals or workouts. The rest will take care of itself.

PRAGMATIC LAZINESS: HOW ONE GRAPH BEATS EXPERT ADVICE

In 2008, a 18.4st (117kg) Phil Libin decided to experiment with laziness.

He wanted to lose weight. This is common. As is also common, he wasn't particularly keen on diet or exercise. He'd tried both off and on for years. The intermittent four- to eight-week programmes helped him drop stones—and then his other behaviours helped him gain them back even faster.

He began to suspect there might be an easier way: doing nothing.

Phil had a simple method in mind: "I wanted to see what effect being precisely aware of my weight would have on my weight."

This is where we depart from the common. Phil lost 2st (12.7kg) in six months without making the slightest attempt to change his behaviour.

First, having arbitrarily decided that 16.4st (104.3kg) was his ideal weight, Phil drew a blue line in an Excel spreadsheet. The downward slope represented his weight decreasing from 18.4 to 16.4st (117 to 104.3kg) over two years. Every day's target weight, which sat on the blue line, was just 0.1% (approximately) lower than the previous day's. Easy peasy. See his graph on the next page, where the "blue" line is the middle dashed line.

He then added in two important lines below and above his "target" blue line: his minimum-allowable weight (green line) and his maximum-allowable weight (red line) for each day. He had no plan to hit his exact target weight each day, as that would be too stressful. He just had to keep between the lines.

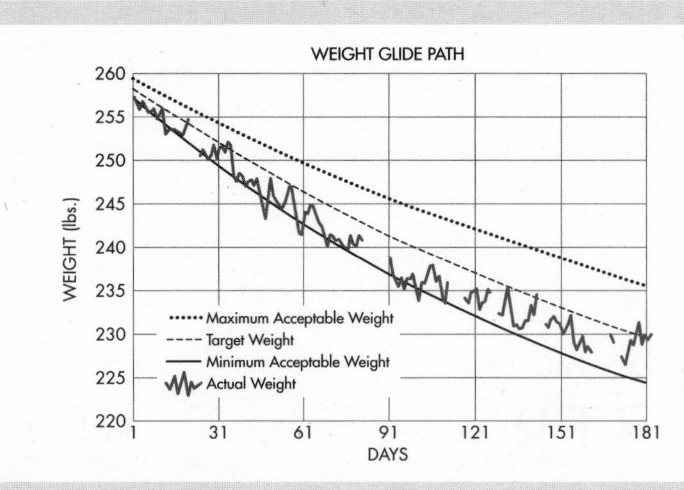

Interested in Phil's Excel spreadsheet? Download a blank version at www.fourhourbody.com/phil. Just input your starting weight and desired ending weight, and you can duplicate his experiment.

How?

He weighed himself naked every morning at the same time before eating breakfast. He stepped on the scale a few times and put the average of the results in his Excel spreadsheet. The jagged line above shows his actual weight changes. Gaps represent periods of travel when he didn't have access to a scale.

Phil kept the spreadsheet in the programme he helped pioneer, Evernote.com, so that he could see it from any computer or phone. It was always at his fingertips.

It was pure 100% awareness training, nothing but tracking.

In fact, Phil made a concerted effort *not* to change:

"I actually made a conscious effort not to deviate from my diet or exercise routine during this experiment. That is, I continued to eat whatever I wanted and got absolutely no exercise. The goal was to see how just the situational awareness of where I was each day would affect my weight. I suspect it affected thousands of minute decisions that I made over the time period, even though I couldn't tell you which."

Oddly, he treated excessive drift upwards (gaining) or downwards (losing) as equally bad:

"The only times I sprang into deliberate action were the few times (seen on the graph) where my weight dipped below the minimum acceptable level. Then I would eat doughnuts or gorge myself to make sure I was back in the 'safe zone' the next day. That was a lot of fun. I suppose I would have done the opposite and eaten less had I ever gone over the maximum weight line, but that never happened. The whole point was not to lose weight *quickly.* It was to see if I could lose weight *slowly* and *without any effort."*

Awareness, even at a subconscious level, beats fancy checklists without it.

Track or you will fail.

SUBTRACTING FAT

Basics

Out of clutter, find simplicity.

—Albert Einstein

THE SLOW-CARB DIET I

How to Lose 1.4st (9kg) in 30 Days Without Exercise

11:34 A.M. SATURDAY, 20 JUNE 2009,
SAN FRANCISCO

Text message from London, eight hours ahead, meant to impress:

> This is my dinner. Happy times!

The accompanying photo: a pepperoni and sausage pizza so large it doesn't fit on the screen.

Chris A., a fellow experimenter, and I were having our weekly virtual date.

Text response from me:

> This is my breakfast. BREAKFAST. Can you hear the insulin pouring out of my eyes? Woohoo! Ante up, fat boy.

My accompanying photo: two doughnuts, two chocolate croissants, grapefruit juice and a large coffee.

Response from Chris:

> LOL . . . please don't make me do this . . .

And so it continued, a text-message eating contest. The truth is, I do some version of this every Saturday, and thousands of people over the last four years have joined me in doing the same. In between pizzas and doughnuts, the net result is that the average follower has lost 8.6kg (19lb) of fat, and a surprising number have lost more than 45.4kg (100lb) total.

This odd approach has produced something of a small revolution.

Let me explain exactly how Chris and I reach and maintain sub-12% body fat, often sub-10%, by strategically eating like pigs.

The Slow-Carb Diet— Better Fat Loss Through Simplicity

It is possible to lose 20lb (9kg) of body fat in 30 days by optimizing any of three factors: exercise, diet or a drug/supplement regimen. Twenty pounds for most people means moving down at least two clothing sizes, whether that's going from a size 16 dress to a size 12 or from an XXL shirt to a large. The waist and hips show an even more dramatic reduction in circumference.

By 6 April, 2007, as an example, I had cut from nearly 12.9st (81.6kg) to 11.8st (74.8kg) in six weeks, while adding about 10lb of muscle, which means I lost approximately 25lb (11.3kg) of fat. The changes aren't subtle.

The diet that I'll introduce in this chapter—the Slow-Carb Diet—is the only diet besides the rather extreme Cyclical Ketogenic Diet (CKD) that has produced veins across my abdomen, which is the last place I lose fat.

There are just five simple rules to follow:

RULE #1: AVOID "WHITE" CARBOHYDRATES.

Avoid any carbohydrate that is, or can be, white. The following foods are prohibited, except for within 30 minutes of finishing a *resistance-training* workout like those described in the "From Geek to Freak" or "Occam's Protocol" chapters: all bread, rice (including brown), cereal, potatoes, pasta, tortillas and fried food with breading. If you avoid eating the aforementioned foods and anything else white, you'll be safe.

Just for fun, another reason to avoid the whities: chlorine dioxide, one of the chemicals used to bleach flour (even if later made brown again, a common trick), combines with residual protein in most of these foods to form alloxan. Researchers use alloxan in lab rats to induce diabetes. That's right—it's used to *produce* diabetes. This is bad news if you eat anything white or "enriched".

Don't eat white stuff unless you want to get fatter.

RULE #2: EAT THE SAME FEW MEALS OVER AND OVER AGAIN.

The most successful dieters, regardless of whether their goal is muscle gain or fat loss, eat the same few meals over and over again. There are 47,000 products in the average supermarket, but only a handful of them won't make you fat.

Mix and match from the following list, constructing each meal with one pick from each of the three groups. I've starred the choices that produce the fastest fat loss for me:

Main Proteins

*Egg whites with 1–2 whole eggs for flavour (or, if organic, 2–5 whole eggs, including yolks)
*Chicken breast or thigh
*Beef (preferably grass-fed)
*Fish
Pork

Legumes

*Lentils (also called "dal" or "daal")
*Black beans
Borlotti beans
Red beans
Soya beans

Supplementary Vegetables

*Spinach
*Mixed vegetables (including broccoli, cauliflower or any other cruciferous vegetables)
*Sauerkraut, kimchee (full explanation of these later in "Damage Control")
Asparagus
Peas
Broccoli
Green beans

Eat as much as you like of the above food items, but keep it simple.

Pick three or four meals and repeat them. Almost all restaurants can give you a salad or vegetables in place of chips, potatoes or rice. Surprisingly, I have found Mexican food (after swapping rice for vegetables) to be one of the cuisines most conducive to the Slow-carb Diet. If you have to pay an extra $1–3 (60p–£1.80) to substitute at a restaurant, consider it your six-pack tax, the nominal fee you pay to be lean.

Most people who go on "low"-carbohydrate diets complain of low energy and stop because they consume insufficient calories. 30g (1oz) of rice is 300 calories, whereas 30g (1oz) of spinach is 15 calories! Vegetables are not calorically dense, so it is critical that you add legumes for caloric load.

Eating more frequently than four times per day might be helpful on higher-carb diets to prevent gorging, but it's not necessary with the ingredients we're using. Eating more frequent meals also appears to have no enhancing effect on resting metabolic rate, despite claims to the contrary. Frequent meals can be used in some circumstances (see "The Last Mile"), but not for this reason.

The following meal schedule is based on a late sleep schedule, as I'm a night owl who gives up the ghost at 2:00 A.M. at the earliest, usually with wineglass or book still in hand, à la heroin addict. Adjust your meals to fit your schedule, but make sure to have your first meal within an hour of waking.

Meals are approximately four hours apart.

10:00 A.M.—Breakfast
2:00 P.M.—Lunch
6:30 P.M.—Smaller second lunch
8:00–9:00 P.M.—Recreation or sports training, if scheduled.
10:00 P.M.—Dinner
12:00 A.M.—Glass of red wine and Discovery Channel before bed

Here are some of my meals that recur again and again:

- Breakfast (home): Scrambled eggs (pourable egg whites with one whole egg), black beans, and mixed vegetables warmed up or cooked in a microwave using Pyrex® containers.
- Lunch (Mexican restaurant): Grass-fed organic beef, borlotti beans, mixed vegetables and extra guacamole.
- Dinner (home): Grass-fed organic beef, lentils, and mixed vegetables.

Just remember: this diet is, first and foremost, intended to be effective, not fun. It *can* be fun with a few tweaks (the next chapter covers this), but that's not the goal.

RULE #3: DON'T DRINK CALORIES.

Drink massive quantities of water and as much unsweetened tea, coffee (with no more than two tablespoons of cream; I suggest using cinnamon instead) or other no-calorie/low-calorie beverages as you like. Do not drink milk (including soy milk), normal soft drinks or fruit juice. Limit diet soft drinks to no more than 450ml (16 fl oz) per day if you can, as the aspartame can stimulate weight gain.

I'm a wine fanatic and have one to two glasses of red wine almost every evening. It doesn't appear to have any negative impact on my rate of fat loss. Red wine is by no means required for this diet to work, but it's 100% allowed (unlike white wines and beer, both of which should be avoided).

Up to two glasses of red per night, no more.

RULE #4: DON'T EAT FRUIT.

Humans don't need fruit six days a week, and they certainly don't need it year-round.

If your ancestors were from Europe, for example, how much fruit did they eat in the winter 500 years ago? Think they had Florida oranges in December? Not a chance. But you're still here, so the lineage somehow survived.

The only exceptions to the no-fruit rule are tomatoes and avocados, and the latter should be eaten in moderation (no more than one cup or one meal per day). Otherwise, just say no to fruit and its principal sugar, fructose, which is converted to glycerol phosphate more efficiently than almost all other carbohydrates. Glycerol phosphate → triglycerides (via the liver) → fat storage. There are a few biochemical exceptions to this, but avoiding fruit six days per week is the most reliable policy.

But what's this "six days a week" business?

It's the seventh day that allows you, if you so desire, to eat peach pancakes and banana bread until you go into a coma.

RULE #5: TAKE ONE DAY OFF PER WEEK.

I recommend Saturdays as your Dieters Gone Wild (DGW) day. I am a-lowed to eat whatever I want on Saturdays, and I go out of my way to eat ice cream, Snickers, and all of my other vices in excess. If I drank beer, I'd have a few pints of Paulaner Hefe-Weizen.[1]

I make myself a little sick each Saturday and don't want to look at any junk for the rest of the week. Paradoxically, dramatically spiking caloric intake in this way once per week increases fat loss by ensuring that your metabolic rate (thyroid function and conversion of T4 to T3, etc.) doesn't downshift from extended caloric restriction.

That's right: eating pure crap can help you lose fat. Welcome to Utopia.

There are no limits or boundaries during this day of gluttonous enjoyment. There is absolutely **no calorie counting** on this diet, on this day or any other.

Start the diet at least five days before your designated cheat day. If you choose Saturday, for example, I would suggest starting your diet on a Monday.

That's All, Folks!

If the founding fathers could sum up our government in a six-page constitution, the above is all we need to summarize rapid fat loss for 99.99% of the population. Followed *to the letter*, I've never seen it fail. Never.

When you feel mired in details or confused by the latest-and-greatest contradictory advice, return to this short chapter. All you need to remember is:

Rule #1: Avoid "white" carbohydrates (or anything that can be white).
Rule #2: Eat the same few meals over and over again.
Rule #3: Don't drink calories.
Rule #4: Don't eat fruit.
Rule #5: Take one day off per week and go nuts.

For the finer points, we have the next chapter.

1. Okay, I did have a few cold ones in Munich. It was one-third the cost of bottled water.

1.34 (83p) PER MEAL?

unity director at TechStars, a well-known start-up incubator in e is also an Internet-famous big bargain hunter. I use "big" in both iteral senses: Andrew is 196cm (6ft 5in) and 17.5st (111kg). that he *was* 17.5st (111kg). In his first two weeks on the Slow-Carb Diet, 0lb (4.5kg) and, perhaps more impressive, racked up incredibly *un*-impressive costs:

Total per-week food cost: $37.70 (£23.53)
Average per-meal cost: $1.34 (83p)

And this was including organic grass-fed beef! If he'd eaten a big salad three times a week instead of a few proteins, his weekly cost would have been $31.70 (£19.79).

He repeated four meals:

BREAKFAST: Egg whites, one whole egg, mixed vegetables, chicken breast
LUNCH: Mixed vegetables, peas, spinach (salad)
SECOND LUNCH: Chicken thigh, black beans, mixed vegtables
DINNER: Beef (or pork), asparagus, borlotti beans

His exact shopping list was simplicity itself. The prices are the per line totals:

1x Eggs (12 pack) $1.20 (75p)
4x Mixed vegetables (1lb bags) $6 (£3.75)
1x Chicken breast $2 (£1.24)
1x Organic peas (2lb bag) $2 (£1.24)
2x Spinach (3lb bags) $6 (£3.75)
3x Chicken thigh $9 (£5.62)
2x Grass-fed organic beef (227g/0.5lb cuts) $4 (£2.50)
2x Pork (1lb cuts) $3 (£1.87)
2x Asparagus bundles $2 (£1.24)
1x Pinto beans (1lb bag) $1.50 (94p)
1x Black beans (1lb bag) $1 (62p)

Getting these prices didn't require a degree in negotiation or dozens of hours of searching. Andrew looked for discounted items near expiry date and shopped at smaller stores, including a Mexican food shop, where he bought all of his dried beans.

Just to restate an important point: Andrew is an active 196cm (6ft 5in), 17.5st (111kg), 26-year-old male, and he exercised three times a week during his Slow-carb Diet experiment. He's not a small organism to feed.

He's also not unique in his experience.

Though you might not get to $1.34 (83p) per meal, his two-week experiment shows what thousands of others have been surprised to learn about the Slow-carb Diet: it's damn cheap.

The myth that eating right is expensive is exactly that: a myth.

THE FORBIDDEN FRUIT: FRUCTOSE

Can fruit juice really screw up fat loss?

Oh, yes. And it screws up much more.

Not to speculate, I tested the effect of fructose in two tests, the first during a no-fructose diet (no juice, no fruit) and the second after one week of consuming 400ml (14fl oz)—about 1.5 large glasses—of pulp-free orange juice upon waking and before bed. The orange juice was the only thing distinguishing diets A and B.

The changes were incredible.

Before (16/10, no fructose) and after (23/10, orange juice):
Cholesterol: 203 → 243 (out of "healthy" range)
LDL: 127 → 165 (also out of range)

There were two other values that shot up unexpectedly:

Albumin: 4.3 → 4.9 (out of range)
Iron: 71 → 191 (!) (out of range aka into the stratosphere)

Albumin binds to testosterone and renders it inert, much like SHBG (discussed in "Sex Machine") but weaker. I don't want either to be out-of-range high. Bad for the manly arts.

If you said "Holy sh*t!" when you saw the iron jump, we're in the same boat. This result was completely out of the blue and is not good, especially in men. It might come as a surprise, but men don't menstruate. This means that men lack a good method for clearing out excessive iron, which can be toxic.[2] The increase in iron was far more alarming to me than the changes in cholesterol.

Here is just one of several explanations from the research literature:

> *In addition to contributing to metabolic abnormalities, the consumption of fructose has been reported to affect homeostasis of numerous trace elements. Fructose has been shown to increase iron absorption in humans and experimental animals. Fructose intake [also] decreases the activity of the copper enzyme superoxide dismutase (SOD) and reduces the concentration of serum and hepatic copper.*

The moral of the story? Don't drink fruit juice, and absolutely avoid a high-fructose diet. It doesn't do the body good.

2. See the "Living Forever" chapter for more on this.

TOOLS AND TRICKS

The Three-Minute Slow-Carb Breakfast (www.fourhourbody.com/breakfast) Breakfast is a hassle. In this video, I'll show you how to make a high-protein slow-carb breakfast in three minutes that is perfect for fat loss and starting the day at a sprint.

Still Tasty (www.stilltasty.com) Not sure if it's safe to eat those eggs or those Thai leftovers? Tired of calling your mum to ask? This site allows you to search the shelf life of thousands of cooked and uncooked foods.

Food Porn Daily (http://www.foodporndaily.com) Need some inspiration for your cheat day? Food Porn Daily provides a delicious and artery-blocking cornucopia of bad (but tasty) eating. Save it for Saturday.

Gout: The Missing Chapter (http://www.fourhourbody.com/gout) Concerned about protein intake and gout? Read this missing chapter from *Good Calories, Bad Calories*, graciously provided by stunning science writer Gary Taubes. It might change your mind.

THE SLOW-CARB DIET II

The Finer Points and Common Questions

As to methods, there may be a million and then some, but principles are few. The man who grasps principles can successfully select his own methods.

—Ralph Waldo Emerson

The system is the solution.

—AT&T

This chapter answers the most common questions related to the Slow-carb Diet, shares real-world lessons learned, and pinpoints the most common mistakes.

I designate Saturday as "cheat day" in all of my answers, but, in practice, you can substitute any day of the week.

Chances are good that at least 50% of the questions in this chapter will come up for you at some point. If you're serious about achieving the fastest fat loss possible, read it all.

Common Questions and Concerns

HOW CAN I POSSIBLY FOLLOW THIS DIET? IT'S TOO STRICT!

Just start with changing your breakfast. You will lose noticeable fat. Be sure to see Fleur B. in "Perfect Posterior", who lost about 3% body fat in four to five weeks with this one substitution. Once you see the results, suck it up and move to 100% slow-carb for six days, after which you can indulge yourself for 24 hours.

Then again, would doing a one-week test from the get-go really be too much? I doubt it. "Pritibrowneyes" developed a simple method for extending self-control:

One thing that worked well for me was keeping a little notepad with me. Everytime I got a craving for something (sweet stuff or just regular food) I added it to the list of things I was going to feast on during my cheat day. This was my way of acknowledging my craving and reminding myself that I could have it, but just not right now. It's like deferred eating.

If that's not enough, don't forget sugar-free jelly. When you are on the verge of self-control breakdown, usually late at night, a few bites will put the demons back in their cages.

BUT EATING THE SAME STUFF IS SO BORING!

Most people vastly overestimate the variety of their meals.

Assuming you're not travelling, what have you had to eat for breakfast for the last week? Lunch? Chances are good that, especially for breakfast, you've repeated one to three meals.

Rotating five or six meals for a few weeks is not hard at all, even though you might imagine otherwise. Feeling awesome and looking better each successive week easily justifies having familiar (tasty) food from Sunday to Friday. Saturday is no-holds-barred. Here's one of hundreds of examples of results trumping variety, this one from Jeff:

I've been going 2 weeks strong, and am down almost 15lbs (6.8kg)! I have this "lose 30 before I'm 30 years old" plan and I'm now halfway there with 4 months to go.

I do egg-whites, lentils and broccoli in the A.M., a burrito bowl (chicken, black beans, veggies) for lunch, then chicken, lentils and assorted veggies for dinner. All followed with some delicious red wine before bed.

I admit I'm already bored with the meals, but the results I'm seeing so far make it a minimal concern. I add some different seasonings or light sauces to the chicken to mix it up....

I've only had one cheat day so far, but am looking forward to my second one tomorrow. I may have overdid it last week, as I consumed almost 5,000 calories, where normally I'm coming in around 1,200–1,300:); Surprisingly, that huge cheat day last week didn't set me back too far, as I was back to my pre-cheat weight by Monday morning.

I don't like exercise, and haven't committed to it as part of my weight loss plan, but some folks at work get me to do 30–45 minutes on a elliptical or bike a couple times a week. Not sure if that's enough that it really has an impact or not, but at least it gets me off my butt.

I'm interested to see how the next 2 weeks go. I'm under 14.2st (90.7kg) for the first time in years, and my goal is 13.2st (84kg).

SHOULD I TAKE ANY SUPPLEMENTS?

I suggest potassium, magnesium and calcium. This diet will cause you to lose excess water, and electrolytes can go along with it.

Potassium can be consumed during meals by using a potassium-enriched salt like "LoSalt" or, my preference, eating extra guacamole with Mexican meals. Avocados, the main ingredient in guacamole, contain 60% more potassium than bananas. Avocados also contain 75% insoluble fibre, which will help keep you regular. If you prefer pills, 99-milligram tablets with meals will do the trick.

Magnesium and calcium are easiest to consume in pill form, and 500 milligrams of magnesium taken prior to bed will also improve sleep.

If you prefer to get your electrolytes through whole foods, here are good slow-carb options, in descending order of concentration. Notice that spinach is the only item on all three lists:

Potassium (4,700 mg per day recommended for an average, healthy 25-year-old male)

1. Butter beans, cooked, 850g (1lb 14oz) (170g/6oz = 969mg)
2. Chard, cooked, 850g (1lb 14oz) (175g/6oz = 961mg)
3. Halibut, cooked, 2.6 fillets (half a fillet = 916 mg)
4. Spinach, cooked, 1kg (2.2lb) (180g/6.3oz = 839mg)
5. Borlotti beans, cooked, 1kg (2.2lb) (170g/6oz = 746)
6. Lentils, cooked, 1.2kg (2.6lb) (200g/7oz = 731mg)
7. Salmon, cooked, 3.4 fillets (half a fillet = 683 mg)
8. Black beans, cooked, 1.3kg (2.8lb) (170g/6oz = 611mg)
9. Sardines, 1.5kg (3.3lb) (190g/6.7oz = 592mg)
10. Mushrooms, cooked, 1.3kg (190g/6.7oz = 555 mg)

Calcium (1,000 mg per day recommended for an average, healthy 25-year-old male)

1. Salmon with bones, 209g (7.3oz) (190g/6.7oz = 919mg) (great-tasting if you're a cat)
2. Sardines with bones, 342g (12oz) (190g/6.7oz = 569mg)
3. Mackerel, canned, 418g (14.7oz) (190g/6.7oz = 458mg)
4. Tofu, firm, 907g (2lb) (252g/8.8oz = 280mg)
5. Collards, cooked, 722g (1.5lb) (190g/6.7oz = 266mg)
6. Spinach, cooked, 738g (1.6lb) (180g/6.3oz = 245mg)
7. Black-eyed peas, cooked, 808g (1.7lb) (172g/6.3oz = 211mg)
8. Turnip greens, cooked, 734g (1.6lb) (144g/5oz = 197mg)
9. Tempeh, 896g (2lb) (166g/5.8oz = 184mg)
10. Agar, dried, 323g (11.4oz) (30g/1oz = 175mg)

Magnesium (400 mg per day recommended for an average, healthy 25-year-old male)

1. Pumpkin seeds (pepitas), 73.7g (2.6oz) (60g/2oz = 300mg)
2. Watermelon seeds, dried, 79g (2.8oz) (60g/2oz = 288mg)
3. Peanuts, 234g (8.2oz) (146g/5oz = 245mg)
4. Halibut, cooked, 1.2 fillets (half a fillet = 170mg)
5. Almonds, 140g (5oz) (60g/2oz = 160mg)
6. Spinach, 450g (1lb) (180g/16.3oz = 157mg)
7. Soya beans, cooked, 464g (1lb) (172g/6oz = 148mg)
8. Cashews, 160g (5.5oz) (60g/2oz = 146mg)
9. Pine nuts, 162g (5.7oz) (60g/2oz = 140mg)
10. Brazil nuts, 6.3 tbsp (2 tbsp = 128mg)

NO DAIRY? REALLY? DOESN'T MILK HAVE A LOW GLYCAEMIC INDEX?

It's true that milk has a low glycaemic index (GI) and a low glycaemic load (GL). For the latter, whole milk clocks in at an attractive 27. Unfortunately, dairy products paradoxically have a high *insulinemic response* on the insulinemic index (II or InIn) scale. Researchers from Lund University in Sweden have examined this surprising finding:

> *Despite low glycaemic indexes of 15–30, all of the milk products produced high insulinemic indexes of 90–98, which were not significantly different from the insulinemic index of the reference bread [generally white bread].... Conclusions: Milk products appear insulinotropic as judged from 3-fold to 6-fold higher insulinemic indexes than expected from the corresponding glycaemic indexes.*

Removing even a little dairy can dramatically accelerate fat loss, as Murph noticed:

> *OK, it's been a week since taking Tim's advice and cutting the dairy. I'm down 6 more pounds. And what's unbelievable to me is that I wasn't even consuming that much beforehand. Maybe a handful of cheese on my breakfast eggs and a glass of milk per day.*

Need something to flavour your coffee? If you must, use cream (not milk), but no more than two tablespoons. I opt for a few dashes of cinnamon and the occasional drops of vanilla extract.

NO FRUIT? DON'T I NEED A "BALANCED DIET"?

No.

To begin with, there is no consensus on what a "balanced diet" is. My researchers and I tried to find an official definition from the U.S. Department of Agriculture or other federal agencies, and we could not. I have not seen any evidence to suggest that fruits are necessary more than once a week on cheat day.

See "The Forbidden Fruit" sidebar in the last chapter for more.

GOD, I F*ING HATE BEANS. CAN I SUBSTITUTE SOMETHING ELSE?

Perhaps you just hate farting and not beans.

First, let's fix that bean issue, then I'll talk about how and when you can omit them.

Lentils seldom cause the gas problem and are my default in the legume category. For beans, purchasing organic will often fix the rumbling trousers effect, and if that doesn't work, soaking the beans in water for a few hours will help break down the offending cause: oligosaccharides. This is one of many reasons I eat canned beans and lentils, disposing of the murky juice in the can and rinsing, instead of purchasing either dry. If all else fails, add some Kombu (type of seaweed) or epazote (available at Mexican food shops or online) to the beans and you're golden.

Is it the blandness that's the problem? That's even easier to fix: add a little balsamic vinegar and garlic powder. I personally love hot sauce (www.cholula.com is my current favourite). Try red beans instead of black or borlotti.

Perhaps it's the beany mouth feel and texture? Try fake mashed potatoes, which slow-carber Dana explains:

Put a little olive oil in a pan... add a can of white kidney beans (or some cauliflower), mash them with a spoon or whatever you choose, add a bit of water to get the consistency you want, season with a little bit of salt, pepper, garlic powder, and some parmesan cheese if you wish... tastes awesome and cooks in no time at all!

The fake mashed potato approach also works well with simple refried beans . . . and don't forget to mix the beans with something else. My breakfast is often a concoction of mixed veggies with lentils and shop-bought, mayonnaise-minimal coleslaw. It's 100 times better-tasting than the three eaten separately.

Do you really have to eat beans every meal? No. Which leads up to the rules of omission.

I do not eat beans with every meal because I eat out almost every lunch and dinner. If I'm cooking, lentils and black beans are my defaults. Outside, I'll order extra protein and vegetables for the entrée and supplement with one or two slow-carb starters, such as unbreaded calamari and a salad with olive oil and vinegar. If you omit legumes in a meal, **you must absolutely** make a concerted effort to eat larger portions than your former higher-carb self. Remember that you're getting fewer calories per cubic inch. Eat more than you are accustomed to.

HOLY FESTIVUS, I GAINED 8LB (3.6KG) AFTER MY CHEAT DAY! DID I UNDO ALL OF MY PROGRESS?

No, not at all. It's common for even a 8.5st (54kg) female to gain up to 8lb (3.6kg) of water weight after 24 hours of increased carbohydrate intake. Larger males can gain 10–20lb (4.5–9kg). Expect MASSIVE weight fluctuations after cheat day. Relax. It will disappear over the next 48 hours.

Mark's experience is typical:

I have been doing this now for about 10 weeks and I have weighed myself daily during the process. I put on up to 4.4lb (2kg) every cheat day, return to my pre-cheat weight by Wednesday at latest, and have been averaging a further 2.2lb (1kg) per week loss by the next cheat day.

To date I have lost 26.5lb/12kg I am fairly strict during the week (protein + beans + veg and that's about it), and I do circuit training and Brazilian Jiu

Jitsu 3–4 times per week. The only variation I have from Tim's guide is a whey protein shake after every hour of training.

Weigh yourself before your first meal on cheat day and ignore the short-term fluctuations, which do not reflect fat loss or gain. *Remember to take circumference measurements on your weigh-in days,* as it is typical to gain some lean muscle while on this diet.

The mitochondria in muscle increase your ability to oxidize fat, so we want to encourage this, but the muscle gain can keep you at the same weight for one to two weeks.

Stones and kilograms can lie, but measurements don't.

Some dieters needlessly fall off the train in frustration. Angel, whom we met once in earlier chapters, didn't. Why not? At the risk of sounding repetitive, let me reiterate, since I know most readers will ignore this:

> [Week one] *Hello all. I just wanted to share my first week with you. I have lost a total of 7 pounds. . . . Mondays are also the day that I take my measurements. I have lost 1 inch from each thigh, 1 inch from my waist, and 1/2 inch from my hips. I already noticed that my pants I haven't worn for a while fit perfect. This is the motivation I need to keep on going.*
>
> [Week two] *After my cheat day on Saturday, I gained 1 pound which is normal for me. The week before I gained pretty much that, but lost it. So week two, I lost that 1 pound. I didn't lose any weight on week two, but I'm not discouraged. I did manage to lose in inches. I lost ½ an inch off my hips which is absolutely great. I lost a total of 1 inch off my thighs. Not so shabby either. So that's a total of 1.5 inches for the week. I'll take the inches. The grand total of inches lost from Day One: 5 inches total. Yippee! No exercise either.*

Enjoy your cheat day guilt-free. Measure the right things at the right times.

CAN I USE SPICES, SALT OR LIGHT SAUCES? WHAT CAN I USE FOR COOKING?

Spices and herbs, but not cream-based sauces, are your friends. Take a trip to Whole Foods with $50 (£31.20) and get educated. That $50 (£31.20) spree will last you at least a few months.

Montreal steak rub, thick salsa without sugar added, garlic salt, white truffle

THE NEW AND IMPROVED OLIVE OIL? INTRODUCING MACADAMIA OIL

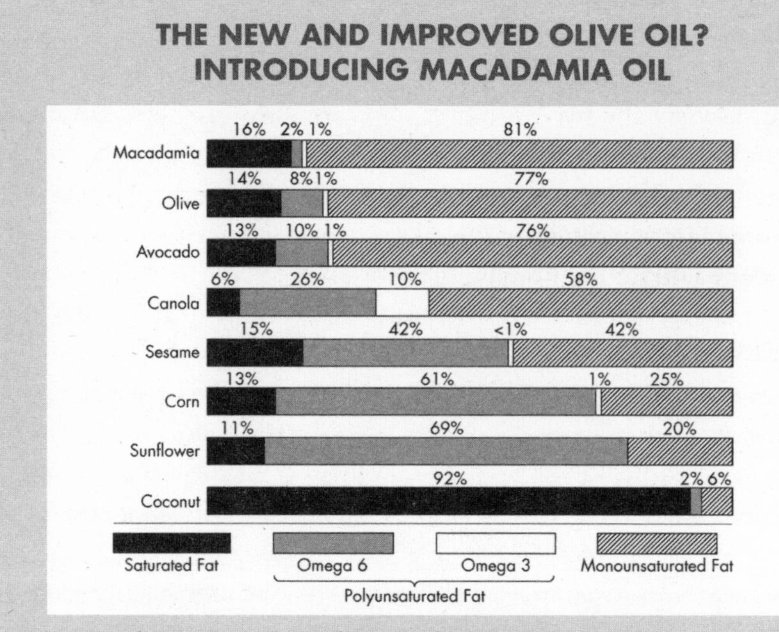

"Comparison of Dietary Fats and Oils", from *Agricultural Handbook*, no. B-4, U.S. Human Nutritional Information Service, http://www.adoctorskitchen.com/about/about-fats. (Courtesy: Deborah Chud MD)

Macadamia oil is the new and improved olive oil. Since several high-level body-building coaches introduced me to this new kid on the block, I've been hooked.

Consider the following:

- It tastes almost like butter. Extra-virgin olive oil is fine alone or on salad, but let's face it—it makes scrambled eggs taste like cat vomit.
- Unlike olive oil, it has a high smoking point (234°C/453°F) and is ideal for sautéeing and all manner of cooking. I now use butter from grass-fed cows, ghee and macadamia oil exclusively for all stove-top action.
- It has a long shelf life and is more stable than olive oil when exposed to light. If you've ever consumed olive oil from a clear container, there is a good chance that you've downed rancid olive oil on at least one occasion. Some industry analysts estimate that more than 50% of all mass-produced olive oil is spoiled when consumed.
- It is the lowest of all cooking oils in omega-6 fatty acids but high in palmitoleic acid, which isn't found in any other plant oil. Because palmitoleic acid is found in the sebum of human skin, macadamia oil can also double as a potent skin moisturizer. Not suggested with olive oil unless you want the sex appeal of a Greek salad.
- The fat in macadamia oil is 80% monounsaturated, the highest percentage among cooking oils.

Sources and Resources: Species Nutrition (http://www.speciesnutrition.com)—President Dave Palumbo was the first to introduce me to macadamia oil and I get mine from his producers.

sea salt (combine this with tarragon on eggs), Thai chilli paste (srichacha)—this is just about all you need to start. For salad dressing, a few drops of a non-sugar sweetener like egave syrup mixed with vinegar and mustard will give you a dressing to satisfy any sweet tooth. My preference, and my go-to restaurant salad dressing, is simply balsamic vinegar and olive oil.

Butter is fine, as long as the only ingredients are butter and salt.

For cooking, you can use olive oil for low heat and either grapeseed oil or macadamia oil for high-temperature cooking.

CAN I DRINK ALCOHOL? WHAT TYPES OF WINE ARE BEST?

On cheat days, all is fair. Have a keg by yourself if the spirit moves you. On diet days, stick to dry wines, "dry" being defined as less than 1.4% residual sugar. The driest red varietals are Pinot Noir, Cabernet Sauvignon and Merlot, whereas the driest whites are generally Sauvignon Blanc and Albariño. This certainly doesn't stop me from enjoying my favourite big reds: Malbec from Argentina and Zinfandel from California. I have found better fat loss results with red wine compared to white.

Though there are exceptions, it is best to avoid Riesling, White Zinfandel and Champagne.

WHAT SHOULD I EAT FOR SNACKS?

There should be no need, or real physical urge, to eat snacks. If you are hungry, you're not eating enough protein and legumes at each meal. This is an uber-common novice screw-up. I've been there too. Eat more.

If you're eating enough and still feel the urge to snack, it's a psychological addiction, one that most often goes hand in hand with procrastination. Some of us go to the bathroom, others go to the water cooler and others eat. I've done all three, so I know the drill.

If all else fails and you *must* have a snack, go for carrots, but a bag of carrots will hit you like a donkey kick in the stomach, so don't binge. If I snack, I'll most often make a small snack—200–300 calories—out of restaurant leftovers like Thai chicken basil with *no* rice. If you're really starving, just eat another slow-carb meal. It won't do any harm.

If you get headaches or have other symptoms of low blood sugar, 90% of the time it will be because you are not eating enough. First-time slow-carbers are accustomed to eating small portions of calorically dense carbohydrates (think bagels or pasta), and they duplicate the portion sizes with the calorically lighter slow-carb foods, resulting in insufficient calories. Expect that you can eat two to three times as much volume, and assume that you should.

Likewise, if you have trouble sleeping due to hunger, you're not eating enough. In these cases, consume a bit of protein prior to bed, which can be as simple as 1–2 tablespoons of almond butter (ideal) or peanut butter with no additives (the only ingredients should be peanuts and perhaps salt). Note to the ladies, for whom peanut butter seems to be like crack: the tablespoon scoop should be no more than a small mound, not half the jar balanced on a spoon.

DO I REALLY HAVE TO BINGE ONCE A WEEK?

It is important to spike caloric intake once per week.

This causes a host of hormonal changes that improve fat loss, from increasing cAMP and GMP to improving conversion of the T4 thyroid hormone to the more active T3.

Everyone binges eventually on a diet, and it's better to schedule it ahead of time to limit the damage. The psychological benefits outweigh even the hormonal and metabolic benefits. I eat like this all the time and have for seven years. Few ways of eating (WOE) are this sustainable and beneficial.

CAN YOU GET AWAY WITH ONE CHEAT MEAL PER WEEK?

Most men can. Some women can't.[3]

Menstruation can stop if leptin levels get too low. This happened to one reader for seven months until she returned to "refeeding", as she called it (binge day), though she only did it once every two weeks. Forced overfeeding can temporarily increase circulating leptin 40%. I still suggest once per week as a default. Bumping up food intake for 12–24 hours, not necessarily to the point of sickness, is an important reset. If you gain too much or plateau and get nervous, eat a good high-protein meal for breakfast on your off day and then binge from lunch to dinner, which is what I now do most of the time.

I don't always splurge to the point of sickness. In a response to one slow-carber, I explained:

> *Yes, you can eat anything you want—in any quantity—on Saturdays. I tend to go nuts every 1 of 4 weeks and eat so much I get nearly sick, which makes me*

3. Especially if consuming less than 30% of calories as fat.

moderate the other 3. I love Snickers, chocolate biscuits, doughnuts (and all pastries), and ice cream. Enjoy.

One more tip: whenever possible, eat out for your cheat meals.

No matter what, throw out all bad food before the next morning. If there is bad food in your house, you will eventually eat it before your "off" day, also called "reverse Lent" by some followers.

WHAT ABOUT BREAKFAST?

My most frequent breakfast consists of eggs, lentils and spinach. I prefer lentils, straight out of the can, to black beans, and hard-boiling a dozen eggs beforehand makes this easy.

Breakfast is the hardest meal for most to modify, as we're a country of toast- and cereal-eating junkies. Moving to slow carbs and protein requires a more lunch-like meal for breakfast. This is easier when you realize that breakfast can be a smaller meal when followed by a lunch three to five hours later. Try it for five days and you'll see the difference. Not only will the increased protein intake decrease water retention, resting metabolism increases about 20% if your breakfast calories are at least 30% protein.

If you want a more typical breakfast, try eggs with turkey bacon (or organic normal bacon)[4] and sliced tomato. Delicious. Cottage cheese, my mother's preference, is also a fine addition. Have you ever cooked eggs with ghee (clarified butter)? Try it and thank me.

Interested in why I specifically choose eggs, spinach and lentils? For those who like to get deep in the weeds, your science fix is on the next page.

4. Residual drugs and environmental toxins are often stored in fat, so you'll want to buy the good stuff when consuming animal fat from higher up the food chain, like pork or beef. Eating larger animals from factory farms is asking for trouble.

GA

In randomized and controlled trials, eating eggs results in more fat loss and increased basal metabolism. In one such trial, overweight women who consumed a breakfast of two eggs a day for eight weeks (at least five days per week) instead of a bagel of equal weight and caloric value lost 65% more weight and—more importantly—had an 83% greater reduction in waist circumference. There were no significant differences between the plasma total-, HDL-, and LDL-cholesterol and triglyceride levels of either group.

Egg yolks also provide choline, which helps protect the liver and increases fat loss as compared to a control. Choline metabolizes into betaine and offers methyl groups for methylation processes. Steven Zeisel from the University of North Carolina–Chapel Hill explains: "Exposure to oxidative stress is a potent trigger for inflammation. Betaine is formed from choline within the mitochondria, and this oxidation contributes to mitochondrial redox status." Guess what another primary source of betaine is? Spinach.

This is where credit is due: Popeye got it right. Spinach is incredible for body recomposition.

The phytoecdysteroids (20HE specifically) in spinach increase human muscle tissue growth rates 20% when applied in a culture (think petri dish). Even if you're not interested in growth, it also increases glucose metabolism. Phytoecdysteroids are structurally similar to insect moulting hormones—finally, an affordable way to eat insect moulting hormones!—and both increase protein synthesis and muscular performance. Even little rats build stronger paw grips. In good news for women, the 20HE ecdysteroid tested demonstrates no androgenic properties. In other words, it won't give you a hairy chest or an Adam's apple.

The Rutgers University researchers responsible for the principal study emphasize, almost as a deterrent, that one would need to eat 1 kilogram (2.2lb) of spinach per day to mimic the administration used. In testing, I've found that it's not hard at all to see a visible effect with smaller amounts. I routinely eat 162–243g (5.7–8.6oz) of spinach per day, which is less than you think. 162g (5.7oz), is about 16% of 1kg (2.2lb). 243g (8.6oz) is almost 25% of 1kg (2.2lb). If the results of the study are dose-dependent, one might expect an increase in muscle fibre synthesis of 3% from 162g (5.7oz) and 5% from 243g (8.6oz), not to mention the effect of increased carbohydrate metabolism. Compounded over time, this is significant. If the effect is not dose-dependent but rather triggered at a dose less than 1kg (2.2lb) per day, it is possible that the 20% increase could be achieved with far less than 1kg (2.2lb). I also believe that spinach increases cAMP, but that's for the geeks to explore.

Lentils, last but not least, are a rich and cheap source of protein (amino acids), isoleucine and lysine in particular. Both lysine and isoleucine, a branched-chain amino acid (BCAA), are noted for their roles in muscular repair, and the latter for its effect on glucose metabolism.

DO I HAVE TO LIMIT VEGGIES TO THOSE LISTED?

There's no need to limit veggies to those I listed, but I've found that the more variety you attempt, the more likely you are to quit, as everything from shopping to cleaning up becomes more complicated.

As I've said before, this diet is not designed to be fun, even though most people end up enjoying it. It's designed to be effective. The vegetables I've listed are those I've found to be most tolerable when eating them again and again. Feel free to substitute whatever you want, but don't forget to include legumes for calories.

One veggie that often gets unnecessarily tossed due to rule #1 (no white foods) is cauliflower. Eat all the cauliflower you like. It's great for making faux mashed potatoes. Otherwise, stick to the no-white rule.

ARE CANNED FOODS ALL RIGHT?

Canned foods are absolutely fine. No problem. Almost all of my vegetables are either frozen (80%) or canned (20%). I'm a huge fan of canned tuna in water mixed with lentils and chopped onions.

CAN I EAT WHOLE GRAINS OR STEEL-CUT OATS?

No.

CAN I DO THIS IF I'M A LACTO-OVO VEGETARIAN?

Lacto-ovo is fine. Meat isn't necessary, but it does make the job easier. Eggs and beans are sufficient to lose weight, but I would avoid most milk products. Cottage cheese is an exception. It doesn't interrupt things, and the high casein content appears to facilitate fat loss.

One reader used veggie sausages and Instone high-protein pudding, in addition to eggs, to satisfy his protein requirements. Brown rice protein, as well as hemp or pea protein, will work if you can stomach it. If possible, I discourage consuming any refined soy products, including all soy milk and isolated soy protein supplements. See the "Meatless Machine" chapter for more warnings on soy and alternatives.

CAN I EAT SALSA?

Salsa is outstanding, especially chunky medium spicy salsa with corn, beans, etc. I can't stand egg whites by themselves, as they're too boring even for me. This is why I almost always eat whole eggs, but if you add a few spoonfuls of salsa on top of either option, it's a delicious little meal. Just don't put the salsa and lentils in the same bowl. The mixture will make you gag like a camel coughing up a hair ball.

CAN I EAT FRIED FOODS?

Stir-fry is ideal for this diet, as are most cuisines (like Thai) that depend on it. Deep-frying should be avoided because of the breading and poor nutrient density for the calories.

Refried beans work just fine, and more than 30 slow-carbers have lost up to 450g (1lb) per day using them as a staple. Reader David C. lost 1.4st (9kg) in 30 days using almost exclusively canned refried beans. In his last update, he'd lost 3st (19kg) and his wife had lost 2.5st (16.3kg).

Refried beans do, however, contain a boatload of sodium, approximately 45% of the daily allowance per serving. If you don't have hypertension, this probably won't kill you, but do your best to include other beans, or mix them together, on occasion. This will result in less water retention. Bloated ain't pretty, no matter how low your body fat.

I love refried beans, too, but try to diversify once you have the hang of the diet.

WHAT IF I'M TRAVELLING AND EATING IN AIRPORTS?

If you're airport-hopping and cannot find a Mexican restaurant or grill, grab a bag of raw almonds or walnuts at a kiosk and commit to consuming no starch for the remainder of your travel time. There are enough calories in that single bag to give you two to three small "meals" and get you through a full 12 hours. Most airports also have chicken salads (omit dressings besides olive oil or vinegar) that you can combine with the nuts.

If it comes down to it, choose mild hunger instead of deviation. If you always eat on the clock, perhaps it's been a few years since you've felt real hunger.

Having followed this diet in 30+ countries, I can state without exception that travel is not a legitimate excuse for breaking the rules.

WHAT ABOUT FAT LOSS DRUGS?

I could recommend several hard-core thermogenics, but the potential for addiction, organ damage, and lesser-known chronic problems (sinusitis, for example) just isn't worth it.

EATING OUT AND THE CHIPOTLE METHOD

Speaking as a cooking-inept bachelor, and as someone who has eaten out an average of twice a day for the last five years, the slow-carb solution in restaurants is eight words:

"I'll just have more vegetables instead of [starch]."

For most places, it's a simple matter of substituting more vegetables—spinach or whatever is available—for the standard rice, bread or potato that comes with the meal. "No substitutions" on the menu? No problem. Add a few more words and it's abracadabra done:

"I'll just have more vegetables instead of the [starch]. If I have to pay a bit extra, that's fine."

If that fails, gird your loins and just order a separate veggie or legume side while omitting the starch. In total, this substituting will average out to less than $3 (£1.80) extra per meal, and it's often free. Consider this your nominal flat stomach tax. If you're eating out to begin with, you can afford an extra $3 (£1.80), so don't be penny-wise and pound-foolish. If you can't afford it, skip a latte or newspaper so you can.

The most cost-effective cuisines I've found for the Slow-Carb Diet are Thai[5] and Mexican, the latter of which leads us to the wonderfully simple example of Eric Foster and his Chipotle® Diet.

Eric lost 6.5st (41.3kg) and went from 44% to 23.8% body fat in less than 10 months adhering to the following menu:

BREAKFAST: One cup of coffee and an egg (scrambled or hard-boiled) [I believe he would have lost significantly more fat by adding even one extra egg each day.]

LUNCH: Fajita bol (peppers, onions, steak, tomato salsa, green tomatillo salsa, cheese, soured cream, guacamole, cos lettuce)

DINNER: Fajita bol (peppers, onions, steak, tomato salsa, green tomatillo salsa, cheese, soured cream, guacamole, cos lettuce)

This diet totals about 1,480 calories and 29 grams of non-fibre carbohydrates daily. Brent, another follower of the Chipotle Diet, lost 8.5st (54kg) in 11 months, bringing him from 300 to 180lb bodyweight.

But doesn't it get boring? Eric suspected it would:

I honestly thought I might get bored of the burritos after a couple months, but it hasn't happened yet. Thank God! Before I started dieting, Chipotle was my favourite place to eat. I made adjustments to the menu items to make it low-carb, and it tasted just as good as if I hadn't made any changes at all.

Losing fat doesn't need to be punishment. It doesn't even need to be inconvenient.

Go slow-carb for a week and you won't go back.

5. I suggest avoiding curries, which can cause intestinal upset without rice.

The most effective, side-effect-minimal "stack" I've found is PAGG, and it's detailed in the chapter entitled "The Four Horsemen".

ISN'T HIGHER PROTEIN HARD ON THE KIDNEYS? WHAT IF I HAVE GOUT?

First, I am not a doctor, nor do I play one on the Internet. If you have medical conditions of any type, consult a doctor. Now, on to my interpretation of the data:

If you don't have a serious pre-existing medical condition, the amount of protein I prescribe should not hurt you. There is no compelling evidence to support the protein-hurts-your-kidneys claim. This is what Michael Eades MD calls a "vampire myth" because it just refuses to die, despite a lack of evidence.

Gout?

Gout is usually blamed on purines and therefore protein, so those diagnosed with it, like my mother, will be put on low-protein, low-legume diets. I ascribe to Gary Taubes's interpretation of the scientific literature, which indicates that fructose (and therefore sucrose, table sugar) and other factors are more likely to be causal agents of gout. Phosphoric acid in carbonated drinks is also to be avoided.

My mother's uric acid levels normalized on the Slow-Carb Diet, despite much higher protein intake. She continued to take low-dose allopurinol during the diet, and the food was the only variable that changed.

This said, no matter what you do with your diet or self-experimentation, do not stop or modify medication without consulting a medical professional.

I'M HITTING A PLATEAU—WHAT SHOULD I DO?

The first three mistakes discussed in the next few pages (eating too late, not eating enough protein, drinking too little water) are the three most common causes.

Nevertheless, the total percentage of body fat lost per month naturally decreases over time. The number of mitochondria in your muscle tissue largely determines your rate of sustained fat loss. Targeted exercise, even just 20 minutes per week, will often double fat loss that's plateaued, and should do so for at least two to four months. The best options are covered in the "Adding Muscle" chapters.

Common Mistakes and Misunderstandings

The first three mistakes in this section cover 90%+ of stalling problems, but the rest are well worth reading. A gram of prevention is worth a lulogram of cure, and a few minutes of education are worth many kilograms of extra fat loss.

MISTAKE #1: NOT EATING WITHIN ONE HOUR OF WAKING, PREFERABLY WITHIN 30 MINUTES

This was my dad's issue and is almost always a show-stopper. Look at what happened once we addressed it:

> 27/12/08
> Beginning weight 17.5st (111kg).
> 30/1/09
> End of month #1 16.2st (103kg).
> 1/3/09
> End of month #2 15.9st (101kg). [Too little protein in morning for last 4 weeks—added 30g (1oz) as a ready-to-drink Myoplex shake within 30 minutes of waking to restart fat loss]
> 2/4/09
> End of month #3 14.5st (92.4kg).
>
> 90 day weight loss = 2.9st (18.7kg).

The first month, his rate of loss was **1.2st (7.7kg) per month**. The second month, when he postponed breakfast, his rate of loss dropped to **0.3st (2.5kg) per month**. The third month, after consuming 30 grams of protein within 30 minutes of waking, that rate more than tripled to **1.3st (8.5kg) per month**!

These numbers don't tell the whole story, of course, as he was adding muscle at the same time, but this type of dramatic acceleration is typical. Skipping breakfast is also closely associated with overeating in the evening. Don't skip. Have no appetite in the morning? No problem. Keep it small and protein-rich, then: two to three hard-boiled eggs sprinkled with white truffle sea salt.

Here's another case study, this time from JayC:

18/10/2008–14/2/2009: Starting weight: 260 lb, Today's weight: 212lb

Wow! This is the first time I've been less than 215 since my freshman year of college! I hit a bit of a plateau after getting down to 220 on Christmas. I was eating the same, drinking the same, etc, and stayed at 220! So how did I get over this plateau?? By eating more! Can you believe the awesomeness of this lifestyle? Tim had posted... to eat at least 30g of protein upon waking, and to up the water even more so. Reluctantly I enlarged my breakfast and lunch portions and BAM!

Skip breakfast, forget to eat within one hour of waking, and you will fail.

MISTAKE #2: NOT EATING ENOUGH PROTEIN

Get at least 20 grams of protein per meal.

This is absolutely most critical at breakfast. Eating at least 40% of your breakfast calories as protein will decrease carb impulses and promote a negative fat balance. Even 20% protein—more than most people consume—doesn't cut it. First choice: down two to three whole eggs at breakfast. Second choice: if that's impossible to stomach, add other protein-rich whole foods, such as turkey bacon, organic bacon, organic sausages or cottage cheese. Third choice: have a 30-gram protein shake with ice and water, as my father did.

The first few days you'll feel like you're force-feeding yourself, and then it will all change and you'll feel incredible. Get at least 20 grams of protein per meal, no matter what.

Related problem: not eating enough food. Do NOT try to restrict portions or calories. Eat until you are full, and eat as much as you like of the approved foods. If you don't, you will either downshift your metabolism or cheat between meals with banned-food snacks.

Kristal wasn't losing weight and was irritable on the diet. Why? Because she was neglecting legumes and focusing on a higher volume of green vegetables, resulting in insufficient calories. There is no need to count calories if you follow the rules, and one of the rules is: get plenty of legumes. Her results multiplied after making one change:

I took your advice and made beans the #1 ingredient this week, and I have a lot more energy and am remarkably less cranky. The first couple weeks I made veggies #1 with a bit of beans and meat tossed in. This week it is beans, beans, beans... and I'm now down 10 pounds. Whoopee!

MISTAKE #3: NOT DRINKING ENOUGH WATER

To ensure optimal liver function for fat loss, increased hydration is a must.

Insufficient water intake ("I just don't like drinking much water") seems to be particularly common among women. My mother plateaued in fat loss and, looking at her water intake, I insisted she add a few more glasses. She immediately started losing fat again and lost 0.2st (1.3kg) in the subsequent week.

Make a special effort to drink more water on your cheat day, as the carbohydrate overload will pull water to your digestive tract and muscle glycogen. If you don't get enough water, headaches will be the result.

MISTAKE #4: BELIEVING THAT YOU'LL COOK, ESPECIALLY IF YOU'RE A BACHELOR

In a sentence: if you don't normally cook, get canned and frozen food for the first few weeks.

Don't buy a bunch of food that requires cooking skills if you don't have them. Don't buy foods that spoil if you've never prepared a proper meal. Unfounded optimism will just result in rotten food and frustration. To the right is a telltale picture of what happens to most onions that live in my refrigerator.

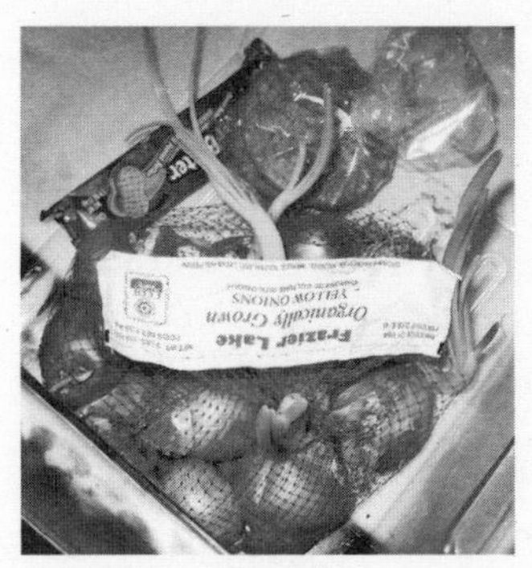

Jack and the onion stalk

I have bags of dried lentils in my cupboard that are now six months old. Why? I'm too lazy to boil and strain them.

Keep it simple. Use frozen and canned stuff for at least the first two weeks. Change one habit at a time: food selection first, food preparation second.

MISTAKE #5: MISTIMING WEIGHINGS WITH YOUR MENSTRUAL CYCLE (NOT A PROBLEM FOR BACHELORS)

Women tend to retain much more water just before their periods. Be sure to take this into account when you start your diet and take measurements.

Ignore scale readings in the 10 days before menstruation. They're not at all a reflection of what's happening. If you are following the diet to the letter, you will lose fat. Treat your first weighing following your period (as soon as one day following is fine) as your "after" measurement.

Don't let short-term water fluctuations discourage you. Be aware of your menstrual timing so you don't mistakenly conclude the diet isn't working.

MISTAKE #6: OVEREATING "DOMINO FOODS": NUTS, CHICKPEAS, HUMMUS, PEANUTS, MACADAMIAS

There are certain foods that, while technically fine to eat on the diet, are prone to portion abuse. I call these "domino foods", as eating one portion often creates a domino effect of over-snacking.

My fat loss has plateaued three times due to almonds, which are easy to consume by the handful and simple to excuse as nutritious. Unfortunately, they also contain 824 calories per serving, 146 calories more than a Whopper from Burger King (678 kilocalories).

A few almonds is just fine (5–10), but no one eats just a few almonds.

Caro learned to avoid domino foods, but lost valuable time in the process, as have dozens of others:

> *I have re-started this eating plan. I started it but wasn't following it exactly how Tim laid it all out.... I added peanuts and I was eating chickpeas and no weight loss, so I thought it was time to get real. I re-started 5 days ago and I am happy to say I have lost 5lb in 5 days by following the plan EXACTLY as Tim says, making no adjustments or substitutes in any way, getting real and honest about what I can and can't eat.*

Think you'll just have one cookie or a couple of potato crisps?

Not if there's a bag of either in the kitchen. Self-discipline is overrated and undependable. Don't eat anything that requires portion control. Get domino foods out of the house and out of reach.

MISTAKE #7: OVER-CONSUMING ARTIFICIAL (OR "ALL-NATURAL") SWEETENERS, INCLUDING AGAVE NECTAR

Even with no calories, most artificial and natural sugar substitutes provoke increased insulin release, though aspartame (Nutrasweet®) shows surprisingly little effect on insulin. Not that this is a free licence to over-consume Nutrasweet®: it's often paired with acesulfame-K, which has a host of negative health effects. Both low-calorie and no-calorie sweeteners have been associated with weight gain. I've seen just about all of them stall fat loss.

Don't think I'm preaching. I'm a total Diet Coke whore. Can't help it.

Indulging my addiction up to 450ml (16 fl oz) a day doesn't seem to interfere with loss. I've found, as have other slow-carbers, that more than 450ml (16 fl oz) interrupts the process at least 75% of the time.

"All-natural" sweeteners are, based on the role of fructose in metabolic disorders, arguably worse for you than even high-fructose corn syrup (HFCS).

So-called "sugar-free" health foods are full of sweeteners such as "concentrated apple and pear juices", which are two-thirds fructose, and the latest and greatest saviours are even worse. Raw agave nectar, for example, is as high as 90% fructose and shows no better antioxidant content than refined sugar or HFCS.

Skip the sweeteners whenever possible. If it's really sweet, it probably spikes insulin or screws up your metabolism. Experiment with spices and extracts like cinnamon and vanilla instead.

MISTAKE #7: HITTING THE GYM TOO OFTEN

One female slow-carber wrote:

> *I have been going to the gym 5x/week, 2 hours on the treadmill plus a one hour spin class 2x a week. . . . I have been doing this for almost three months. In the first 3 weeks I lost almost 20 pounds but since have regained about 7 pounds. I also complete a variety of exercises targeting various muscles groups (2x/week for my legs, hips, arms, etc)*

The 3.1kg (7lb) could have been muscular gain, which is good, but she was spending more than 12 hours a week in the gym. I suspected her problem, which I'd seen in others, was unsustainable over-training and related "reward" eating:

> *I suspect you are over-training and actually losing muscle, given your description. This will lower your basal metabolic rate and then cause you [to] stall with fat loss. Try the diet with no more than 2–3 short weight training workouts per week [if you even choose to exercise; it's not mandatory] and remember to track body fat % and not just weight.*

Doing too much will not only *not* help, it will reverse your progress, as it also leads to overeating, sports drinks, and other assorted self-sabotage.

Remember the MED. Less is more.

DAMAGE CONTROL

Preventing Fat Gain When You Binge

Life itself is the proper binge.

—Julia Child

Doughnuts are a normal part of a healthy, balanced diet.

—Brooke Smith, Krispy Kreme spokeswoman

I was on a first date at Samovar Tea House in San Francisco.

The incense, subdued global music and meticulous track lighting made us feel like we were somewhere between a Buddhist-inspired Last Dragon and a Dutch coffee shop. Then, as if on cue, both of us ordered Schizandra berry tea. The description?

> *2000 years ago Shen Nong first identified this potent elixir as an "adaptogenic tonic" (i.e., it gives you whatever you need: energy, relaxation, beauty, sexual prowess).*

Things were off to a good start.

After some flirting and playful verbal sparring, I made my move.

"Don't let this weird you out."

I took an electronic food scale out of my man-purse,[6] which I use to carry odd items, and began separating all of my food so I could weigh the individual pieces. This was, of course, the beginning of the end.

6. Strange enough to begin with.

Ah, l' amor . . . It is fickle and not fond of serial-killer-like behaviour.

But love could wait. I had other things on my mind.

It was just the beginning of a 12-hour quest for fatness, and it was my second attempt. The first attempt, done with more than 4.5kg (10lb) of fatty cuts of grass-fed beef, had failed. That is, I could consume only 2.72kg (6lb) without vomiting, and I didn't gain one gram of fat.

Why the hell do a quest for fatness at all, you ask?

Because I wanted to prove, once and for all, that the calories-in-calories-out model was plain wrong, or at least incomplete. The easiest way I could do this was by consuming a disgusting number of calories in a short period of time and documenting the after-effects.

This time, I had a different approach.

At 11:43 P.M. that evening, with two minutes remaining, I struggled to choke down a final package of Nutter Butters. I had polled my then 60,000 or so Twitter followers the previous night for their favourite calorically dense foods, and I had committed to consuming as many as possible. Everything I ate or drank would be photographed and either measured or weighed.

Here's how it added up, with non-eating but important events indicated with an asterisk:

11:45 A.M. start

- 180g (6.3oz) steamed spinach (30 kcal)
- 3 tbsp almond butter on one large celery stick (540 kcal)
- 2 heaped tbsp All-in-one superfood supplement in water (86 kcal)
- Chicken curry salad, 195g/6.8oz (approximately 350 kcal)

  Total = 1,006 kcal

12:45 P.M.

- Grapefruit juice (90 kcal)
- Large coffee with 1 tsp cinnamon (5 kcal)
- 2% milk fat milk, 315ml/10 fl oz (190 kcal)
- 2 large chocolate croissants, 168g/6oz (638.4 kcal)

  Total = 923.4 kcal

2:00 P.M.

- Citrus kombucha, 454kg/16oz (60 kcal)

*2:15 P.M.

- Poo

- AGG (discussed later)
- Butter fat and fermented cod liver

*3:00–3:20 P.M.

- 15 repetitions x 3 sets each:
  1. Bent row
  2. Incline bench press
  3. Leg press

3:30 P.M.

- 1l (1.75 pints) Straus cream-top organic whole milk (600 kcal)

*4:00 P.M.

- Probiotics
- 20-min. ice bath

4:45 P.M.

- Quinoa, 230g/8oz (859 kcal)

5:55 P.M.

- Nougat and caramel chocolate bar (216 kcal)
- Yerba maté (30 kcal)
  Total = 246 kcal

*6:20 P.M.

- Poo

*6:45 P.M.

- 40 air squats and 30 wall tricep extensions

6:58 P.M.

- Assorted cheeses, 33g/1oz (116 kcal)
- Honey, 30g/1oz (90 kcal)
- Medium apple (71 kcal)
- Crackers, 8g/ ¼oz (30 kcal)
- Chai tea with soy milk (not my choice),350ml/12fl oz (175 kcal)
  Total = 482 kcal

*9:30 P.M.

- 40 air squats in men's room

9:36 P.M.

- Pizza (nettles, red onion, provolone, mushroom, pancetta and olive oil with one whole egg), 8 pieces (64g/2.2oz each) (1,249 kcal)
- 1 small glass red wine, Nero d'Avola, 150ml/5fl oz. (124 kcal)
- Vanilla ice cream, 59g/2oz (140 kcal)
- Double espresso (0 kcal)
  Total = 1,513 kcal

10:37 P.M.

- 2 heaped tbsp all-in-one superfood supplement in water (86 kcal)

*10:40 P.M.

- PAGG (discussed later)
- 60 standing band pulls

*11:10 P.M.

- Poo

11:37 P.M.

- Peanut cookie, 40g/1.5oz (189 kcal)
- Peanut butter cookies packet, small (250 kcal)

  Total = 439 kcal

2:15 A.M.

- Bedtime/face plant

For a grand total of. . . drum roll, please . . . 6,214.4 calories in 12 hours.

Based on basal metabolic rate (BMR) calculations that took into account my lean mass v. fat mass at the time, my BMR for 24 hours was approximately 1,764.87 calories, which would make my 12-hour BMR 882.4 calories.

There are two things we need to add to this: the 20-minute moderate-intensity weight-lifting session (80 calories maximum, which we'll use here) and walking.

I walked approximately 16 flat blocks and one mild uphill block during that period of time, which adds no more than 110 calories in this case, given the 2.25km (1.4-mile) distance at 3.2km (2 miles) per hour speed and 12st (76.2kg) bodyweight. I otherwise avoided movement and standing whenever possible, with the exception of the brief air squats. Twenty minutes of lifting + walking = 190 calories. Let's call it 200.

Using this maths, **I still consumed 6.8 times my resting metabolic rate in my 12-hour quest for fatness.**

So what happened? Let's look at my body fat and weight measurements, which were taken using the BodyMetrix ultrasound device, and the average of three separate weighings:

Saturday, 29 August 2009 (the morning of the binge): 9.9% body fat at 12st (76.6kg)

Monday, 31 August 2009 (48 hours later): 9.6% body fat at 9.7st (61.6kg)

WTF?

Now let's look at how I did it.

The Lost Art of Bingeing

Sitting down for Christmas dinner or butter cookies at Christmas?

Sounds like a binge. That, in and of itself, doesn't need to mean horrible guilt and extra fat rolls afterwards. If you plan ahead of time and understand a little science, it's possible to minimize the damage. I eat whatever I want every Saturday, and I follow specific steps to minimize fat gain during this overfeeding.

In basic terms our goal is simple: to have as much of the crap ingested either go into muscle tissue or out of the body unabsorbed.

I do this by focusing on three principles:

PRINCIPLE #1: MINIMIZE THE RELEASE OF INSULIN, A STORAGE HORMONE.

Insulin release is minimized by blunting sharp jumps in blood sugar:

1. Ensure that your first meal of the day is not a binge meal. Make it high in protein (at least 30 grams) and insoluble fibre (legumes will handle this). The protein will decrease your appetite for the remainder of the binge and prevent total self-destruction. The fibre will be important later to prevent diarrhoea. In total, this can be a smallish meal of 300–500 calories.
2. Consume a small quantity of fructose, fruit sugar, in grapefruit juice before the second meal, which is the first crap meal. Even small fructose dosing has an impressive near-flat-lining effect on blood glucose.[7] I could consume this at the first meal, but I prefer to combine the naringin in grapefruit juice with coffee, as it extends the effects of caffeine.
3. Use supplements that increase insulin sensitivity: AGG (part of PAGG) and PAGG (covered in the next chapter). The example intake in this chapter is quite mild, so I dosed only twice. If I'm going the whole hog, I will have another PAGG dose upon waking. This reduces the amount of insulin the pancreas releases in spite of mild or severe glucose surges. Think of it as insurance.

7. See "The Glucose Switch" for more on this.

4. Consume citric juices, whether lime juice squeezed into water, lemon juice on food, or a beverage like the citrus kombucha I had.

PRINCIPLE #2: INCREASE THE SPEED OF GASTRIC EMPTYING, OR HOW QUICKLY FOOD EXITS THE STOMACH.

Bingeing is a rare circumstance where I want the food (or some of it) to pass through my gastrointestinal tract so quickly that its constituent parts aren't absorbed well.

I accomplish this primarily through caffeine and yerba maté tea, which includes the additional stimulants theobromine (found in dark chocolate) and theophylline (found in green tea). I consume 100–200 milligrams of caffeine, or 450ml (16 fl oz) of cooled yerba maté, at the most crap-laden meals. My favourite superfood supplement (mentioned in the schedule) doesn't contain caffeine but will also help.

Does this really work? Taking the goodies from taste buds to toilet without much storage in between?[8]

More than a few people have told me it's pure science fiction.

Too much information (TMI) warning: I disagree, and for good reason. Rather than debate meta-studies, I simply weighed my poo. Identical volumes of food on and off the protocol. On protocol = much more poo mass (same consistency, hence the importance of fibre) = less absorption = fewer chocolate croissants that take up residence on my abs. Simple but effective? Perhaps. Good to leave out of first-date conversation? Definitely.

On to one of the cooler aspects of this whole craziness: GLUT-4.

PRINCIPLE #3: ENGAGE IN BRIEF MUSCULAR CONTRACTION THROUGHOUT THE BINGE.

For muscular contractions, my default options are air squats, wall presses (tricep extensions against a wall), and chest pulls with an elastic band, as all three are portable and can be done without causing muscle trauma that screws up training. The latter two can be performed by anyone, even those who have difficulty walking.

But why the hell would you want to do 60–90 seconds of funny exercises a few minutes before you eat and, ideally, again about 90 minutes afterwards?

Short answer: because it brings glucose transporter type 4 (GLUT-4) to the surface of muscle cells, opening more gates for the calories to flow

8. It's true that increasing the speed of gastric emptying can increase the glycaemic index of meals; that makes it all the more important to blunt that response with a small dose of fructose.

into. The more muscular gates we have open before insulin triggers the same GLUT-4 on the surface of fat cells, the more we can put in muscle instead of fat.

Longer answer:

GA GLUT-4 has been studied most intensely for the last 15 years or so, as it became clear around 1995 that exercise and insulin appear to activate (translocate) GLUT-4 through different but overlapping signalling pathways. This was exciting to me, as it meant it might be possible to use exercise to beat meal-induced insulin release to the punch—to preemptively flip the switch on the biological train tracks so that food (glucose) is preferentially siphoned to muscle tissue.

But how much contraction is enough? It turns out, at least with animals, that much less is needed than was once thought. In one fascinating Japanese study with rats, high-intensity intermittent exercise (HIT) (20-second sprints × 14 sets, with 10 seconds of rest between sets) was compared to low-intensity prolonged exercise (LIT) (six hours of extended exercise) over eight days.

The surprising result? Bolding is mine:

> *In conclusion, the present investigation demonstrated that 8 days of **HIT lasting only 280 seconds** elevated both GLUT-4 content and maximal glucose transport activity in rat skeletal muscle to a level **similar to that attained after LIT ["Low-Intensity Training" of six hours a session],** which has been considered a tool to increase GLUT-4 content maximally.*

Compared to a control, GLUT-4 content in the muscle was increased 83% with 280 seconds of HIT v. 91% with six hours of LIT.

Now, of course, animal models don't always have a direct transfer to humans. But I wondered: what if 280 seconds was all it took? This thought produced even more questions:

Do we have to get the 280 seconds all at once, or can they be spread out?

Is 280 seconds really the magic number, or could even fewer seconds trigger the same effect?

Is it even plausible that 60–90 seconds of moderate contractions could have a meaningful impact?

To attempt to answer these questions, I contacted researcher after researcher on three continents, including GLUT-4 specialists at the Muscle Biology Laboratory at the University of Michigan at Ann Arbor.

The short answer was: it did appear plausible.

The most important research insight came from Dr. Gregory D. Cartee and Katsuhiko Funai:

> *The insulin-independent effect of exercise begins to reverse minutes after exercise cessation with most or all of the increase lost within 1–4 hours. A much more persistent effect is improved insulin sensitivity that is often found approximately 2–4 hours and as long as 1–2 days after acute exercise.*

I started with 60–120 seconds total of air squats and wall tricep extensions immediately prior to eating main courses. For additional effect, I later tested doing another 60–90 seconds approximately one and a half hours after finishing the main courses, when I expected blood glucose to be highest based on experiments with glucometres.[9]

Exercises are best done in a toilet stall and not at the table. If you can't leave the table, get good at isometric (without moving) contraction of your legs. Try to look casual instead of constipated.

It takes some practice.

In China, I was taught a rhyming proverb: *Fàn hòu bǎi bù zǒu, néng huó dào jiǔ shí jiǔ* [飯後百步走，能活到九十九]. If you take 100 steps after each meal, you can live to be 99 years old.

Could it be that the Chinese identified the effect of GLUT-4 translocation hundreds, even thousands, of years before scientists formalized the mechanism? It's possible. More likely: they just liked rhyming.

In all cases, if you do 60–90 seconds of contraction after each meal (and a bit before, ideally), you might live to see your abs.

Don't forget the air squats.

9. Again, see "The Glucose Switch" for more tricks along these lines.

STALLING MANOEUVRES: AIR SQUATS, WALL PRESSES AND CHEST PULLS

I aim for 30–50 repetitions of each of the following:

Air Squats

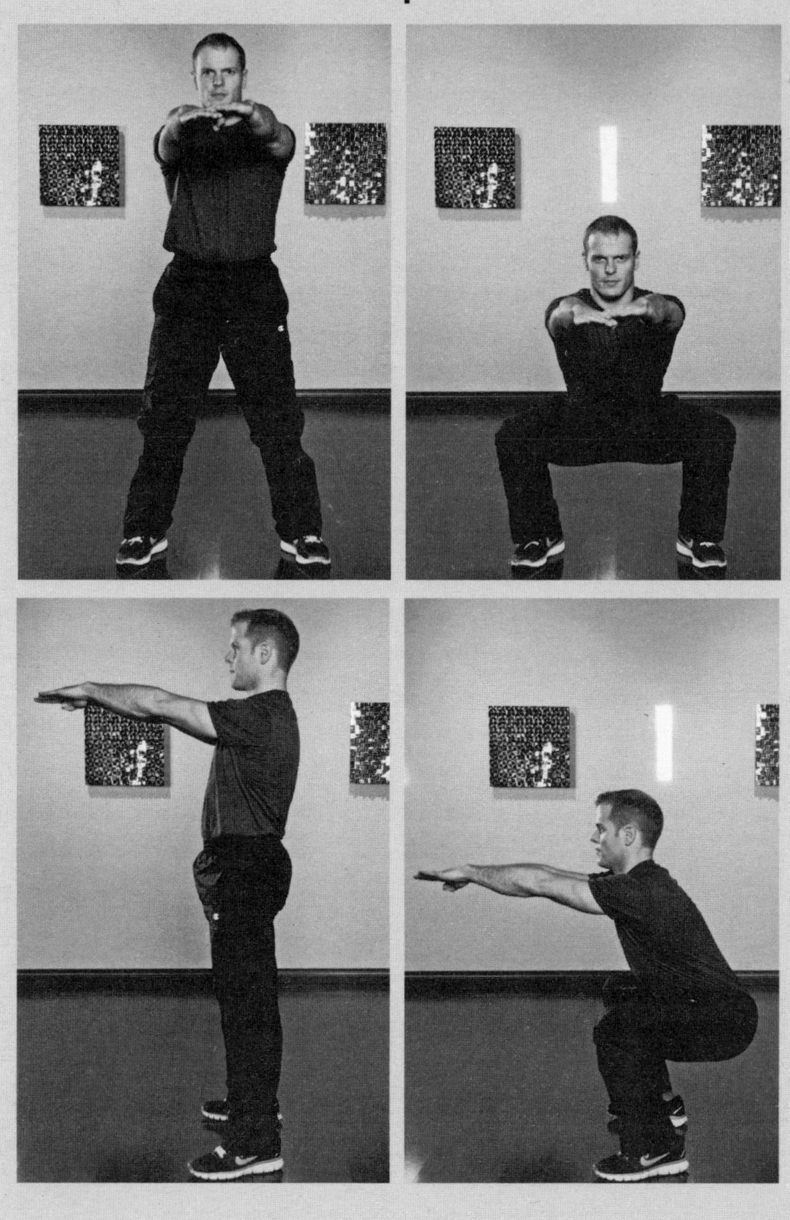

Wall Presses

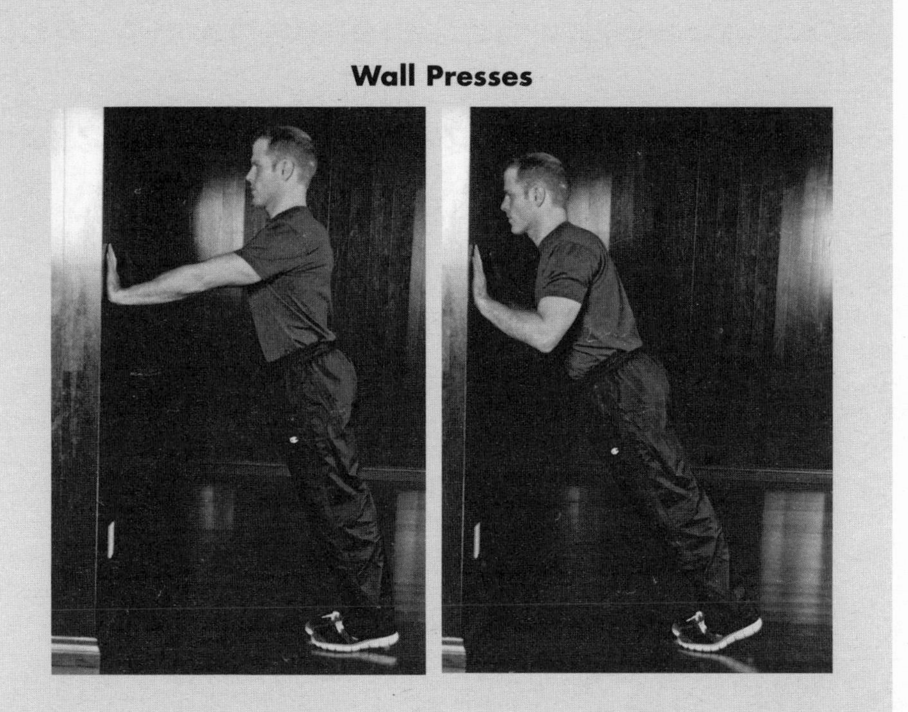

Chest Pulls

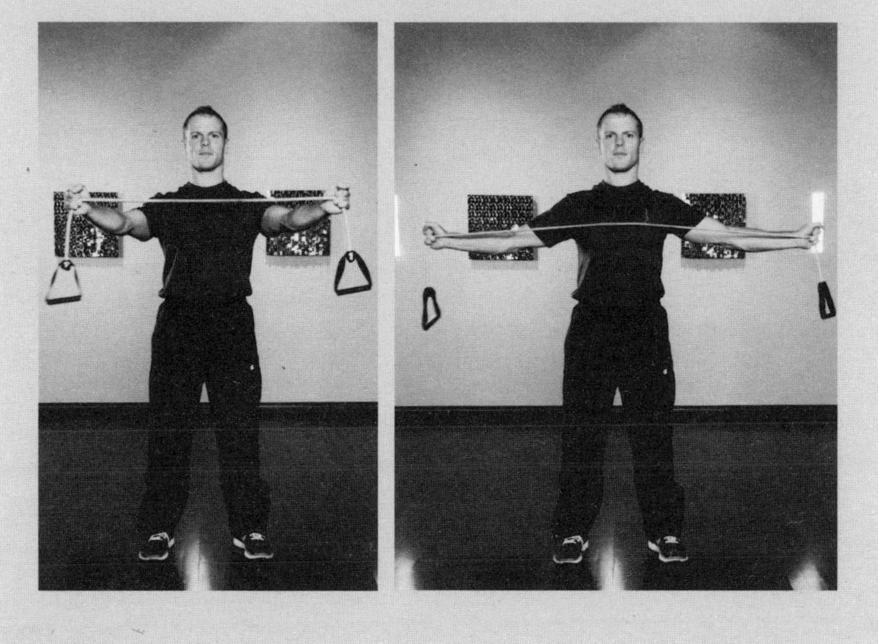

X-FACTOR: CISSUS QUADRANGULARIS

Cissus quadrangularis (CQ) is an indigenous medicinal plant of India.

It is a newcomer in mainstream supplementation, usually prescribed for joint repair. In July 2009, I experimented with high-dose CQ following elbow surgery due to a staph infection. Unexpectedly, used in combination with PAGG, it seemed to have synergistic anti-obesity and anabolic (muscle growth) effects. Upon performing a second literature review of its use in Ayurvedic medicine and fracture repair, it became clear that there were implications for preventing fat gain during overfeeding.

Rural China, where I continued experimentation with CQ, provided high-volume rice meals combined with sweets at mandatory sit-down meals, 3–5 times per day. It was the perfect fat-gaining environment.

CQ preserved my abs. I saw measurable fat loss and anabolic effects once I reached 2.4 grams (2,400 milligrams), three times per day 30 minutes prior to meals, for a total of 7.2 grams per day. Is that the magic dose? I had approximately 11.4st (72.7kg) of lean bodymass, so there might be a trigger at 45 milligrams per kilogram lean bodymass, or it could be an absolute effective dose regardless of bodyweight. Until long-term side-effect studies are done at these higher doses, I don't suggest exceeding 7.2 grams per day.

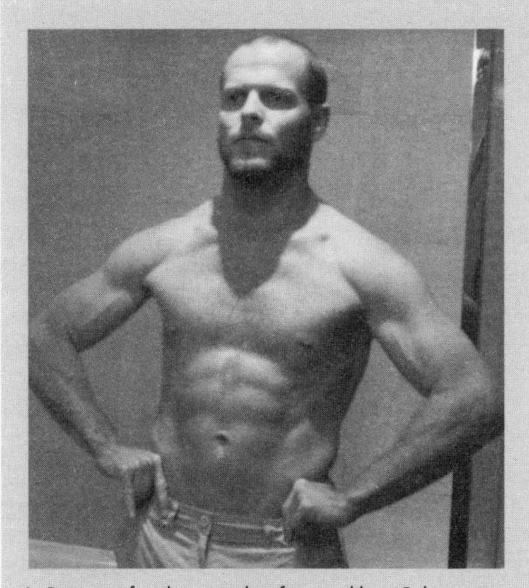

In Beijing, after three weeks of eating like a Peking pig.

For those who can afford it, I believe CQ is very effective for minimizing unwanted fat gain while overfeeding. Until more human studies are done, I don't plan on continuous use, but I will use it during 8–12 week growth cycles, on "off" days, or after joint sprains.

Kevin Rose, one of my travelling companions during our three-week trip, lamented, "Glenn and I were getting fatter and fatter, while this f*cker was getting ripped. What the hell?!"

One friend, a serial CTO, referred to cissus quadrangularis as the "morning-after pill" for diet after seeing me chase peanut butter ice cream and brownies with it.

CQ works.

INSIDE THE MICROBIOME: BALANCING BACTERIA FOR FAT LOSS

Why is obesity so much more common today than it was even a few decades ago?

Researchers are starting to find bacterial clues that may point to an answer. There has been a profound shift in our populations of gut bacteria—the little creatures that live in our digestive tracts—and studies show the changes as correlated with increased fatness.

There are actually 10 times more bacterial cells in your body than human cells: 100 trillion of them to 10 trillion of you. For the most part, these bugs help us, improving our immune system, providing vitamins, and preventing other harmful bacteria from infecting us. These bacteria also regulate how well we harvest energy from our food.

So far, two primary strains of bacteria have been found to influence fat absorption, almost regardless of diet: Bacteroidetes and Firmicutes. Lean people have more Bacteroidetes and fewer Firmicutes; obese people have more Firmicutes and fewer Bacteroidetes. As obese people lose weight, the ratio of bacteria in their gut swings confidently over to more Bacteroidetes.

This finding has significant enough implications for national health that the National Institutes of Health (NIH) launched the multi-year Human Microbiome Project in late 2007. It is like a Human Genome Project for bacteria and intended to explore how some of the 40,000+ species of micro-friends (and fiends) are affecting our health and how we might modify them to help us more.

This could take some time, but you don't need to wait to act. There are a few things you can do now to cultivate healthy and fat-reducing gut flora:

1. **Get off the Splenda.** A 2008 study at Duke University found that giving Splenda to rats significantly decreased the amount of helpful bacteria in the gut. Once again, the fake sugars turn out just as bad as, if not worse than, the real deal.
2. **Go fermented.** Dr. Weston Price is famous for his studies of 12 traditional diets of near-disease-free indigenous communities spread around the globe. He found that the one common element was fermented foods, which were consumed daily. Cultural mainstays varied but included cheese, Japanese natto, kefir, kimchi (also spelled "kimchee"), sauerkraut and fermented fish. Unsweetened plain yogurt and fermented kombucha tea are two additional choices. Fermented foods contain high levels of healthy bacteria and should be viewed as a mandatory piece of your dietary puzzle. I consume five forkfuls of sauerkraut each morning before breakfast and also add kimchi to almost all home-cooked meals.

3. **Consider probiotics and prebiotics.** *Probiotics* are bacteria. I've used Sedona Labs iFlora probiotics both during training (to help accommodate overfeeding) and after antibiotics.

   Prebiotics are fermentable substrates that help bacteria grow and thrive. In this category, I've experimented with organic inulin and fructo-oligosaccharides, commonly referred to as FOS. For a host of reasons, I prefer inulin, which I get through the superfood supplements mentioned previously. Inulin is about 10% the sweetness of sugar, but unlike fructose it's not insulinemic. In the whole-foods realm, garlic, leeks and chicory are all high in inulin or FOS content.

Though the research is preliminary, introducing pre- and probiotics together in the diet could have beneficial effects on allergies, ageing, obesity and a range of diseases from AIDS to type 2 diabetes. I found one potential benefit particularly fascinating, given our focus on GLUT-4: both inulin and FOS improve calcium absorption, and calcium absorption promotes the contraction-dependent GLUT-4 translocation!

If the anti-obesity effects weren't enough, consider bacterial balance a crucial step in supporting your "second brain".

Most of us have heard of serotonin, a wide-acting neurotransmitter that, when deficient, is intimately linked to depression. Prozac and other selective serotonin reuptake inhibitors (SSRIs) act to increase the effects of serotonin. Despite the label "neurotransmitter", which leads most people to visualize the brain, only 5% of serotonin is found in your head. The remaining 95% is produced in the gut, sometimes referred to as "the second brain" for this reason.

In a randomized, double-blind, placebo-controlled study of 39 patients with chronic fatigue syndrome, *Lactobacillus casei* strain Shirota was found to significantly decrease anxiety symptoms. Probiotics (bifidobacteria is one example) have also been shown as an effective alternative treatment for depression because of their power to inhibit inflammatory molecules called cytokines, decrease oxidative stress, and correct the overgrowth of unwanted bacteria that prevents optimal nutrient absorption in the intestines.

Give your good bacteria an upgrade and get your microbiome in shape. Faster fat loss and better mental health are just two of the benefits.

TOOLS AND TRICKS

Twelve Hours of Bingeing in Photos (www.fourhourbody.com/binge) See the binge from this chapter as I captured it in real time and posted the photos on Flickr. It will give you an appreciation for the quantity.

Super Cissus Rx (www.fourhourbody.com/cq) This is the brand of CQ I used during the experimentation.

Athletic Greens (www.athleticgreens.com) This is my all-in-one greens insurance policy. It contains 76 ingredients, including inulin for improving bacterial balance.

Escali Cesto Portable Nutritional Scale (www.fourhourbody.com/cesto) This is the 450g (1lb) scale I carried around in my man-purse to measure the weight and nutritional composition of my meals. The Escali Cesto display shows calories, sodium, protein, fat, carbohydrates, cholesterol and fibre for almost 1,000 different types of food. May the force be with you, fellow OCDers.

Nutrition Data (www.nutritiondata.com) Want to find out how many calories are in your favourite splurge meal or family recipe? Just use the "Analyse Recipe" Nutrition Management Tool on this site to calculate the nutritional value of the dish. You can also save your recipes and share them with others. I use this site often, including for the calculations in this chapter.

Thera-Bands (www.fourhourbody.com/thera) I started doing standing chest pulls with Thera-Bands (primarily grey), which are popular among physical therapists for rehab exercises. Once I got up to 75 reps per set without fatigue, I upgraded to the mini-bands below.

Mini-bands (www.fourhourbody.com/minibands) I now use these for standing band pulls. Made famous by Louie Simmons of the Westside Barbell gym, these bands are often used by powerlifters to add resistance to deadlifts, bench presses, and squats in the upper ranges of motion. On a related note, think age is an excuse? Tell Louie. He squatted 417kg (920lb) at age 50.

THE FOUR HORSEMEN OF FAT LOSS

PAGG

Without garlic, I simply would not care to live.

—Louis Diat, First Chef de Cuisines of the New York Ritz-Carlton

SUMMER 2007, NORTHERN CALIFORNIA

The smoke wisped into the air amid the sounds of summer eating: laughter, beer bottles clinking, and the undeniable sizzle of rump steak on three enormous outdoor barbecues. All was well in Willow Glen, San Jose, where my parents were visiting me. I was at home, but they had ventured out to explore downtown Lincoln Avenue on a beautiful afternoon, which led them to La Villa Italian restaurant.

My father was standing on the corner admiring the barbecue work when a thin homeless man sauntered up to his side. After a minute or two of silence and staring at meat and tongs, the homeless man made this opening:

"You know how I lost all my weight? More than 7.14st (45.4kg)?"

My dad was 168cm (5ft 6in) and almost 17.9st (113kg) at the time. Silence followed for several seconds, and my father—amused by the approach and more than a bit curious—finally relented: "How?"

"Garlic. Clove after clove. It's that simple."

The homeless man didn't want anything and never asked for anything. He was earnest. After sharing his advice, he just walked away.

As unusual as this encounter was, I had, in fact, been looking at garlic for some time. This was just the final anecdotal push I needed to begin experimenting at much, much higher doses. The homeless man's contribution to my latest cocktail made it all come together.

The final feedback from one guinea pig, a semi-professional athlete with approximately 9% body fat at 14.3st (90.7kg), was representative: "I've lost 6lb (2.72kg) of fat in the last week. This is un-freaking-believable."

Allicin, one component of garlic, appeared to be the missing fourth ingredient in a supplement stack I'd been refining for two years: PAGG.

Before: ECA

From 1995 to 2000, I experimented with a fat loss cocktail that comprised ephedrine hydrochloride, caffeine and aspirin—the famed and research-proven "ECA" stack. This was the mixture I used three times per day when on the Cyclical Ketogenic Diet to produce veins on my abdomen for the first time in my life, all in less than eight weeks.

Ephedrine hydrochloride: 20 mg
Caffeine: 200 mg
Aspirin: 85 mg

The biochemistry was spot-on, and dozens of studies supported the effects. If E = 1, C = 1, and A = 1, the three combined have a synergistic effect of 1 + 1 + 1 = 6–10.[10]

Sadly, the ECA stack is not a free ride. The effects are beautiful and predictable, but there are prices to be paid: side effects.

Tolerance to the upper-like effects[11] develops quickly and cessation can cause severe headaches. The withdrawal pains lead to a domino effect of stimulant use. Either people never stop taking ECA or they substitute in equally strong drugs to avoid chronic fatigue. I suspect there is an entire

10. The ephedrine increases cAMP levels, the caffeine slows cAMP breakdown, and the aspirin further helps sustain increased cAMP levels by inhibiting prostagladin production.

11. In over-the-counter drugs, ephedrine is generally mixed with guafenesin (an expectorant), as it can otherwise be freebased with basic lab supplies into methamphetamine.

generation of strength and endurance athletes with ECA-induced adrenal fatigue who now depend on stimulants for normal everyday function. Some I know opt for 6–10 double espressos per 24 hours. Used in high doses or in high-humidity/high-heat conditions, ephedrine and ephedra have also both been associated with heart attack and death.

I suffered so many sinus infections post-ECA that I visited a Stanford-trained specialist who, after reviewing a cranial MRI, asked without a second of hesitation: "Do you drink much caffeine or take other stimulants?" Almost all of my sinal cavities were completely blocked with compressed, dried matter. She was amazed that I was able to get out of bed in the morning.

From that point onward, I removed stimulants for brief but increasing periods, as painful as it was, until I had re-established basic adrenal function. It was clear that another fat loss approach was needed, something more sustainable.

I wanted to find a non-stimulant stack that used different pathways altogether.

After: PAGG

The end result was PAGG.

Policosanol: 20–25 mg
Alpha-lipoic acid: 100–300 mg (I take 300 mg with each meal, but some people experience acid reflux symptoms with even 100 mg)
Green tea flavanols (decaffeinated with at least 325 mg EGCG): 325 mg
Garlic extract: at least 200 mg (I routinely use 650+ mg)

Daily PAGG intake is timed before meals and bed, which produces a schedule like this:

Prior to breakfast: AGG
Prior to lunch: AGG
Prior to dinner: AGG
Prior to bed: PAG (omit the green tea extract)

AGG is simply PAGG minus policosanol.

This dosing schedule is followed six days a week. Take one day off each week and one week off every two months. This week off is critical.

Let's look at our new cast of characters.

POLICOSANOL

Policosanol, an extract of plant waxes, often sugar cane, is the most controversial element in the PAGG stack. I originally experimented with policosanol at low and high doses to increase HDL cholesterol and decrease LDL cholesterol. Used in combination with time-release niacin, one orange before bed, and chromium polynicotinate (*not* picolinate) during the four-week "Geek to Freak" project detailed in later chapters, I lowered my total cholesterol from 222 to 147 while almost doubling HDL.

There was a pleasant side effect: an unintended but significant reduction in body fat. I isolated the policosanol over several weeks of further testing. The research studies are far from conclusive regarding policosanol's effects on cholesterol; most show no effect whatsoever. This could be due to not dosing policosanol before peak cholesterol production between midnight and 4:00 A.M. Regardless, the addition of policosanol (10–25 milligrams before bed) to the PAGG (then AGG) stack produces, in my experience and that of my guinea pigs, far superior effects for fat loss vs. AGG alone. This was tested with three brands and three dosages (10, 23, and 40 milligrams per day). I found 23 milligrams per day to be optimal for fat loss, with little additional benefit from higher doses.

ALPHA-LIPOIC ACID (ALA)

Alpha-lipoic acid (ALA) is a potent antioxidant and free radical scavenger that has been proven to regenerate vitamin C and vitamin E; restore levels of intracellular glutathione, an important antioxidant that declines with age; and increase excretion of toxic heavy metals such as mercury.

It was first synthesized and tested in the 1970s for the treatment of chronic liver diseases. The intravenous interventions reversed disease in 75 out of 79 subjects.

Given its impressive effects, the most remarkable feature of ALA is its apparent lack of toxicity in humans.[12] It's NOAEL (No Observable Adverse Effect Level) is 60 milligrams per kilogram of bodyweight, which would

12. Except for those predisposed to Insulin Autoimmune Syndrome (IAS).

make up to 4,091 milligrams per day safe for a 10.7st (68kg) person. Our dosing will be 300–900 milligrams total per day.

Though lipoic acid naturally occurs in some organ meats and vegetables, including spinach and broccoli, the amounts are trace. I didn't want to consume 10 tons of liver for 30 milligrams of lipoic acid, so I began using synthetic alpha-lipoic acid in 1995.

GA

I began taking ALA for its impressive impact on glucose uptake and reduced triglyceride production.

First and foremost, I wanted to increase muscular absorption of the calories (and supplements) I consumed, and ALA turned out to be the perfect force multiplier. More calories absorbed into muscle meant fewer calories deposited as fat and faster strength gains.

ALA accomplishes this, in part, by recruiting GLUT-4 glucose transporters to the muscular cell membrane. This both mimics insulin and increases insulin sensitivity, and ALA is therefore being explored as an "insulino-mimetic" that can be used to treat type 2 diabetes and metabolic syndrome.

Not only does ALA increase glucose and nutrient absorption, but it also demonstrates triglyceride inhibition and—through extrapolation—fat storage. Here is an abstract from a 2009 article from the *Archives of Biochemistry and Biophysics* that drives the point home:

> *Livers from LA [lipoic acid]-treated rats exhibited elevated glycogen content, suggesting dietary carbohydrates were stored as glycogen rather than becoming lipogenic substrate.*

In one sentence, here is why alpha-lipoic acid is kick-ass for our purposes: **ALA helps you store the carbohydrates you eat in muscle or in your liver as opposed to in fat.**

GREEN TEA FLAVANOLS (EGCG)

Epigallocatechin gallate (EGCG) is a catechin and flavanol found in green teas.

It has been researched for a wide range of applications, including decreasing the risk of UV-induced skin damage, inhibiting cancer growth, and reducing mitochondrial oxidative stress (anti-ageing).

I tested green tea and EGCG, once again, for the underreported "off-label" benefits. Specifically, two related to body recomposition:

- Much like ALA, EGCG increases GLUT-4 recruitment to the surface of skeletal muscle cells. Of equal interest, *it inhibits GLUT-4 recruitment in fat cells.* In other words, it inhibits the storage of excess carbohydrates as body fat and preferentially diverts them to muscle cells.
- EGCG appears to increase programmed cell death (apoptosis) in mature fat cells. This means that these hard-to-kill bastards commit suicide. The ease with which people regain fat is due to a certain "fat memory" (the size of fat cells decreases, but not the number), which makes EGCG a fascinating candidate for preventing the horrible rebounding most dieters experience. Super cool and important.

Human studies have shown some potential fat loss with as little as a single dose of 150 milligrams of EGCG, but we will target 325 milligrams three to four times per day, as the fat loss results seem to "hockey-stick"—go from a mild incline to a sharp rise—between 900 and 1,100 milligrams per day for the 10.7 to 14.3st (68 to 90.7kg) subjects I've worked with. I suggest decaffeinated green tea extract pills as the source, unless you want to be stuck to the ceiling and feel ill. Using tea leaves and steeping cup after cup is too imprecise and too caffeinated.

If you are undergoing cancer treatment, please consult your doctor before using EGCG, as it can increase the effects of some drugs (the oestrogen antagonist tamoxifen, for example) while decreasing the effects of others,[13] such as the drug Velcade®, to which it binds. If you are undergoing treatment for multiple myeloma or mantle cell lymphoma, likewise avoid EGCG.

GARLIC EXTRACT (ALLICIN POTENTIAL, S-ALLYL CYSTEINE)

Garlic extract and its constituent parts have been used for applications ranging from cholesterol management to inhibiting lethal MRSA staph infections.

Strangely, test subjects and I have had the best fat loss results with extracts designed to deliver relatively high doses of allicin. Allicin, if delivered in a stable form, appears to have the ability to inhibit fat regain. The reason our results were "strange" relates to the "stable form" bit. Most research indicates that allicin should have almost zero bio-availability more than six days after extraction from garlic cloves, particularly after exposure

13. If you're a male bodybuilder, this effect on tamoxifen can be a good thing, but watch your HDL, which can drop like a stone.

to stomach acid. Our confounding results could be due to a combination of other organic components, most notably one precursor to allicin: S-Allyl cysteine (alliin). S-Allyl cysteine exhibits outstanding oral bio-availability, near 100% in large mammals.[14]

Until further research concludes otherwise, I suggest using an aged-garlic extract (AGE) with high allicin potential that includes all constituent parts, including S-Allyl cysteine. If AGE isn't available, unaged garlic extract appears to work at slightly higher doses.

I've tried consuming it fresh, chomping on cloves, and it isn't kind to your digestive tract. If you are going the whole-food route, use it in your cooking to prevent stomach self-destruction.

For precision and convenience, I use supplements to reach my target baseline in dosing, and I use extra garlic in food for delectable (but not necessary) insurance above that baseline.

Warnings

Ensure adequate consumption of B-complex vitamins while using PAGG and consult your doctor before use if you have a medical condition (e.g., hypertension, hypoglycaemia, diabetes) or are taking any medications in particular, blood-thinning medications (e.g., warfarin, aspirin, etc.), thyroid medications, or anti-anxiety drugs like clozapine.

If you are pregnant or breastfeeding, do not use PAGG. Blood-thinning compounds ain't for babies.

TOOLS AND TRICKS

I used the following products for my testing, but I'll update the links based on availability and reader feedback. I have no financial interest in any of them:

Allicin 6000 Garlic—650 mg, 100 caplets (www.fourhourbody.com/garlic)

Mega Green Tea Extract—325+ mg EGCG, 100 capsules (www.fourhourbody.com/greentea)

Vitamin Shoppe—Alpha-Lipoic Acid, 100 mg, 60 capsules (www.fourhourbody.com/ala)

Nature's Life—Policosanol, 60 tablets (www.fourhourbody.com/policosanol)

14. Though S-Allyl cysteine (SAC) is an easier molecule to get into your bloodstream and has been implicated in minimizing the damage of glycation and free radicals in diabetes, it would be premature to label this the single component responsible for lipid changes or fat loss. The fat loss could well be due to several synergistic compounds in garlic that activate phase I and II detoxification enzymes.

Advanced

ICE AGE

Mastering Temperature to Manipulate Weight

Don't tell me it's impossible, tell me you can't do it. Tell me it's never been done . . . the only things we really know are Maxwell's equations, the three laws of Newton, the two postulates of relativity, and the periodic table. That's all we know that's true. All the rest are man's laws.

—Dean Kamen, inventor of the Segway and recipient of the National Medal of Technology and Lemelson-MIT Prize

"Michael Phelps eats 12,000 calories a day . . ."

That was all Ray Cronise heard from across the room. He jerked his eyes up from the spreadsheet and reached for the TiVo to pause the television.

Twelve thousand calories.

Ray Cronise had been a high-ranking material scientist at NASA for almost 15 years, and his specialities included biophysics and analytical chemistry. He'd been in mission operations and seen—hell, helped *produce*—research the public wouldn't see for decades.

But spending half of his life behind a computer had taken its toll. The creeping 2 to 4lb (900g to 1.8kg) per year had added up and left him weighing 16.4st (104kg) at 175cm (5ft 9in).

It was now a much-improved 15st (95kg) Ray Cronise who sat with a spreadsheet in front of him and his eyes on the paused television. He still had more than 2.14st (13.6kg) to lose. It would take at least 18–24 weeks at his current rate.

The spreadsheet was designed to fix this by comparing all the human activities he could isolate, each correlated to its caloric expenditure per hour for his weight. He was tired of being fat and hoped the numbers would provide a faster solution. Instead, they painted a futile picture: even if he ran a 42km (26 mile) marathon he would only burn around 2,600 calories, or approximately 340g (¾ lb) of fat.

How could Phelps eat an *extra* 9,000 calories per day? Ray scanned his finger through the columns, jotted down a few notes and defaulted to the calculator. It made no sense.

"In order for Phelps to burn those kinds of calories above and beyond what his resting metabolic rate [RMR] was," Ray recalls, "keeping in mind that I had the calculations in front of me, and it's about 860 calories an hour at competitive swimming rates, he would have to sustain more than 10 hours of continuous butterfly every day. Not even he can do that."

So what was going on? Was Phelps misinforming journalists during his Olympic quest? Sabotaging competitors foolish enough to mimic him based on interviews?

The physics didn't work.

Then, in an instant, paused over the spreadsheet, after 15 years of frustration, it all became crystal clear:

"It was the thermal load of the water. Water is 24 times more thermally conductive than air. Phelps spends three or four hours a day in the water."

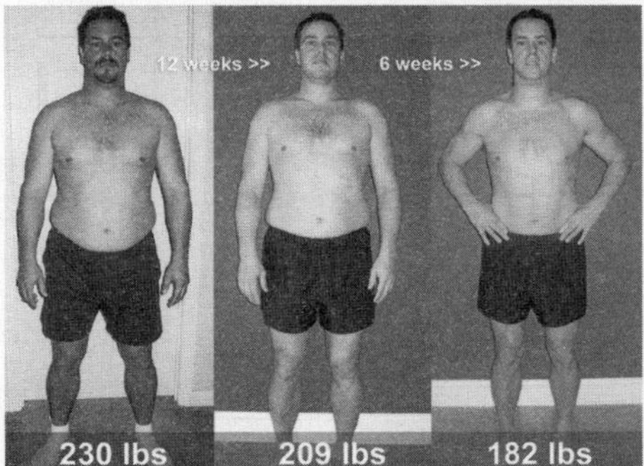

The first 12 weeks *without* cold exposure vs. the second 6 weeks *with* cold exposure.

The effect was the same as pouring hot coffee into a metal cup instead of a ceramic mug; the former loses calories (heat) much faster. Ray did the maths with this new variable, and, amazingly, it seemed to add up.

In the six weeks that followed, from the weekend of 27 October to 5 December, he would lose 13kg (28.6lb) of fat and never regain them.

The game had changed.

From NASA to Everest: Correcting the Metabolism Equation

It seemed too good to be true. So, as any good scientist would, Ray tried to disprove himself.

In the studies and science he reviewed, what struck him most was not evidence that contradicted his conclusions, but rather the near-complete omission of heat as a factor in fat loss.

The common equation in the literature was simple: weight loss or gain = calories-in – calories-out. ΔWt = kcal in – kcal out.

This wasn't the problem.

The problem was that every table for calories-out (caloric expenditure) immediately fixated on activity level. Thermodynamics—*thermo*dynamics—had somehow been robbed of heat. In Ray's world of space shuttles and atmospheric re-entry, heat was king. The laws of thermodynamics were being cited by people who didn't understand them. Take the first law as an example. In simple terms:

Energy can neither be created nor destroyed. It can only change forms.

The misquoters were limiting the ways ingested calories could change form. They treated exercise and storage as the only two options. In fact, the human body is an *open* thermodynamic system and has a number of other options. Ray's then-15st (95kg)-meat-frame could exchange energy with his environment in the form of work (exercise), heat or matter (excretion).

Running a marathon might burn 2,600 calories, but working out in an 27.7°C (82°F) pool for four hours could burn up to an *extra* 4,000 calories, if one considered thermal load.

How else could people like Scott Parazynski, a friend of Ray's, eat can after can of Spam and other high-fat foods? Scott was an MD and former astronaut who had attempted to summit Everest twice, losing about 1.79st (11.3kg) on each attempt. He was successful on his second ascent. His troupe ate lard and 115g (4oz) butter to prevent excessive weight loss. The workload of the climb alone could not account for the caloric expenditure, a 5,000-calorie deficit. It was the cold. Lots of cold.

So Ray began to treat himself like a human space heater.

He tried everything: he drank a gallon of ice water between waking and 11 A.M.; he slept with no covers; he took midwinter "shiver walks" of 20–30 minutes with nothing but a T-shirt, earmuffs and gloves on his upper body.

He later found less painful options, but the results were undeniable. He lost almost 2.7kg (9lb) in the first week.

It Gets Better—The Devil's in the Details

This was not the first time Ray had tried to lose weight.

In 2006, he lost a respectable 1.4st (7kg) following the Body-for-Life (BFL) exercise and diet plan, designed by Bill Phillips. BFL performed as advertised, and Ray lost 17.8lb (8kg) of fat in 12 weeks, for an average weekly fat loss of **1.8lb (834g)**. This was, by all conventional measures, a huge success. Unfortunately, in a pattern familiar to millions, he then gained it all back, plus interest.

In the second experiment, however, repeating BFL with intermittent cold exposure, Ray lost 2st (13kg) in six weeks, for an average weekly fat loss of **4.77lb (2.16kg)**. The addition of cold exposure alone increased fat loss per week more than three times. This added up to 61% *more* total fat lost in *half* the time.

I found Ray's results both incredible and believable. But something seemed to be missing.

First of all, he had also gained more muscle with cold exposure. Losing more heat couldn't account for that. Though the muscle gain could have been accounted for by the slight inaccuracies of home-use calipers (plus or minus 900g/2lb), I suspected there was more to the story.

Second, looking at the research, the maths didn't add up quite as neatly as I'd hoped.

It's been shown that you can burn almost four times more fat than usual with two hours of cold exposure[15] (176.5 milligrams per minute instead of 46.9 milligrams per minute). This is great, but percentage changes can be deceptive. If there are nine calories in one gram of fat, and assuming the effect lasts for the time you are in the water, then this exposure would burn an extra 139 calories,[16] or *15.5 grams of fat.*

15.5 grams?! That's about 11 paper clips. . . for two hours of torture.

Ray was losing more than three additional pounds (approximately 1.36kg) of fat per week with cold exposure. To achieve that with water immersion

15. Men acutely exposed to cold for two hours (in a liquid-conditioned suit perfused with 10°C [50°F] water) have been observed to increase heat production by 2.6-fold and increase the oxidation rate of plasma glucose by 138%, of muscle glycogen by 109%, and of lipids by 376%. Raising the body's heat in response to cold exposure is done mostly by burning lipids (50%), then glycogen from muscles (30%), then blood glucose and proteins (10% each).

16. (176.5 – 46.9)/1,000 g/min * 120 min * 9 cal/g.

	BFL		BFL + COLD	
	7/10/2006	10/2/2006	10/27/2008	12/8/2008
MEASUREMENT	START	WEEK 12	START	WEEK 6
Right Arm	14.50	14.0	14.25	13.75
Left Arm	14.25	14.0	14.25	14.00
2" Above Navel	39.00	34.0	39.00	33.25
Navel	40.00	36.0	40.50	36.00
2" Below Navel	41.00	37.3	41.00	37.00
Hips (Widest Point)	42.25	40.0	42.25	39.50
Right Thigh	25.25	22.0	25.25	21.75
Left Thigh	24.75	22.3	24.75	21.75
Total Inches	241.00	219.50	241.25	217.00
INCHES (LOSS)	NA	21.50	NA	24.25
Skinfold (mm)	20.0	13.0	20.0	7-8
Bodyfat % (Accu-Measure)	**24.70%**	**17.80%**	**24.70%**	**12.65%**
Total Bodyfat (lbs.)	51.5	33.7	51.6	23.1
Total Lean Mass	156.9	155.6	157.4	159.2
Weight	208.4	189.3	209.0	182.3
Total Weight Loss	NA	**19.1**	NA	**26.7**
Total Fat Loss	NA	**17.8**	NA	**28.6**
Total Lean Mass Gain	NA	**−1.3**	NA	**1.9**

Ray Cronise's fat loss spreadsheet. 12 weeks without cold vs. 6 weeks with cold.

alone, looking at the same studies, he'd need to spend 174.2 hours per week in 10°C (50°F) water. It seems unlikely that Ray spent more than 24 hours per day in water. In fact, he didn't spend two hours per day swimming in, or consuming, 10°C (50°F) water.

Something else needed to be happening. It could have been the other thermic loads he experimented with: cold walks, sleeping without sheets, etc.

Digging deeper still, I now believe that the "something else" involves two players you'll hear much more about in the next few years: adiponectin and BAT.

Adiponectin is a cool little hormone, secreted by fat cells, that can both increase the oxidation ("burning") of fatty acids in mitochondria and increase uptake of glucose by muscle tissue. I believe adiponectin is largely to thank for Ray's muscle gain.[17] Speculation notwithstanding, the research is in its early

17. Shivering also contributes to increased muscular GLUT-4 activity, just like air squats.

stages, so I'll reserve adiponectin as an intellectual dessert for the geeks. My forays into its potential can be found in the online resources.

BAT and my related torture experiments, on the other hand, are worth taking a closer look at.

If the science gets too dense and you want the index card version, skip to "Ice Age Revisited—Four Places to Start" on page 130. I won't be offended.

GA

Fat-burning Fat

Not all fat is equal. There are at least two distinct types: white adipose tissue (WAT) and brown adipose tissue (BAT).

WAT is what we usually think of as fat, like the marbling on a steak. A WAT cell—an adipocyte—is composed of a single large fat droplet with a single nucleus.

BAT, in contrast, is sometimes referred to as "fat-burning fat" and appears to be derived from the same stem cells as muscle tissue. A BAT cell is composed of multiple droplets that are brown in colour because of a much higher volume of iron-containing mitochondria. Normally associated with muscle tissue, mitochondria are best known for producing ATP and oxidizing fat in muscle tissue. BAT helps dissipate excess calories as heat. These excess calories would otherwise be stored in the aforementioned WAT and end up in your beer gut or muffin top.[18]

In a nutshell: cold stimulates BAT to burn fat and glucose as heat. Cold, as well as drugs called beta-adrenergic agonists,[19] can also make BAT appear within WAT in mice and rats. In other words, cold might help you increase the amount of your "fat-burning" fat. This has tremendous implications.

18. This energy "wasting" is possible due to an uncoupling protein called UCP1, also known aptly as *thermogenin*.

19. Ephedrine and clenbuterol, neither of which I recommend, are two examples of b-agonists. According to reliable sources interviewed for this book, several infomercial fitness celebrities achieved their amazing transformations with abuse of clenbuterol, not the exercise they claim responsible. "Clen" works, but don't count on your endocrine system working properly after megadoses.

MY EXPERIENCE

In 1995, I began conducting experiments on myself using the powerful "ECA stack" discussed in the last chapter.

It was an effective thermogenic cocktail. So effective, in fact, that I suffered heat exhaustion three times and should have been hospitalized on two of those occasions. It doesn't matter how ripped you are if you're dead.

In 1999, four years of experimentation later and much the wiser, I had eliminated the contributing factors that led to heat stroke conditions (in my case, all exercise or sun exposure at 70%+ humidity) and began to combine ECA with timed cold exposure.

The outcome: in four weeks, I lost what usually took up to eight weeks with ECA alone, and I did it without the side effects. I used two different protocols, both of which worked:

PROTOCOL A

1. I consumed the ECA stack 45 minutes prior to cold-bath immersion on an empty stomach. Though the metabolism of caffeine (caffeine clearance) varies from person to person, I assumed that blood concentration would peak between 60 and 90 minutes post-oral consumption, which was based on the average *pharmacokinetics* of caffeine in white male subjects. Pharmacokinetics, usually in graph form, show the relative blood concentrations of a specific drug over time after administration. Caffeinated gum, for comparison with pills, shows peak levels at 15 minutes. Delivery mechanisms matter.
2. I placed two 4.5kg (10lb) bags of ice in a cold-water bath and submerged myself for a total of 20 minutes. Those 20 minutes were phased as follows:

   00:00–10:00 minutes: Up to mid-waist, legs submerged, torso and arms not submerged.

   10:00–15:00 minutes: Submerged up to neck with hands out of the water (sitting cross-legged then reclining makes this easier in a standard bathtub).

   15:00–20:00 minutes: Submerged up to neck, hands underwater.

Sound painful? It is.

The second protocol, performed without ECA and tested separately, activated BAT and was far easier.

PROTOCOL B

1. I placed an ice pack on the back of my neck and upper trapezius area for 30 minutes, generally in the evening, when my insulin sensitivity is lower than in the morning.[20]

That's it.

I tested protocol A three times per week (on Monday, Wednesday and Friday) and protocol B five times per week (Monday through Friday). The former caused grand mal-like shivering and the latter caused no shivering.

Nonetheless, looking at the body fat results, Protocol B appeared to be around 60% as effective as the torture baths in Protocol A.

Not a bad yield, considering that no convulsing is involved.

In 1999, amusingly, most researchers firmly believed that BAT, while abundant in infants, was non-existent or negligible in adults. I was in the midst of my Guantanamo Bay baths[21] at this time, and these conclusions did not square with my experience. It wasn't until years later that better tools, most notably positron-emission topography (PET), became more widespread and were used to demonstrate that BAT is most certainly present in adults, particularly in the neck and upper chest areas.

That explains why the ice packs on my neck and upper trapezius worked.

In the May 2009 issue of *Obesity Review*, a paper was published titled "Have we entered the BAT renaissance?" I'd say the answer is yes. The abstract concludes: "These recent discoveries should revamp our effort to target the molecular development of brown adipogenesis in the treatment of obesity."

Let's start with cold. It isn't fancy, but it works well.

20. This evening decline is largely true only for non-obese people; obese individuals tend to have uniformly depressed insulin sensitivity at all times.

21. Nickname courtesy of one test subject in 2009.

Ice Age Revisited—Four Places to Start

If we combine the research with data from self-trackers like Ray and his 50+ informal test subjects, there are four simple options you can experiment with for fat loss:

1. Place an ice pack on the back of the neck or upper trapezius area for 20–30 minutes, preferably in the evening, when insulin sensitivity is lowest. I place a towel on the sofa while writing or watching a film and simply lean back against the ice pack.
2. Consume, as Ray did, at least 500ml (18 fl oz) of ice water on an empty stomach immediately upon waking. In at least two studies, this water consumption has been shown to increase resting metabolic rate 24–30%, peaking at 40–60 minutes post-consumption, though one study demonstrated a lower effect of 4.5%. Eat breakfast 20–30 minutes later à la the Slow-carb Diet detailed in earlier chapters.
3. Take 5–10-minute cold showers before breakfast and/or before bed. Use hot water for 1–2 minutes over the entire body, then step out of water range and apply shampoo and soap to your hair and face. Turn the water to pure cold and rinse your head and face alone. Then turn around and back into the water, focusing the water on your lower neck and upper back. Maintain this position for 1–3 minutes as you acclimatize and apply soap to all the necessary regions. Then turn around and rinse normally. Expect this to wake you up like a foghorn.
4. If you're impatient and can tolerate more, take 20-minute baths that induce shivering. See protocol A earlier in this chapter but omit the ECA. For extra thermogenic effect, consume 200–450 milligrams of cayenne (I use 40,000 BTU or thereabout) 30 minutes beforehand with 10–20 grams of protein (a chicken breast or protein shake will do). I do not suggest consuming cayenne or capsaicin on an empty stomach. Trust me, it's a bad idea.

SIX REASONS TO TAKE A COLD SHOWER

1. Short-term cold exposure (30 minutes) in humans leads to fatty acid release to provide fuel for heat production through shivering. This same shivering could be sufficient to recruit GLUT-4 to the surface of muscle cells, contributing to increased lean muscle gain.
2. Even at shorter durations, cold exposure with shivering could increase adiponectin levels and glucose uptake by muscle tissue. This effect could persist long after the cold exposure ends.
3. In the absence of shivering, it is still possible to capitalize on "fat-burning fat" through the stimulation of BAT thermogenesis. Curiously, even without shivering, there are small but unaccounted increases in lean muscle tissue when comparing underwater (superior) v. land-based exercise.
4. Cold water improves immunity. Acute cold exposure has immuno-stimulating effects, and preheating with physical exercise or a warm shower can enhance this response. Increases in levels of circulating norepinephrine may account for this.
5. Not germane to fat loss, but another reason to use cold exposure: cold showers are an effective treatment for depression. One study used showers at 20°C (68°F) for two to three minutes, preceded by a five-minute gradual adaptation to make the procedure less shocking.
6. The visible results, of course:

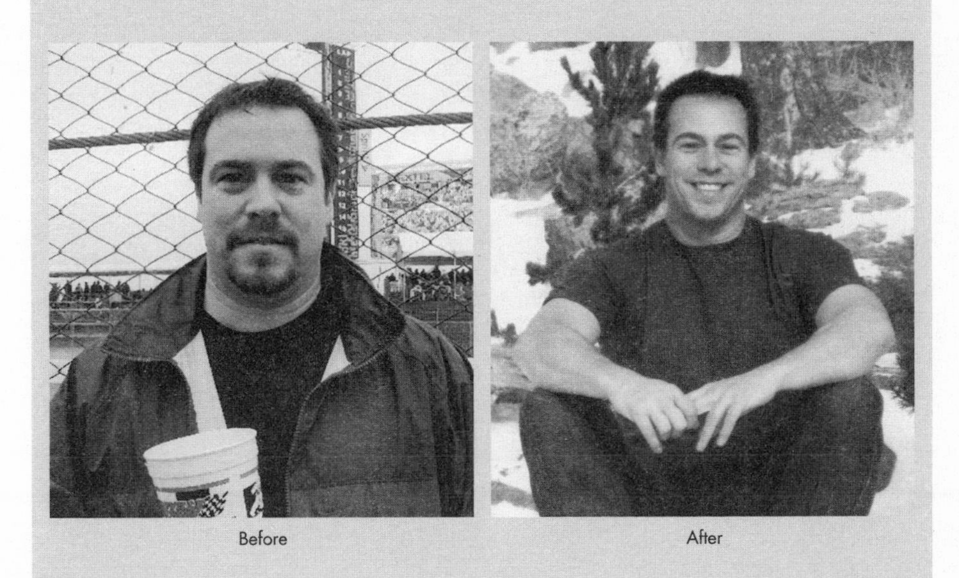

Before After

TOOLS AND TRICKS

ColPaC Gel Wrap (www.fourhourbody.com/colpac) These pliable wraps, used in physical therapy clinics, can be cooled quickly and applied to any body part, including the back of the neck, for BAT activation.

"How to Make a Real Ice Pack for $0.30" (www.fourhourbody.com/diy-ice) If you prefer the frugal approach, this article will show you how to quickly and easily make your own reusable ice packs at a fraction of the cost of shop-bought packs.

"TED Talks Lewis Pugh Swims the North Pole" (www.fourhourbody.com/pugh) Lewis Pugh is known as the human polar bear. Why? He swam across the icy waters of the North Pole in a Speedo and regularly swims in freezing cold water. Watch this TED speech for astonishing footage and blunt commentary on super-cold swims.

Ray Cronise Cold Experiments (www.raycronise.com) Explore Ray's experiments in cold exposure to find additional options for accelerating fat loss. If he can keep NASA shuttles from incinerating, he can help you lose heat.

THE GLUCOSE SWITCH

Beautiful Number 100

DISCLAIMER:
This chapter discusses the use of medical devices. Speak with your medical professional before jabbing such gadgets in your flesh.

Everything is a miracle. It is a miracle that one does not dissolve in one's bath like a lump of sugar.

—Pablo Picasso

7:00 A.M. PST, SECURITY LINE, DELTA AIRLINES

My hands were sweating.

Rehearsing one-line explanations in my head was getting tiring, and the queue ahead of me wasn't getting shorter. I started shifting impatiently from foot to foot, like a boxer waiting for the bell, or a three-year old preparing to wee himself.

Understandably, this behaviour made the older midwestern couple to my right nervous. I considered telling them, "Just be glad I didn't go with plan A," but I had a feeling this would make things worse.

Plan A, to be clear, was awesomely stupid.

Plan A was to wear a 22.7kg (50lb) weighted vest through security and onto the plane headed for Central America.

Two days earlier, I'd explained the rationale to a friend:

"I don't know if the gyms will have what we need, so I would at least have the vest."

"Hmmmm . . . okay."

"But it's too heavy to check as luggage, so I'll just wear it. The only downside is it might be impossible to get in the overhead locker, so I'd have to wear the damn thing for the whole flight. The 900g (2lb) bricks are clearly made of dense black plastic, though, so security shouldn't be an issue."

"Bricks? Ha ha ha . . . yes, a great idea. Well, give me a call once you have a security boot on your head and an assault rifle in your eye. Dude, that's a TERRIBLE idea."

"You think?"

"Suicide bomber jacket? Yes, I think."

So the vest remained at home.

But that was just one carry-on item. Fortunately, the metal detectors didn't pick up plan B, which wasn't *on* me but *in* me. This required some tact. I moved to a restaurant near to my gate to check on things. Something was wrong.

Sitting in the darkest corner I could find, I pulled up the side of my shirt and surveyed the damage. The sensor wasn't working.

"Motherf*cker," I muttered as I winced and slowly pulled it out of my abdomen. I held up the two metal prongs I'd inserted under my skin the night before and looked at them from all angles like a diamond. No visible problem. Perhaps the metal detectors screwed it up.

The Nicaraguans at the closest table had stopped eating and were all staring at me with mouths agape.

"No pasa nada. Soy diabético." *Nothing's wrong. I'm a diabetic.* That was the easiest explanation I could offer, even though I wasn't a diabetic. They nodded and went back to eating.

I ordered coffee and pulled out a notebook. Despite this minor glitch, I already had some fantastic data.

I would put in a new implant as soon as I landed in Managua.

Two Months Earlier—Firefly Restaurant, San Francisco

"Is this really interesting to you?"

It was a group dinner, and the man across from me thought I was just being polite. I'd asked what he did nine-to-five, and his answer was: medical device designer. In the span of "Oh, really?!" I was on him like a two-year-old Labrador on someone's leg. The 20 questions were just getting started, and the wine hadn't even arrived yet.

His cousin, a close friend of mine, chimed in, as I was already plotting experiments in my mind:

"Trust me. He's interested. This is all he thinks about. It's weird."

And that is how I first heard the name "DexCom". I jotted it down and did my best to act normal. It was hard to contain my excitement.

Soon thereafter, I knew all about DexCom. I called their headquarters, I called the head of marketing, I called the head of education, I spoke with the chief scientific officer, and I read about Charlie Kimball, over and over again.

Charlie Kimball is a type 1 diabetic. Unlike type 2 diabetics, he needs to inject insulin multiple times per day. He also happens to be a professional racing car driver.

In 2006, Charlie became the first American to ever win an F3 Euroseries race. Then, in 2007, at age 22, he went to the doctor for a small skin irritation and left the office with a diagnosis of type 1 diabetes. Tragically, this meant he was forced to abandon racing altogether. Pricking your fingers to take blood sugar readings just isn't possible when flying around curves at 240km per hour (150 miles per hour).

In 2008, Charlie returned to the wheel and claimed a podium finish in his first race. How?

He was the first racing car driver in the world to have a strange device strapped to his steering wheel: the DexCom SEVEN continuous glucose monitor (CGM).

I check it like it's one of my race car gauges as I'm driving around the track. It's my body's data. And it's not information overload. It's perfect.

In more tangible form, it's a receiver that looks like this:

Current Glucose Level
updates every 5 minutes
Trend-Arrows tell you
where you're headed and
how fast you're moving
Trend Screen Views
with options of 1, 3, 6, 12,
and 24 hours of continuous
glucose information
Glucose Trend-Wave
shows you where you've been
Customizable Low Glucose Alert
notifies you when you are going low
Customizable High Glucose Alert

Charlie has an implant in his side (as I did) that samples his blood glucose levels[22] every five seconds. These data are then transmitted to the receiver, a palm-sized device with a screen, where Charlie can see his blood glucose levels in a graph. It displays updates every five minutes, shows his ups and downs, tells him when he's falling too fast, and alerts him when he's at risk of hypoglycaemia (low blood sugar).

So why on earth would I want to use this device as a non-diabetic? Why might you?

What if you could tell which meals were most likely to make you fat?

What if you could predict when food would hit your bloodstream and schedule exercise to optimize fat loss or muscular gain?

What if, as an endurance athlete, you could eat carbs only when you most needed them instead of guessing with a timer?

The wish list went on and on. Now I just needed to check them off, one by one.

Making a (Wish) List. . . And Checking It Twice

After my dinner at Firefly, I immediately started jotting down dream tests, as this little gizmo seemed capable of clearing up some long-standing theoretical bullsh*t.

I'd long been fascinated by the glycaemic index (GI) and glycaemic load (GL) index, both of which reflect how much certain foods raise blood sugar levels as compared to a control (usually white bread or glucose with a designated value of 100). The higher the GI or GL value (the latter takes into account portion size),[23] the more a food causes blood sugar to jump. The more a food causes blood sugar to jump, in general, the fatter you will get.

There are two problems with these indices. The first is that real-world meals seldom resemble laboratory meals. When's the last time you ate 100g (3.5oz) of potato starch by itself? Second, the indices are one-size-fits-all.

Reality isn't one-size-fits-all. If someone of baguette-eating European descent eats white bread, will his blood response be the same as someone

22. Technically, interstitial fluid levels, from which the blood glucose is extrapolated.
23. GL = (GI x amount of carbohydrate in grams)/100.

from a pastoral bloodline that historically fed off of livestock and little starch? Not likely, as members of the former group often have higher levels of amylase enzyme, which breaks starch down into sugar.

Blood sugar is a very personal thing.

There are some predictable results—eating doughnuts will spike blood sugar more than an equal volume of melon—but what of the more subtle choices? What of the old folk remedies and bodybuilding anecdotes? Here's a short list of questions the DexCom allows us to put to the test:

Does lemon or vinegar really decrease the GL of a meal?
Which lowers glucose response more, if either: protein or vegetables and fibre?
Does eating fat and protein *with* a high-carb meal lower GL more than eating either *before* the meal?
Does drinking water with a meal increase or decrease its GL?

How I Used It and What I Learnt

23 September was one of the first test days with the implant.

I tried everything, as I wanted to see highs and lows. The following graphs show my data for that 24-hour period, and the downward arrows in the first graph indicate where I inputted glucometer readings.

Taking the blood glucometer readings is the only pain-in-the-arse part.

The SEVEN is designed to show trends and alert you when the upward or downward changes are too dramatic. To ensure that the displayed number is close to accurate, you need to calibrate with a glucometer at least twice a day.

Don't want to become diabetic? Want to curb things like eating sweets, which can lead to adult-onset diabetes? Try using a glucometer for 24 hours. For each glucometer calibration, you stick a lancet (needle) into your finger and put a drop of blood on a test strip, which is read by a hand-held device (the glucometer) to display your number. Many type 1 diabetics prick their fingers more than four times per day.

I started off using a OneTouch UltraMini® glucometer, one of the most popular glucometers in the United States, but abandoned it after three weeks. It was so erratic as to be unbelievable. For each calibration, I wanted

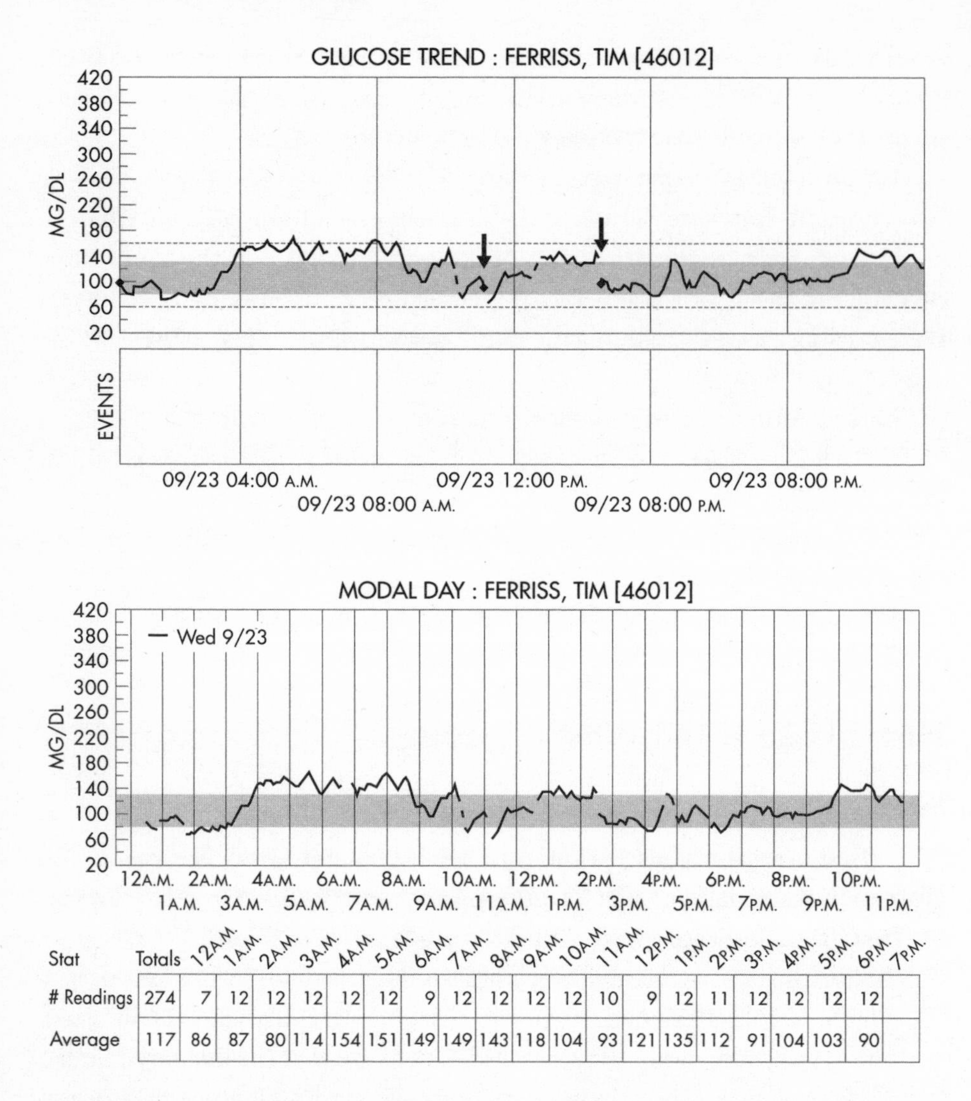

Stat	Totals	12A.M.	1A.M.	2A.M.	3A.M.	4A.M.	5A.M.	6A.M.	7A.M.	8A.M.	9A.M.	10A.M.	11A.M.	12P.M.	1P.M.	2P.M.	3P.M.	4P.M.	5P.M.	6P.M.	7P.M.
# Readings	274	7	12	12	12	12	12	9	12	12	12	12	10	9	12	11	12	12	12	12	
Average	117	86	87	80	114	154	151	149	149	143	118	104	93	121	135	112	91	104	103	90	

to get two readings within five points (milligrams per decilitre [mg/dL]) of each other, and then input the average in the DexCom device. This would minimize the likelihood of using an error for calibration. I expected this process to take two or three jabs, but it often took more than eight needle sticks. DexCom recommends calibrating twice daily, but I tended to do it at least three times daily (meaning up to 24 needle sticks). Not fun if you have to use your hands for anything.

Everything from humidity and sweat to temperature and air exposure can screw up readings. I ended up depending on the WaveSense® Jazz glucometer, the best device I could find that corrected for these variables. It brought the number of sticks per calibration from 8+ down to two to three sticks. I recommend this device.

But tracking glucose levels 24/7 was just one half of the puzzle.

I recorded everything I ate, and just about everything I did, in a Moleskine journal, which I then had transcribed.

Here is 23 September, verbatim with comments in brackets, which corresponds to the graphs on the previous page. I used the OneTouch here, and finger names followed by numbers indicate repeated glucometer jabs:

Wednesday 23/9
12:22 am
Glucometer: [I would often swab multiple fingers with alcohol, wait 30 seconds, then go down the line with multiple lancets]
Middle 102
Ring 88
Pinky 94
Index 95
1:42 am rib-eye steak 227g (8oz)
1:54 am 74 glucose (CGM)
1:40–2:30 am 3 glasses wine (Stag's Leap red)
2:13–2:30 am 200g (7oz) steak
Sleep
10:57 am Er 5 [this was a glucometer error]
Pinky 90 (air exposed 5 sec.)
Index 96
Index 114 (same needle)
Mid 93 (new needle)
11:11 am 20 almonds
11:16 am 67 glucose
11:19 am 2 tbsp superfood supplements + 2g vit. C
Break: 11:37 am:
2 scrambled eggs
4 tbsp olive oil
hot sauce
11:56 am:
30g (1oz) spinach
133g (5.2oz) lentils (first legumes since 9/5, 18 days)[24]
12:10 pm: 2–2.5 tbsp almond butter with celery
1:10 pm: 400ml (14 fl oz) cold water
1:54 pm: 40 air squat
Out of range 10 mins [I left the receiver on a table and wandered off]
2:35 pm: 128 dexcom ——>94–96 glucose
2:37 pm: Lipo-6 1 pill [a thermogenic] + 2g vit. C
3:50 pm: Kombucha
Lunch: 4:06 pm: hot & sour beef with aubergine
4:46 pm: yerba mate (20g/ ¾oz sugar)
7:09 pm: unsweetened yerba mate
7:25 pm: 15 almonds + 2g vit. C
9:00 pm: workout start
9:30 pm: workout end
9:35 pm: protein shake
10:00 pm: seaweed salad (huge)
10:15 pm:
12–15 pieces sashimi
1.75 bowl rice
3 cups green tea
11:05 pm: 300 ALA
11:33 pm: 50 air squat

24. I was looking at artificially creating food allergies and then removing them, an experiment that didn't make it into this book.

Compare the jagged graph for 23 September on page 138 with the following graph for 25 September, which is a near flatline. On the 25th, I deliberately consumed high-fat meals and snacks for pre-sex testosterone (see "Sex Machine" for how to do this).

It's important to note that, at 10:15 P.M. the evening before (24 September), I also consumed two rib-eye steaks (200g/7oz each) with sides of broccoli and spinach, which explains the flatline even before breakfast.

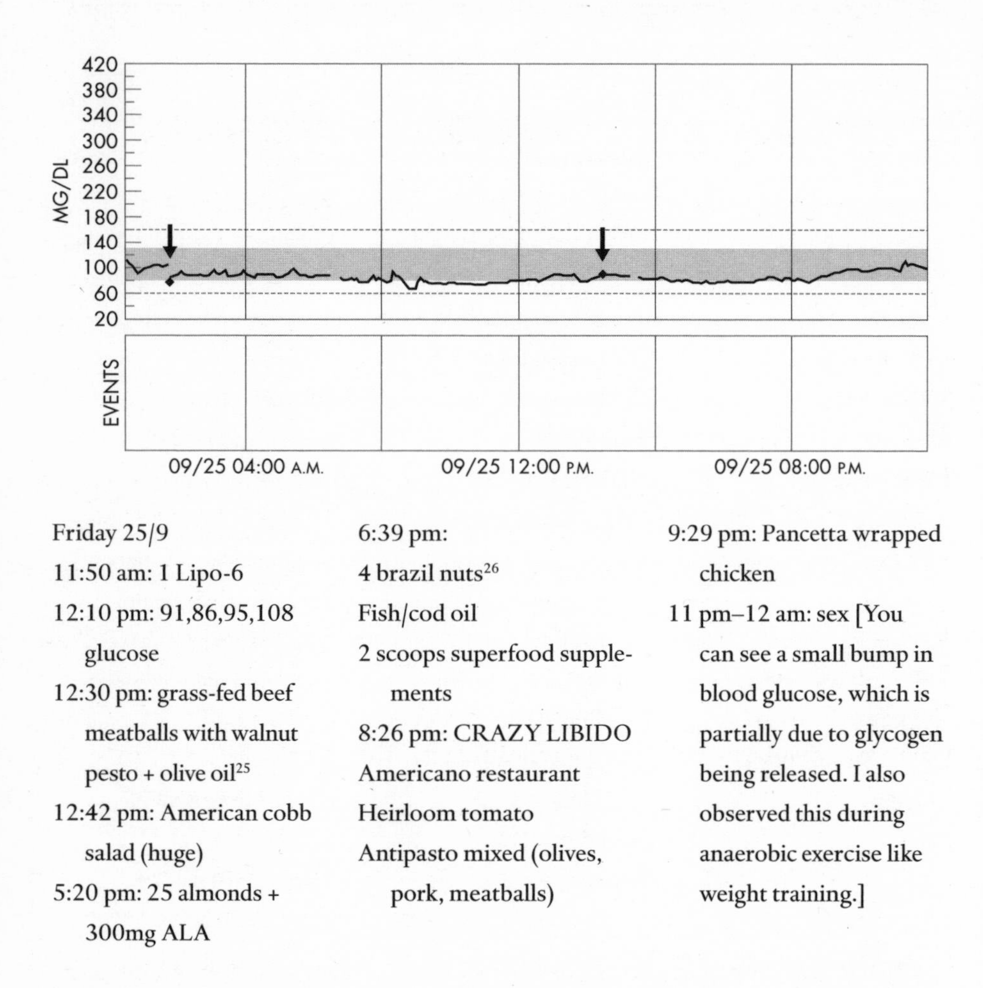

Friday 25/9
11:50 am: 1 Lipo-6
12:10 pm: 91,86,95,108 glucose
12:30 pm: grass-fed beef meatballs with walnut pesto + olive oil[25]
12:42 pm: American cobb salad (huge)
5:20 pm: 25 almonds + 300mg ALA
6:39 pm:
4 brazil nuts[26]
Fish/cod oil
2 scoops superfood supplements
8:26 pm: CRAZY LIBIDO
Americano restaurant
Heirloom tomato
Antipasto mixed (olives, pork, meatballs)
9:29 pm: Pancetta wrapped chicken
11 pm–12 am: sex [You can see a small bump in blood glucose, which is partially due to glycogen being released. I also observed this during anaerobic exercise like weight training.]

26 September, a Saturday, and my weekly binge day, produced a unusually flat graph considering the jamming of chocolate croissants and other goodies down the gullet:

25. If you're ever in Mill Valley, California, go to Small Shed Flatbreads and get this dish.
26. Eaten for specific non-slow-carb reasons. See the "Sex Machine" chapter for more.

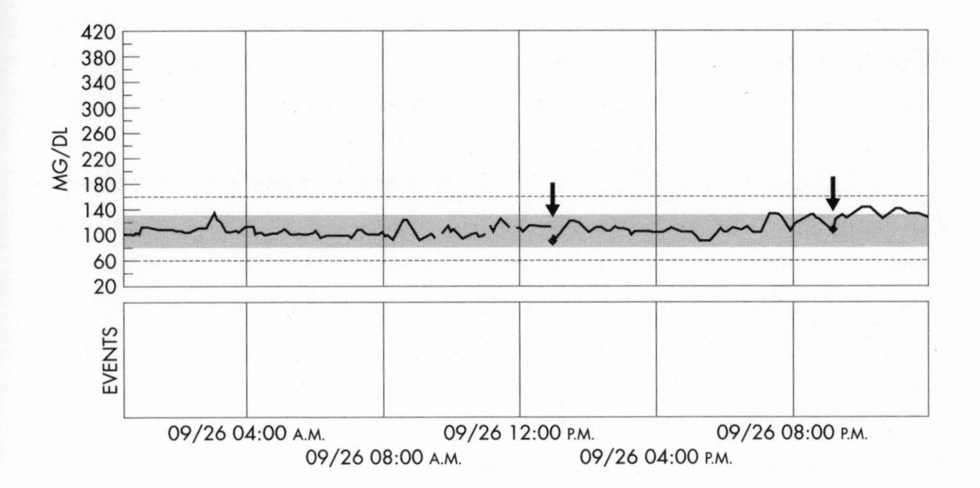

Saturday 26/9
10:40–11:40 am: sex
12:40 pm:
4 brazil nuts
2 cod caps
1 adrenal recovery pills, 3 desiccated liver ["liver"]
12:50 pm: 225ml (8 fl oz) orange juice
1:03 pm:
2 chocolate croissants (3)
Doughnut (1)
Coffee with cinnamon (3)
1:13 pm: done [I sometimes noted when I finished meals for duration]
1:44 pm:
Carrot juice
Almond croissant
3:45 pm: Kombucha
4:08–4:35 pm:
Hot & sour beef + aubergine
150g (5.8oz) brown rice
5:45 pm:
20 almonds
115g (4oz) liver
6:45 pm: Protein vanilla shake
7:30 pm:
2 brazil nuts
227g (8oz) chicken curry salad
181g (6.3oz) quinoa
AGG
+ 40 mini-band chest pulls
10:04 pm: 1 glass red wine [started drinking here and sipped]
10:45 pm:
spinach salad + oyster starter
11pm: Hanger steak

How is such a flat graph on 26 September possible when I was consuming such obvious garbage? Several of the tricks were covered in "Damage Control", but there were other patterns that emerged over the weeks of testing with my implant. Patterns that you can use to your advantage.

The Results

The data set, small as it was, allowed me to form some preliminary personal conclusions that others were able to replicate. Here are a few worth considering:

IT'S NOT WHEN YOU PUT IT IN YOUR MOUTH THAT COUNTS. IT'S WHEN IT GETS TO THE CELLS.

Food doesn't move to the bloodstream nearly as quickly as I thought.

When I first implanted the SEVEN sensor, I was as giddy as a 10-year-old birthday girl and compulsively checked the values every five minutes during meals. I ended up misattributing all over the place. My blood glucose hit 200 during sex, and I thought it was the horizontal gymnastics that caused it, not taking into account the enormous sushi plate I ate two and a half hours earlier. It was probably 80%+ due to the latter.

It turned out that food and liquids took much, much longer to get to my bloodstream than one would expect. In most cases, I peaked one and a half to two and a half hours after food consumption, even with yogurt. Orange juice peaked 40 minutes after drinking.

This has profound implications and made the entire experiment worth the hassle.

Think you'll have a quick bite for energy 20 minutes before going to the gym? It might not be available to your muscles until an hour after the gym. The solution: eat it an hour earlier.

Think that protein shake is getting to your muscles in the valuable 30-minute post-workout window? In my case, if I drank the "post-workout" shake post-workout, it didn't. I needed to have it before my workout and then sit down to a large meal almost immediately after the workout. Doing it one and a half hours after the workout, as commonly suggested, just wouldn't get the goods to my muscles in time.

INCREASING FAT CONTENT IN MEALS BLUNTS JUMPS IN GLUCOSE MUCH MORE THAN LEAN PROTEIN.

The more fat, and the earlier in the meal, the less the glycaemic response. Eat good fat, preferably as a starter before the main course. I now eat four Brazil nuts and one tablespoon of almond butter first thing upon waking.

FRUCTOSE HAS A LARGE AND VERY EXTENDED GLUCOSE-LOWERING EFFECT, BUT THIS DOESN'T MEAN YOU SHOULD CONSUME IT. LOW BLOOD GLUCOSE DOES NOT ALWAYS = MORE FAT LOSS.

For one week of my testing of the SEVEN device, I drank 400ml (14 fl oz) of orange juice first thing in the morning as my benchmark instead of white bread or glucose. Once I'd established my typical response to 400ml (14 fl oz) of one brand of OJ, I could isolate one variable (like vinegar or lemon juice) and measure the deviation from my usual morning response.

OJ helped me to maintain much lower average glucose values throughout the day.

Does this mean you should eat more fructose? Not necessarily.

My fat loss plateaued as soon as I introduced fructose (the 400ml/14 fl oz of orange juice), even though it created a pleasant flat line around the 100 mg/dL mark.[27] In future tests, I would like to see if a much smaller amount of fructose in whole fruit form, probably berries, could be used to blunt glucose response without stalling fat loss or causing fat gain. I think this would ideally be limited to a 24-hour period like a binge day and consumed 30 minutes prior to the one or two highest-GL meals, similar to how I used a *small* amount of OJ before croissants on 26 September.

It's easy to get fixated on one measurement, whether the number on a scale or the number on a glucometer. But, as Warren Buffett, the richest investor in the world, is fond of emphasizing: it's not enough to simply measure things—you have to measure what matters.

If your goal is fat loss, before-and-after body fat percentages determine pass or fail, not glucose measurements alone. Keep your eye on the right ball.

VINEGAR, COUNTER TO EXPECTATIONS, DIDN'T LOWER GLYCAEMIC RESPONSE. LEMON JUICE, ALSO COUNTER TO EXPECTATIONS, DID.

There's a great deal of evidence for vinegar lowering the glycaemic index of a meal by more than 25%. It seems as reliable as any food "rule" could be.

Both white vinegar and apple cider vinegar were used in the literature. But acetic acid is acetic acid, so any kind of table vinegar that has at least 5% acetic acid should work[28] if you consume at least 20 millilitres (1.5 tablespoons).

27. The reasons for this are explained in "The Slow-carb Diet I."

28. Or a serving of any unsweetened table dressing that amounts to the equivalent of 20 milliliters of 5% acetic acid.

In my trials, neither white vinegar nor balsamic vinegar had a lowering effect on blood sugar. I even drank 3 tbsp+ of vinegar before my meals as a last-ditch attempt. Unhappy times in stomach-ville and no discernible benefit.

Why no effect? There are a few possible explanations, but the most likely are: I need a higher dose, or vinegar doesn't affect fructose metabolism and showcases its effects in a high-starch meal. Recall that, owing to the problems of standardizing true real-life mixed meals, I used changes in responses to OJ as a benchmark.

Lemon, however, showed its merits without fail.

There are anecdotes and websites galore that claim lemon juice lowers glycaemic index. Neither my researchers nor I could find any controlled studies showing evidence of a GI-lowering effect for lemon, lime or citric acid. The closest was citrate, a salt or ester of citric acid in combination with other things like insoluble calcium. In my personal trials, three tablespoons of fresh-squeezed lemon juice just prior to eating (not shop-bought with preservatives and artificial additives) appeared to lower blood sugar peaks by approximately 10%.

CINNAMON, EVEN IN SMALL DOSES, HAS A SUBSTANTIAL EFFECT ON GLUCOSE LEVELS.

There is ample evidence that cinnamon can be used to reduce the glycaemic index of a meal up to 29%. At four grams per meal or even six grams per day, it can lower not only blood glucose but also LDL cholesterol and triglycerides. Cinnamon weighs in at 2.8 grams per teaspoon, **so four grams of cinnamon is about one and a half teaspoons.**

Cinnamon's effect on glucose levels seems partially due to the fact that it slows the rate at which food exits the stomach (gastric emptying), which means that you also feel full faster with cinnamon.

I tested three species of cinnamon: **Ceylon cinnamon** (*Cinnamomum verum* or *zeylanicum,* also referred to as "true cinnamon"), **Cassia cinnamon** (*Cinnamomum cassia* or *aromaticum*) and **Saigon cinnamon** (*Cinnamomum loureiroi,* also known as Vietnamese cinnamon).

Though Cassia is thought inferior to Ceylon or completely ineffective in some bodybuilding circles, it has lowered glycaemic response in both published studies and in my experience. This is fortunate, since Cassia is what is most often found at coffee shops and restaurants if you ask for "cinnamon". I found Saigon cinnamon to be most effective, with Cassia in close second place and Ceylon in much further third place.

In terms of reducing glycaemic response, I found the following, from largest to smallest effect, effective:

1. **Get freshly ground cinnamon or grind it yourself.** If you, like me, have a bachelor-special spice rack that's three years old, toss it and get new raw materials. The polyphenols and active ingredients degrade over time and with air exposure.
2. **Learn how to spot species.** Unfortunately, U.S. packagers are not legally required to specify the type of cinnamon species on the label. Not sure which raw "cinnamon" sticks are Cassia? They will roll up from both sides, like a scroll. Ceylon will roll up from one side, as if you had rolled up a bath towel. Distinguishing powder is harder, as age plays a part, but Cassia tends to be a darker reddish-brown and Ceylon a lighter tan colour.
3. **Don't use too much.** It's easy to get overambitious with cinnamon, but there are active substances that can hurt you if consumed in excess. Coumarin, as just one example, is a potent blood-thinner and some cinnamon in Europe has a warning label for this reason. Use no more than four grams per day. I use a few dashes in coffee and limit myself to two to three cups of coffee throughout the day.

To reiterate, based on material bulk density reference charts, cinnamon weighs in at 0.56 grams per cubic centimetre, one cubic centimetre = 0.2 teaspoon, and so there are **2.8 grams of cinnamon per teaspoon.**

So four grams of cinnamon = 4 divided by 2.8, or just about one and a half teaspoons. Don't consume more per day.

MORE THAN QUALITY, IT'S THE SIZE AND SPEED OF MEALS THAT DETERMINED GLYCAEMIC RESPONSE.

Even on protein and vegetables alone, I could bump glucose as high as 150 mg/dL without much effort. Granted, I eat like a starving dog. In Whym restaurant in Manhattan, one friend nicknamed me "Orca" after watching me nonchalantly swallow a piece of ahi-tuna the size of my fist. To him, this was unusual. To me, it was the only way I'd ever eaten: fast.

The easiest thing you can do to decrease glucose spikes is slow down.

I had to methodically finish my plate in thirds and train myself to wait five minutes between thirds, usually with the help of iced tea and slices of lemon. It also helps to drink more water to dilute digestion (I'm fantastic at this), eat smaller portions (not so good at this), and chew more (Orca is *terrible* at this).

All four strategies serve to decrease the amount of food that gets digested per minute, which will determine the size of your glucose arc.

Two real-world examples:

1. Matt Mullenweg, lead developer of the WordPress blogging platform, lost 1.3st (8.2kg) with one change: chewing each mouthful of food 20 times. The exact number wasn't important. It was having a precise number that helped. Counting slowed him down and made him aware of portion size, which made him less likely to overeat. I don't have the patience for chewing like normal humans, but Matt did.
2. Argentine women are famous for being gorgeous and eating crap. In total, I've spent about two years in Buenos Aires, and the female Argie diet appears to consist of little more than cappuccino, biscuits and scones, a super-sweet caramel called *dulce de leche*, ice cream, and—for dinner—meat and salad with a side of pasta. Is it just fantastic genetics? I don't think so. Several male friends have travelled with petite Argentine girlfriends, who, once in the United States or Europe, immediately put on 0.7–1.4st (4.5–9kg). The reason? The girls themselves admitted it: increased portion size and increased speed of eating. The beautiful people of Buenos Aires might eat a wide spectrum of rubbish calories, but they tend to do it in small bites and over a long period of time.

Slow down and smell the roses.

Make 30 minutes the minimum for a meal.

FOR FASTEST FAT LOSS, MINIMIZE YOUR BLOOD SUGAR BUMPS ABOVE 100 TO NO MORE THAN TWO PER DAY.

I was able to sustain rapid fat loss if I didn't jump above 100 mg/dL more than twice daily. Fat loss was marginally greater when I remained under 90, but this was difficult to achieve without omitting legumes and following more of a ketogenic diet. For convenience and socializing, I prefer the slow-carb approach unless I'm dieting to below 8% body fat.

The 100-mg/dL rule excludes binge day, where all is allowed. On non-binge days, using fructose or semi-starvation to remain under 100 mg/dL is counterproductive and considered cheating.

But how to keep yourself under 100 mg/dL if you don't have an implant in your side?

Just follow a handful of simple rules based on the literature and my personal tracking, in addition to the basic tenets of the Slow-carb Diet:

- Eat decent quantities of fat at each larger meal. Saturated fat is fine if meat is untreated with antibiotics and hormones.
- Spend at least 30 minutes eating lunch and dinner. Breakfasts can be smaller and thus consumed more quickly.
- Experiment with cinnamon and lemon juice just prior to or during meals.
- Use the techniques in "Damage Control" for accidental and planned binges. Keep in mind that the techniques in that chapter will help you minimize damage for about 24 hours, not much more.

TOOLS AND TRICKS:

DexCom Seven Plus (www.dexcom.com) The DexCom Seven Plus is the continuous glucose monitor I used and abused. It is an implant that gives you the approximate data of 288 fingertip blood samples per day. I found it invaluable, even as a non-diabetic.

WaveSense Jazz Glucometer (www.fourhourbody.com/jazz) This is, by orders of magnitude, the best glucometer I found. It's small, simple to use, and incredibly consistent, as it accounts and corrects for environmental factors. For those who don't want an implant but want an actionable glimpse of how they respond to foods, this is a great option.

Glucose Buddy (www.fourhourbody.com/app-glucose) Glucose Buddy is a free iPhone app for diabetics that allows you to manually enter and track glucose numbers, carbohydrate consumption, insulin dosages and activities.

Juliet Mae Fine Spices & Herbs (www.julietmae.foodzie.com) This is where you can buy Juliet Mae's delicious cinnamon. I used her sampler for all testing, which includes Cassia, Ceylon, and Saigon cinnamon.

MiR 50-Lb. Short Adjustable Weighted Vest (www.fourhourbody.com/vest) The best weighted vests in the business. This is what I almost wore through airport security. If you want a rifle butt in the head at customs, it's the perfect choice.

THE LAST MILE

Losing the Final 5–10lb (2.3–4.5kg)

I saw an angel in the block of marble and I just chiselled until I set him free.

—Michelangelo

I looked down at my pad of paper and read the first question: "What's the biggest mistake that drug-free 'natural' bodybuilders make?"

"Natural bodybuilders?" John Romano laughed. "The biggest mistake 'natural' bodybuilders make is thinking they're natural. Eating 20 chicken breasts a day isn't natural. The best I'll give them is 'over-the-counter'."

And so our conversation began. It was going to be a fun interview.

Romano had his finger on the pulse of physique augmentation for more than two decades as the editor in chief of *Muscular Development* (*MD*) magazine. *MD* is the one mainstream magazine that serves as an intersection between published research and experimentation in the wild world of bodybuilding. *MD* wasn't enough for John, so he left to push the boundaries even further on a site called RX Muscle.

I reached out to him about specifics of drug-assisted and drug-free approaches for achieving sub-10% body fat, as he's observed thousands of guinea pigs and their results. John is a testament to his findings: he looks like he's in his thirties though he just turned 50, which he credits to infrequent HIT-style resistance training (see "From Geek to Freak"), a simple decision-free diet and a "modicum of the right drugs".

The diet he follows for fat loss, and the one he prescribes to competitors, is also that of his business partner, whom we'll meet later: Dave "Jumbo" Palumbo. It is an elegant and effective means for losing the last 5–10lb (2.3–4.5kg) that seem resistant to everything else.

The following menu is for a 14.3st (90.7kg) male at 10–12% body fat, and the ounces of protein (225g/8oz for a 14.3st/90.7kg male) should be adjusted up or down 30g (1oz) per 4.5kg (10lb) of *lean* bodyweight (e.g., 200g/7oz for 86kg (190lb), 250g/9oz for 95kg/210lb) with a minimum per-meal intake of 115g (4oz). In other words, even if you weigh 7.2st (45.4kg), you will not decrease the ounces of protein below 115g (4oz).

For sizing: 75g (3oz) of almonds is about 60 almonds, and 225g (8oz) of lean protein is approximately the size of your fist.

Here's the kicker: **One of these meals has to be eaten every three hours while you're awake, and you must eat within one hour of waking and one hour of bed.** Hunger is no longer the driver for food intake. Tupperware is your friend, and the clock is your drill sergeant. Skipping meals is not permitted, so purchase in bulk and prep food in advance if needed.

If you weigh less than 10.7st (68kg), use the lower end of protein intake at 115g (4oz) protein (or 30g/1oz for protein shakes) and have smaller portions for the add-ons: 37.5g (1.3oz) of nuts *or* one tablespoon of peanut butter *or* one tablespoon of extra-virgin olive oil (EVOO) or macadamia oil.

Eat one of these meals every three waking hours:

Option 1: 50g (1.7oz) of whey protein isolate + 75g (3oz) of nuts or two tablespoons of peanut butter

Option 2: 225g (8oz) of cooked, white, non-fatty fish (no salmon, mackerel, etc.) + 75g (3oz) of nuts or two tablespoons of peanut butter. Acceptable fish include, but are not limited to, lean tuna, white fish, bass, whiting and plaice.

Option 3: 225g (8oz) of cooked turkey or chicken + 75g (3oz) of nuts or two tablespoons of peanut butter

Option 4: 225g (8oz) of cooked fattier protein: red meat (à la flank), minced beef, fatty fish, or dark poultry + one tablespoon of olive oil or macadamia oil

Option 5: five whole eggs (easiest if hard-boiled)

Unlimited quantities of the following are allowed at each meal:

Spinach
Asparagus
Brussels sprouts
Kale
Collard greens
Broccoli rabe
Broccoli and other cruciferous vegetables

One tablespoon of olive oil or macadamia nut oil can be included as dressing, as long as you have not included the 75g (3oz) of nuts or two tablespoons of peanut butter in that meal. In the lower-fat meal options, you may make a salad dressing using slightly more oil: two tablespoons olive oil or macadamia oil.

No sweetcorn, beans, tomatoes or carrots are permitted, but one cheat *meal* is encouraged every seven to ten days.

Simple and effective.

WHAT THE BODYBUILDERS ADD THAT YOU SHOULDN'T

The above diet can get you to 8% body fat or even less. Needless to say, there is a point of diminishing returns when each additional 1% drop is more difficult than the preceding 5%.

If training and diet hit a ceiling, how on earth do bodybuilders get to less than 4% subcutaneous body fat?

In a word: drugs.

Romano's pre-competition schedule on the following page assumes a well-trained 175cm (5ft 9in), 14.3 to 15.7st (90.7 to 99.8kg) bodybuilder at 10–12% body fat who gets down to 12.8–13.6st (81.6–86kg) at 6–8% body fat before implementing the drug regimen. On contest day, he should end up at 14.3–14.6st (90.7–93kg) pounds at less than 4% body fat.

Almost all of the drugs listed can have serious side effects when misused. Google "Andreas Munzer autopsy" to see what can happen when you make mistakes.[29] Do not try this at home.

29. Munzer added many other drugs that probably contributed to his organ failure and death, including EPO, Cytadren and diuretics.

"This is really, in my opinion, the best way to prepare," Romano says, "but you need patience, and that is usually more difficult to build than the muscle. Train with super-high intensity (one body part per day, five days a week) and do cardio (30–40 minutes per day). Continue this regime during your 'pre-diet' phase. You will want to whittle your body fat down VERY low with a no-carb diet—under 8%. You have to keep up the intensity and the cardio. This is probably going to take 10–12 weeks. Crazy as it sounds, you want to break down some of the muscle you just built and deplete yourself as much as possible.

"Then you add the juice. One Sustanon every other day with 75 milligrams trenbolone (Tren) or 200 milligrams Deca-Durabolin (Deca). Two IU Growth Hormone (GH) every day. Add 75 grams of carbs to your first three meals. Drink 40g (1.4oz) of whey protein isolate before bed. Wake up four hours later and drink another 40g (1.4oz). Back the cardio off to 30 minutes, four times a week, and keep upping your training intensity.

"After eight weeks, switch from Sustanon and Tren to Equipoise (EQ)—150 milligrams every other day, and Primo Depot, 400 milligrams once a week. Up the GH to 4 IU every day. Back your carbs down gradually to zero by the end of the first week. Switch your training to lighter weights and higher reps, but still with high intensity. Bring your cardio up to 30 minutes a day, six days a week. Start practising mandatory poses 30 minutes every night. Work up to holding each pose for one minute.

"After four weeks, add 100 milligrams of Masterone every other day, 100 milligrams of Winstrol (Winny) every day, two Clenbuterol (Clen) every four hours, 25 micrograms of T-3 every morning and a cap of GHB before bed. Increase posing to 30 minutes in the morning and 30 minutes at night. You can stay on this for four to six additional weeks.

"Two weeks out: Stop Clen. Add 25 micrograms of T-3 before bed. Cut fat out of diet.

"One week out: Go back on Clen as before. Stop GH.

"Three days out: Cut sodium, add 50 grams of carbs to first meal, stop cardio, increase water consumption to at least 9 litres (288 fl oz) a day.

"Two days out: Last training session—full body, high rep with super-high intensity. Add 50 grams of carbs to first two meals. Stop middle-of-the-night protein shake.

"One day out: Add 75 grams of carbs to last two meals. Stop drinking water at 8:00 P.G.—only little sips after that, as few as possible. Cut Clen. No shake before bed.

"There will be a few tweaks to this system during its progression, as every person will respond differently. But this should give you a good platform."

Aesthetics are one thing, therapeutics are quite another. For a glimpse of the latter, we must learn from Nelson Vergel.

STEROIDS 101: FACT V. FICTION

In 2001, Lee Brown, the mayor of Houston, proclaimed 13 September "Nelson Vergel Day".

Diagnosed as HIV-positive in 1987, Nelson has dedicated his life to furthering HIV research in both prevention and treatment. For two years, he was a member of the Metabolic Disorders Committee at the AIDS Clinical Trials Group (ACTG) in Washington, the largest HIV/AIDS research organization in the world.

He is best known for simple interventions that have helped save many lives and improved thousands more. He describes the results of one such approach, used personally, in his own words:

> *My CD8 cells, which may be one of the most important barometers for longevity for PWA's [people with AIDS], went from 900 to 2500 cells [per millimetre squared], and my symptoms disappeared! I never felt or looked better in my entire life, even when I was HIV-negative!*

Jeff Taylor, who's been HIV-positive for more than 25 years, had two collapsed lungs and just two T-cells remaining when he began a similar treatment. Six weeks later he had 300 T-cells. It saved his life.

The mystery treatment wasn't a new antiviral cocktail. In fact, it wasn't new at all.

It was anabolic steroids. Specifically, Nelson used testosterone cypionate and Deca-Durabolin® (nandrolone decanoate), and Jeff used Anavar® (oxandrolone).

This is confusing to most people. Aren't steroids supposed to kill you, or, at the very least, cause cancer or liver failure?

How can it be that the very same oxandrolone Jeff used "has been found to be one of the most cost-effective and least-toxic therapies to date" for treating male burn victims?

After doing an exhaustive review of the literature and interviewing scientists and actual users, Bryant Gumbel, the host of *Real Sports with Bryant Gumbel*, concluded the following on 21 June 2005:

> *As frequently evidenced by officials nationwide, Americans, when drugs are concerned, rarely choose logic when they can opt for hysteria. Case in point: the recent hoopla over steroids. In light of the media excess, the public pronouncements, and the wailing in Washington, one would assume that the scientific evidence establishing the health risk of steroids is overwhelming. But it's not. On the contrary, when it comes to steroid use among adult males, the evidence reveals virtually no fire, despite all the smoke.*

This summation, needless to say, ran counter to expectations.

What Are Steroids Exactly?

Did you know that birth control drugs are technically steroids?

This is also true of the cortisone shots that future baseball Hall of Famer Curt Schilling used in the 2004 World Series, the same anti-inflammatory injections Andre Agassi used during his final U.S. Open.

Steroids represent an incredibly broad and important class of hormone, and there are hundreds of variations in plants, fungi and animals. If you eliminated steroids from your body, you would die.

The term "steroid" is most often used in the media to refer to anabolic-androgenic steroids (AAS), more commonly called anabolic steroids. These compounds are variations of the hormone testosterone or are intended to mimic the effects of testosterone.

Nandrolone, for example, is testosterone that has been chemically modified to minimize its conversion to oestrogen or DHT, the latter change making it less *androgenic*—that is, it will have less of an amplifying effect on secondary male characteristics like hair growth (or loss from the scalp) or the thickening of the vocal chords.

Below is a side-by-side comparison of normal testosterone and the most commercially popular form of nandrolone, Deca-Durabolin® ("Deca"), which Nelson used. Deca is also one AAS that Barry Bonds and Roger Clemens are alleged to have used.

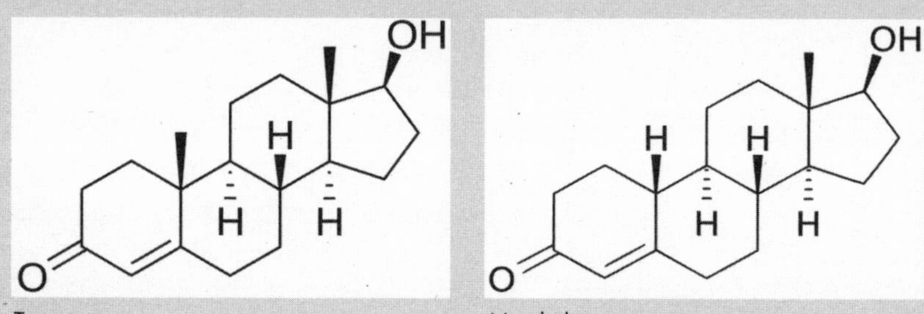

Testosterone

Nandrolone

I have legally used low-dose anabolic steroids and other growth agents under medical supervision both before and after joint surgeries. Multiple MDs reviewed blood tests every two to four weeks to ensure there were no complications. These drugs are specifically designed to increase protein synthesis; in the case of my surgeries, it was moderated and a proper use of the appropriate tools.

Do I encourage recreational or cosmetic use without medical supervision or without legal prescriptions? No. Anabolic steroids are Class C controlled substances, and you can receive up to three years' imprisonment for possession and up to 10 years' imprisonment if convicted of trafficking or intent to traffic.

Do I think that healthy children, adolescents or women should use powerful male hormones? Absolutely not.

Do I think that athletes should be disqualified if they break the rules of their sport? Most definitely.

But the science shouldn't be distorted. These are valuable drugs with real applications.

The Dose Makes the Poison

Here is a small sample of well-documented side effects, provided by the U.S. National Institutes of Health:

- Swelling of the eyes, face, lips, tongue or throat
- Wheezing or difficulty breathing
- Fast heartbeat
- Fast breathing
- Cold, clammy skin
- Ringing in the ears
- Loss of hearing
- Bloody vomit
- Bright red blood in stools

This list should scare you.

It should scare you because these aren't side effects of anabolic steroids. These are common side effects of aspirin.

First Rule of Drug Use: There Is No Safe Drug

Some drugs are safer than others, but almost anything will kill you at a high enough dose. It's the dose that makes the poison.

Never forget this, and don't confuse the effects of moderate use with those of outright abuse.

It's the difference between a single 8–12-week cycle of low-dose injectable testosterone for surgery, on the one hand, and uncycled megadoses of the oral steroid Anadrol-50® for elite bodybuilding, on the other. It's the difference between a baby aspirin (75–85 milligrams) and half a bottle of aspirin. It's the difference between having a glass of wine before bed and drinking bottles until you wake up in the intensive care unit.

Sensationalism is more common than good science, and the two are not the same.

TOOLS AND TRICKS

RXMuscle with John Romano and Dave Palumbo (www.rxmuscle.com) If you have drug questions, don't ask me. I'm neither a doctor nor an expert. John Romano and Dave Palumbo, on the other hand, have been on the inside of professional bodybuilding and physique enhancement for decades. Both have seen the best and the worst outcomes in athletic chemical warfare. RXMuscle is where you can ask professionals your questions related to AAS and other performance-enhancing drugs (PED).

Bigger, Stronger, Faster **DVD (www.fourhourbody.com/bigger)** From the producers of *Bowling for Columbine* and *Fahrenheit 9/11*, this outstanding documentary explores steroid use in the biggest, strongest, fastest country in the world: America. The cast of characters ranges from Carl Lewis and MDs to Louis Simmons of Westside Barbell. It has an astounding 96% positive rating on Rotten Tomatoes.com.

Medibolics (www.medibolics.com) This site, published by Michael Mooney, provides a wealth of information on the medical use of anabolic steroids, growth hormone and unorthodox supplementation for the prevention of lean-tissue loss in persons with muscle-wasting diseases, including HIV.

Anabolics, **9th ed. (www.fourhourbody.com/anabolics)** This 800-page book is the #1 bestselling anabolic reference guide worldwide. It features: reviews of nearly 200 pharmaceutical compounds, detailed explanations of the real risks of anabolics, prevention and harm reduction strategies, steroid cycling and stacking sections to take the guesswork out of cycle construction, and approximately 3,000 colour photographs of legitimate, counterfeit and underground drug products.

ADDING MUSCLE

BUILDING THE PERFECT POSTERIOR

(OR LOSING 7+ST/45+KG)

I am my own experiment. I am my own work of art.

—Madonna

Backs are to lifters what biceps are to bodybuilders.

—Randall J. Strossen PhD, editor of *MILO* magazine

This chapter will teach both men and women how to build a superhuman posterior chain, which includes all the muscles from the base of your skull to your Achilles tendons.

In the process, it will also teach women how to build the perfect bum and lose dramatic amounts of fat.

For maximum strength and sex appeal in minimal time, the posterior chain is where you should focus.

The Bet

"We have a bet going."

Tracy Reifkind walked into work that evening expecting a normal shift. But six of her female co-workers had reached critical mass and created a betting pool. Each had put in $100 (£62), and the $600 (£375) would go to whoever lost the highest percentage body fat in 12 weeks. Tracy was lucky number seven, upping the ante to $700 (£437).

It was good timing.

Tracy had been a chubby kid when kids weren't chubby. She'd continued to gain throughout life and ended up weighing 17.5st (111kg) at age 41. She had resigned herself to a dismal fate: she would never be able to enjoy certain basics, like wearing a tank top. That was just the hand she'd been dealt.

But her weight was creating health problems. She'd become a gourmet cook with the dream of visiting Italy, and that trip—almost within reach—was now jeopardized by her obesity. She was experiencing gastrointestinal problems that made it impossible to travel.

"Everything wrong with me had to do with the fact that I was fat. Every day, I felt like I was dodging a bullet. I didn't want to go to the doctor because I didn't want to find out I was pre-diabetic or that I had heart disease. I just liked eating and wasn't ready to stop. I, of course, knew what I had to do. But that bet, that event, gave me the reason and the timing."

Tracy responded well to challenges. She was somehow confident that she would win. The real question was: how?

The answer came, most unexpectedly, from strong men.

Michelle Obama's Arms

Tracy was dumbstruck as she looked at the fitting room mirror in San Jose. She pulled up the new pair of jeans and turned around. Then she turned around again. No matter how many times she spun, the image didn't compute.

"What? That's me?!" She saw arms she'd never seen before. She also had her tank top.

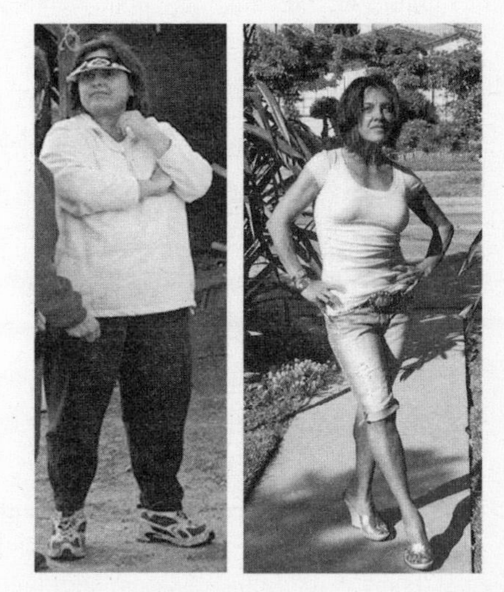

Tracy Reifkind had lost more than 7.1st/45.1kg (45lb/20.4kg) of fat in the first 12 weeks) and won her bet. But the numbers alone don't do her physique justice: this mom of two from a two-income family looked 10 years younger at 9.3st (59kg).

The secret wasn't marathon aerobics sessions, nor was it severe caloric restriction. It was the Russian kettlebell swing, twice a week for an average of 15–20 minutes. Her peak session length was 35 minutes.

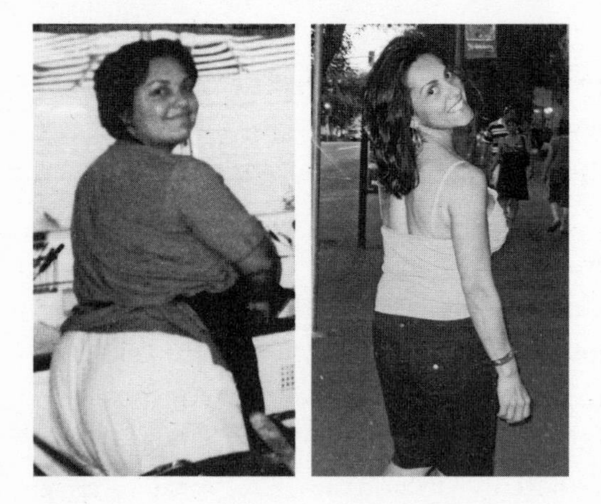

She was introduced to kettlebells by her husband, Mark Reifkind, a former national team coach in powerlifting who also competed against Kurt Thomas in Olympic gymnastics.

"Every woman wants Michelle Obama's arms. The truth is that you can have them, and a new body, in four weeks. The two-handed swing is the jewel. If you could only do one movement for the rest of your life, do the kettlebell swing."

I agree with Tracy 100%, though the path that led me to the swing was quite different.

In 1999, I made three-weekly pilgrimages from Princeton to Philadelphia where I trained at a gym called Maxercise. For the 45-minute workout that justified the trip, I was commuting more than two hours. Steve Maxwell, the owner of Maxercise, was a six-time Pan-American gold medallist in Brazilian jiu-jitsu (two world championships came later) and held a master's degree in exercise science. His clients ranged from the FBI and Secret Service to the Phillies and the Dodgers. His singular focus was on measurable results. If something didn't work, it didn't last long with Maxwell.

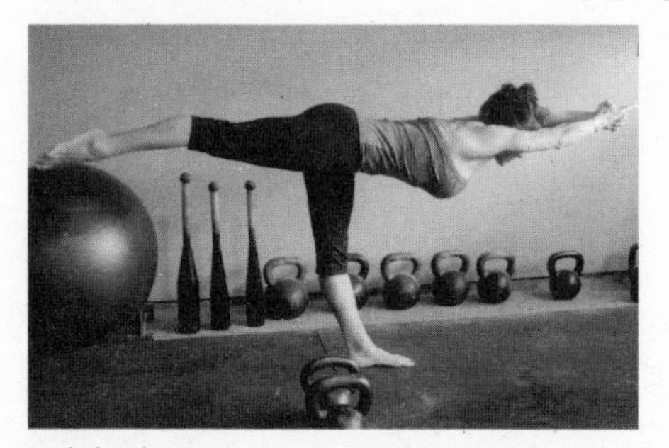

Body by design: Tracy removed the curves she didn't want and added the curves she did. Notice the kettlebells, which look like cannonballs with handles, lined up against the wall.

I first met kettlebells on a frigid winter evening in Maxercise's second-floor torture chamber. They were generally reserved for fighters and aspiring strong men. Most of the high-velocity kettlebell movements like "the snatch",[1] considered standard for training programmes, didn't combine well with my injured shoulders. I abandoned kettlebells after two sessions.

It wasn't until six years later that I realized how simple kettlebells could be. One move: the swing.

1. Even better, kettlebells are weighed in Russian "poods".

From Jiu-Jitsu to New Zealand: The Kettlebell Swing

Long before I met Tracy, I met "The Kiwi" in Buenos Aires, Argentina.

In early 2006, he happened to be taking a private Spanish lesson in the same café where I was finishing the manuscript for *The 4-Hour Workweek*, and we quickly became close friends. He had competed in elite-level rugby in New Zealand but was equally proud, I soon learned, of applying his BSE in exercise physiology to perfecting the female posterior.

He told me the story over a bottle of Catena Malbec. His obsession started when he saw a professional samba dancer in Brazil balance tequila shots on top of each bum cheek in a dance club. Lamenting the lack of similar scenes in his own country, he set off on a mission to isolate the best exercises for creating buttocks worthy of tequila shots.

By 2000, he had refined his approach to a science. In four weeks, he took his then-girlfriend, an ethnic Chinese with a surfboard-like profile, to being voted one of the top 10 sexiest girls out of 39,000 students at the University of Auckland. Total time: four weeks. Other female students constantly asked her how she'd lifted her glutes so high up her hamstrings.

If The Kiwi could have answered for her, he would have said, "Add reps and weights to the swings."

In 2005, my interest in kettlebells reinvigorated, I returned to the United States from Argentina and purchased one 24kg (53lb) kettlebell. I did nothing more than one set of 75 swings one hour after a light, protein-rich breakfast, twice a week on Mondays and Fridays. In the beginning, I couldn't complete 75 consecutive repetitions, so I did multiple sets with 60 seconds between until I totalled 75.

Total swing time for the entire week was 10–20 minutes. I wasn't trying to balance tequila shots on my buttocks. I wanted abs. In six weeks, I was at my lowest body fat percentage since 1999.

My weekly training schedule was so light as to be laughable by conventional standards. I also took 10–20-minute ice baths (two bags of ice bought at a gas station) on Mondays, Wednesdays and Fridays.

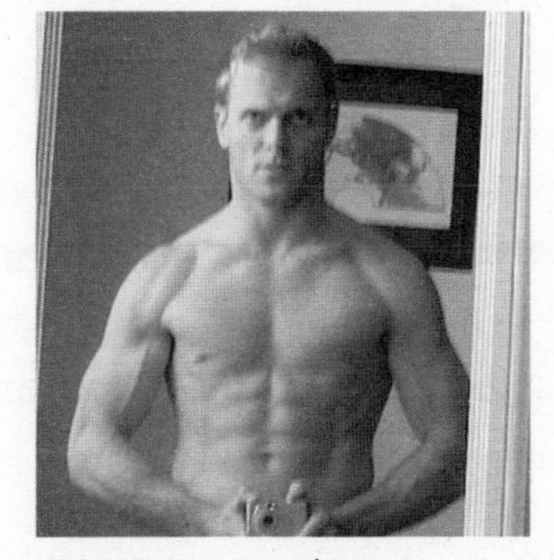

2005: Swing minimalism.

DAY 1 (MONDAY)

- High-rep kettlebell (24kg/53lb) swings to at least 75 reps (ultimately, I got to 150+ reps in a single set)
- Slow myotatic crunch (next chapter) with max weight x 10–15 slow reps

DAY 2 (WEDNESDAY)

I alternated these two exercises for a total of 3 sets × 5 reps for each. I took two minutes between all sets and therefore had at least four minutes between the same exercise (e.g., dumbbell [DB] press, wait two minutes, row, wait two minutes, DB press, etc.):

- Iso-lateral dumbbell incline bench press
- "Yates" bent rows with EZ bar (palms-up grip and bent at the waist about 20–30 degrees)

Then:

- Reverse "drag" curls using a thick bar twice the diameter of a standard Olympic bar (I put plates on metal piping I bought from a DIY shop, secured with $5/£3.10 pinch clamps): 2 sets of 6 reps, three minutes' rest between sets

DAY 3 (FRIDAY)

- High-rep kettlebell (24kg/53lb) swings to 75-rep minimum
- Slow myotatic crunch (next chapter) with max weight x 12–15 reps
- Every other week: single-arm kettlebell swings to 25 minimum reps each side

I should add that I was negligent, often adding one to three additional rest days between sessions. It didn't matter. The training volume needed for head-turning changes was lower than even I thought possible.

Though I added in a few extras for other reasons, the king of exercises—the two-arm kettlebell swing—is all you need for dramatic changes. Here are a few guidelines (more later):

- Stand with your feet 15–30cm (6–12in) outside of shoulder width on either side, each foot pointed outwards about 30 degrees. If toes pointed straight ahead were 12:00 on a clock face, your left foot would point at 10:00 or 11:00, and your right would point at 1:00 or 2:00.

- Keep your shoulders pulled back (retracted) and down to avoid rounding your back.
- The lowering movement (backswing) is a sitting-back-on-a-chair movement, not a squatting-down movement.
- Do not let your shoulders go in front of your knees at any point.
- Imagine pinching a penny between your buttocks when you pop your hips forward. This should be a forceful pop, and it should be impossible to contract your bottom more. If your dog's head gets in the way, it should be lights out for Fido.

The Minimal Effective Dose—How to Lose 3% Body Fat in One Hour a Month

Fleur B. didn't have as much weight to lose as Tracy.

Fleur was, like many people, simply unable to lose those last few kilograms of extra fat, no matter how hard she tried. She'd hit the wall.

Running a few miles three times per week had no effect: "For the amount of exercise I do, the results should be much better." She was, however, against crash dieting and wanted to keep the curves she loved.

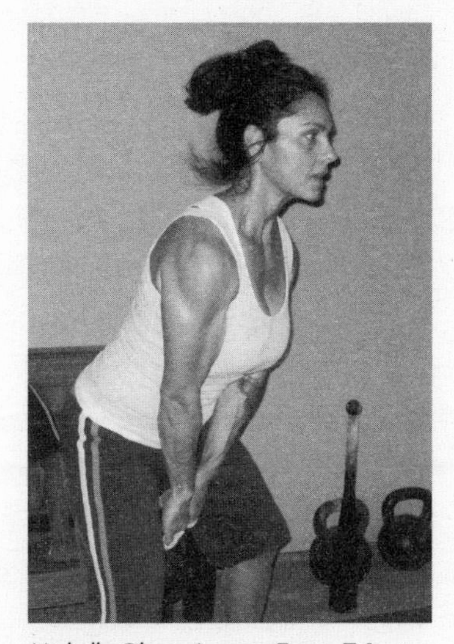
Michelle Obama's arms: Tracy, 7.1+st (45+kg) lighter, showing perfect form on the downswing of the kettlebell swing.

How to cross the last mile of fat loss?

Fleur was a major breadoholic by culture (European) and a workaholic by training (journalist). I purposefully set the expectation that it would be difficult and that she would need to commit to exercising militant self-control for the first two weeks until her cravings disappeared. This way, she would be doubly encouraged when it didn't prove hard after the first 72 hours. Setting the expectation that things will be easy results in disappointment and quitting at the smallest hiccup. If you prepare yourself for massive challenges and no such challenges crop up, it will be a pleasant surprise. This encourages you to be even more aggressive with changes.

Remember: body recomposition depends more on behavioural modification (reread "From Photos to Fear" if needed) than on memorizing the right list of instructions.

I proposed a four-week test focusing on the swing and minuscule dietary changes, which Fleur agreed to:

1. She switched her breakfast to a high-protein meal (at least 30% protein) à la the Slow-carb Diet. Her favourite: spinach, black beans and egg whites (one-third of a carton of scrambled liquid egg whites) with cayenne pepper flakes.
2. Three times a week (Monday, Wednesday, Friday), she performed a simple sequence of three exercises *prior* to breakfast, all of which are illustrated in the next few pages:

One set: 20 two-legged glute activation raises from the floor

One set: 15 flying dogs, one set each side

One set: 50 kettlebell swings (For you: start with a weight that allows you to do 20 perfect repetitions but no more than 30. In other words, start with a weight, no less than 9kg (20lb), that you can "grow into".)

That's it. Total prescribed exercise: about 5 minutes per session × 3 sessions = 15 minutes per week. One hour over the course of a month.

Fleur's before-and-after measurements were separated by five weeks because she was travelling. Even if we increase the estimated exercise time to 75 minutes total, the results are impressive.

BEFORE AND AFTER

Total weight: 9.9st (63kg) → 9.7st (61.7kg).

Body fat %: 21.1% (13.3kg/29.33 lb) → 18% (11kg/24.48 lb—**almost 450g/1lb of fat lost per week**)

Thigh fat thickness: 10.4 mm (0.4in) → 10.2 mm (0.4in)

Tricep fat thickness: 9.7 mm (0.4in) → 7.7 mm (0.3in)

Waist fat thickness: 7.0 mm (0.27in) → 4.1 mm (0.16in)

THE KETTLEBELL SWING

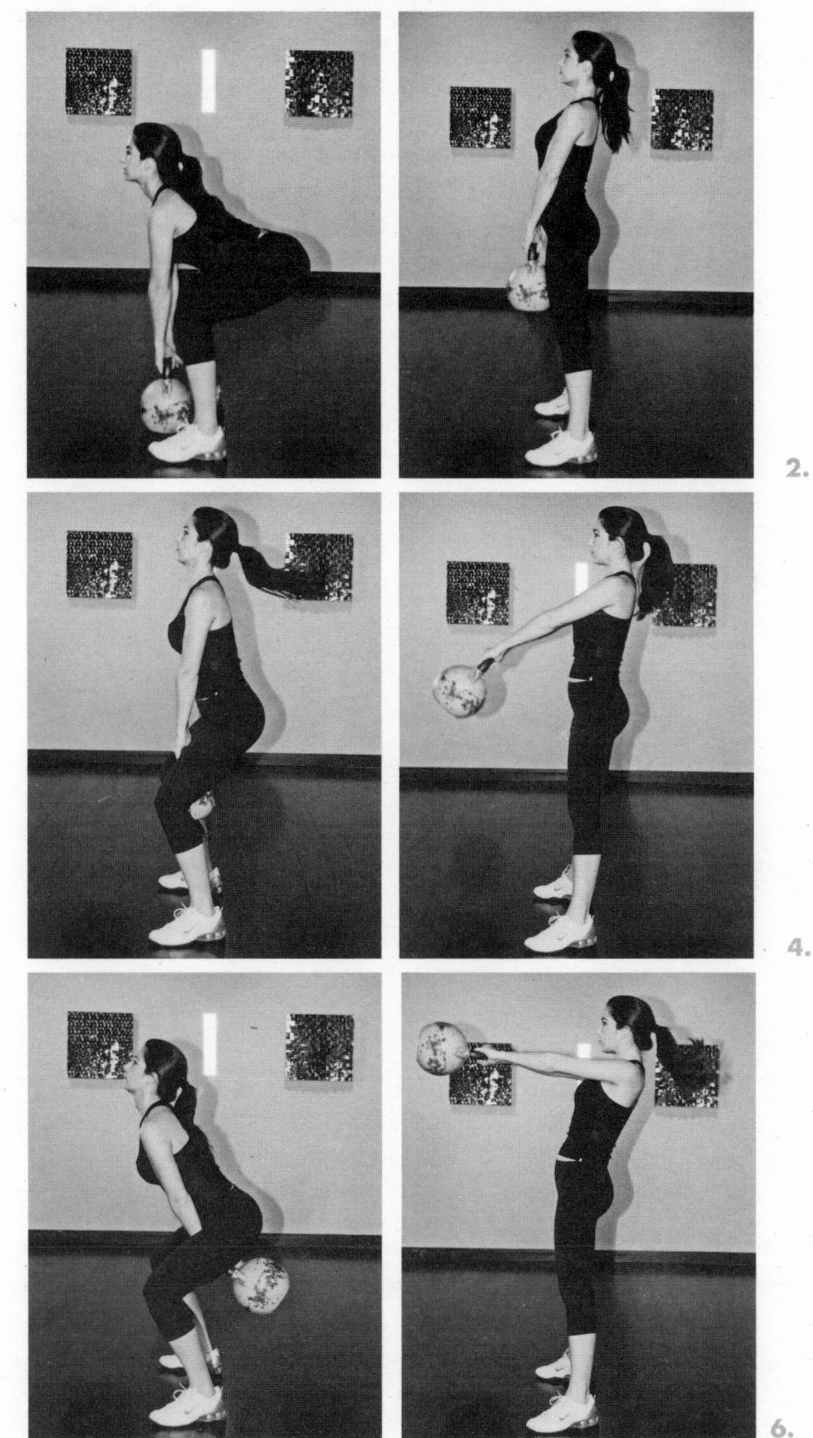

Once you achieve the proper height (the last picture), each rep is alternating between the last two photos.

LEARNING THE SWING

The easiest way to learn the swing is based on a method developed by Zar Horton:

1. Touch-and-Go Deadlifts from Point A (Three Sets of Five Reps)

Stand with the kettlebell directly between the middle of your feet. Bend down and do deadlifts (head up, eyes straight ahead), first slowly, then in a "touch-and-go" fashion, picking up the kettlebell explosively as soon as it touches the ground. It is critical that you touch the same spot on the ground every time. This spot between your insteps is point A.

I strongly suggest doing this facing a wall with your toes about 15cm (6in) from the wall. This will force you to keep your head up and use the proper deadlift motion: hinging at the hip and sitting back, instead of squatting down. Keep any bending at the ankle minimal or non-existent.

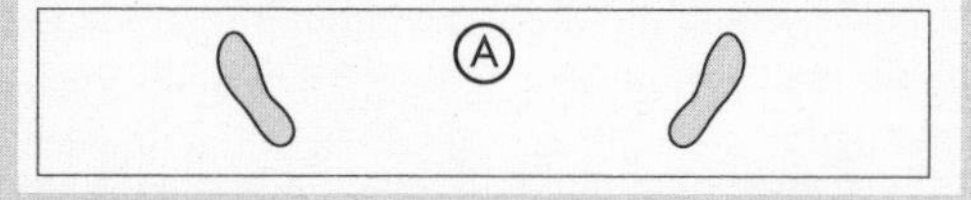

2. Touch-and-Go Deadlifts from Point B (Three Sets of Five Reps)

Repeat the above touch-and-go deadlift, but use point B: place the kettlebell on the floor between your feet but this time further back, with the front of the kettlebell aligned just behind your heels. You must return the kettlebell to exactly this spot every time:

Now when you come up and explosively pop your hips forward (think "violent hips"), the angled rise of the kettlebell will give it a pendulum-like swing.

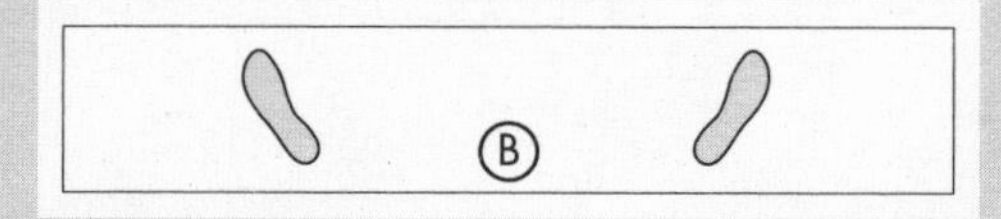

3. Swings from Point C (start with sets of 10)

Now place the kettlebell back at point A and follow the pictures of Marie on the previous page. Pick the kettlebell up off the floor, start a small swing by first "sitting back" with the hips and then popping forward, and make the movement larger while maintaining your balance.

The entire time, focus on getting the kettlebell back to point C, which is in the air behind the hamstrings (back of legs) and tucked right up under the buttocks, as seen in picture 5.

That's it: you are doing the two-handed kettlebell swing.

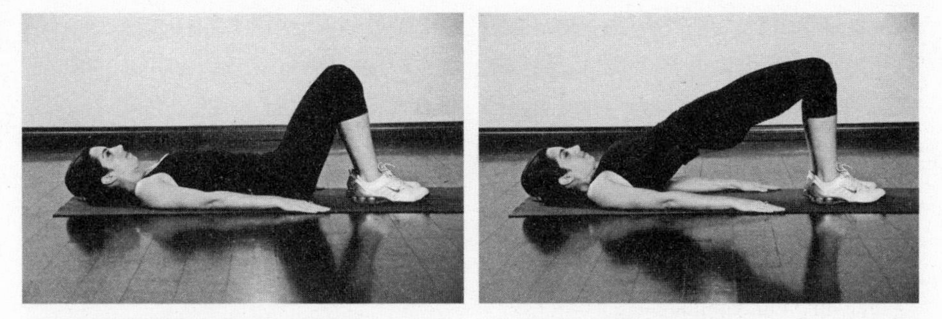

Two-legged glute activation raises. Pull the toes up as you drive off of your heels.

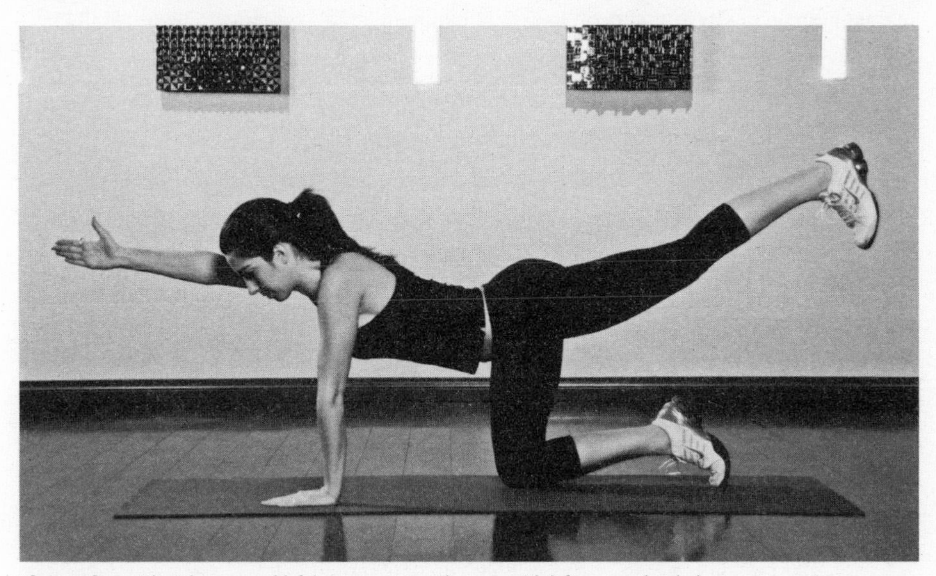

Flying dog with right arm and left leg extension. Alternate with left arm and right leg.

Fleur's resulting numbers demonstrate the difference between scale weight—a blunt instrument that tells you little—and body fat percentage or tape measure. Do not neglect to include at least one of the latter two in your measurement tool kit.

The 75 minutes of exercise had a number of important effects on Fleur's physique that went beyond fat loss and bottom building.

Most important, it fixed her kyphosis (from the Greek *kyphos*, meaning "hump"), a postural problem common to millions of computer users. From desk work and muscular imbalance, she had a shoulders-forward, concave-chest slouch before beginning the programme. Five weeks later, she stood and walked with shoulders back, which created the perception of both a smaller rib cage and larger breasts. Good posture is hot.

Here is Fleur's first e-mail to me, edited for length:

> Hey,
>
> I'm doing well . . . much better than I could have imagined. . . .
>
> There are [a] few things I've noticed about the diet that I think you'll be very interested to learn.
>
> Firstly, I can't imagine why you say it's not supposed to be fun? I'm loving it! . . . There's tons of ways you can make the same foods taste totally different each meal just by adding a different herb or spice.
>
> I'm eating so much better. My diet was not great before, mostly because I just wasn't making the time, and I was too lazy.
>
> Eating the way you suggest has changed my hunger even; I never get that strange cramp-hunger feeling that sugar and "bad" carbs create. It's maybe also because I'm eating more, and more regularly. Just eating breakfast early in the morning instead of coffee and toast or a pastry at 11 am has made a huge difference.
>
> I'm thinking about fueling my body, not restricting it.
>
> I ate really well all last week and then assigned Sunday as my "free day". I ate pancakes and an omelet at the IHOP (very healthy). Then I felt like crap. All the cheese made me want to throw up. [Tim: Cheese was one of Fleur's domino foods before the programme.]
>
> But I literally had to force myself to eat some chocolate later on in the day, just because I'd told myself I could. I then realized that I hadn't even thought once about chocolate all week, hadn't once craved for it. Then I bought a croissant (just because I could), took one bite and threw it away. Sunday night I had a beer and couldn't finish that either (very unlike me). I found myself desperate to go to sleep so I could wake up Monday morning and go back to feeling healthy again.
>
> Is this normal?! . . .
>
> One thing I did really want on Sunday though was fruit. That's ok right? As much of any type that I want? [Answer: On binge day and on binge day only, yes. Nothing is forbidden.]
>
> In general, so far, I'm not missing or craving anything I'm not supposed to have. . . . I have noticed I have more energy, and it's real energy, not just an hour hit from a double cappuccino and a snack-bar that then turns into

a slump. I'm not really drinking coffee much either, just lots of water and green tea.

I know it's only been a week, but I feel fantastic. Thank you!

New behaviours aren't that hard once you start them.

Critical (M)Ass: The Kiwi's Complete A/B Workout

For those who want a more extended bottom programme, here is The Kiwi's complete sequence.

He advocates three to four circuits of these exercises, in the order provided. I believe the MED is two circuits and will deliver 80–90% of the benefits for most women and men. Men can use these sequences to develop stronger hip drive, which translates to better performance in almost all sports and power lifts.

If you try this but start to miss workouts or postpone them, revert to the basic swings twice per week, as I do, which will still guarantee faster progress than most exercise programmes.

To mimic The Kiwi, perform A on Monday and B on Friday, and glute activation raises (seen earlier) are performed before each.

Workout A

All exercises, except for kettlebell swings, are performed for 10 repetitions using a 13-Repetition Max[2] (RM) weight.

1. Heavy dumbbell front squat to press (bottom to heels)—squeeze glutes at bottom for one second before rising
2. One-arm, one-leg DB row
3. Walking lunges with sprinter knee raise
4. Wide-grip push-ups[3]
5. Two-arm kettlebell swings × 20–25

Repeat sequence 2–4 times.

2. This means you are doing 10 reps with a weight that would allow you to complete 13 but not 14 reps. Approximate is fine, but you shouldn't have more than 3 or so reps left in the tank when you finish the set.

3. Men can use any hand position. Wide-grip is recommended for women who want to avoid tricep (back of the upper arm) growth. If you can't do ten push-ups on the floor, they can be performed with the hands on a low bench, or—if still impossible—against a table or wall.

Workout B

1. One-leg Romanian Deadlift (RDL)[4] (10–12 reps each side)
2. Chin-up (four-second negative lowering portion only) × 10 or until you cannot control descent[5]
3. One-leg hamstring curls on a Swiss ball—6–12 reps each leg
4. Plank for abs (and gluteus medius on sides) → Progression: start with 30 seconds front, 30 seconds each side, working up to 90 seconds maximum
5. Reverse hyper × 15–25

Repeat sequence 2–4 times.

See the www.fourhourbody.com/exercises for photos of all The Kiwi's exercises.[6] Written descriptions alone will confuse more than help.

TOOLS AND TRICKS

Kettlebells (www.fourhourbody.com/kettlebells) Most men should start with a 20kg (44 lb) or 24kg (53 lb) kettlebell and most women should start with a 16-kg (35 lb) or 20kg (44 lb) kettlebell. I suggest using a T-handle (see page 172) to determine your 20-rep swing weight before spending too much.

4. Effectively the same as the 2SDL described in "Pre-Hab".
5. Expect severe soreness the day after the first two workouts.
6. One of them is my favourite indirect abdominal/core exercise (one-arm, one-leg row), and two are excellent for travel for both genders (one-leg hamstring curls and reverse hyper on Swiss ball).

TRACY'S DIET: THE LUXURY OF NO CHOICE

Tracy never hit a fat loss plateau.

She credits her success to two things: cheat meals and kettlebells. The cheat meals allowed her to remain strict more than 95% of the time, and the kettlebells allowed her to accelerate progress when diet-driven fat loss slowed.

She scheduled one cheat meal per week, most often on Friday night, which was also date night with the husband. Her diet is otherwise the epitome of simplicity: eat the same meals each day, at least five days per week. She refers to her meal plans as "the luxury of no choice":

"Especially if you have 3.6–7st (22.7–45kg) or more to lose, you have enough stress. You won't be able to stop thinking about how overweight you are, but you can stop thinking about what to eat."

Her advice and observations should sound familiar:

2lb (900g) per week isn't the limit. "If you have 5.7–7st (36.3–45kg) to lose and aren't losing 5lb (2.3kg) per week for at least the first few weeks, you are doing something wrong."

Avoid domino foods: "If I liked to eat a cookie here, a chocolate bar there, I could fit sweets into my daily menu from a caloric standpoint, but my sweet tooth has no 'shut-off sensor'. Once I get started, I have a hard time stopping. I can consume 1,200–1,800 calories of dense sweets in no time flat. If I start to eat sweets, I know I will not be happy until I get my fill. And 'my fill' is way more full than the average person. It is not a serving of cookies or cake, it's an entire bag of cookies, or half a cake. . . and that's no joke. This I know. So I don't try and fool myself into thinking I can eat just one cookie or just two chocolate bars. If I could eat two pieces of bread, as another example, I'd be fine, but I have to have four, so I don't eat it at all."

Organic food—good but not necessary: "I lost 7st (45kg) never eating a single organic vegetable. Do it if you can, but if you can't—for budgetary reasons or otherwise—don't create more stress because you can't go to the farmers' market or a high-class grocery store. Eat the right foods and you'll be fine."

Vegetables and protein: "The only reason I'll never be fat again is because I start each meal with a base of vegetables that taste good. Then I add my protein. I don't discriminate against protein, though my favourites are lamb, pork, chicken and beef. I'll eat an entire cow before I eat powdered protein. Blech."

THE COMPLETE GYM FOR $10(£6.20)—THE T-HANDLE

Kettlebells are not inexpensive.

If you can't afford them, or to determine your ideal swing weight (what you can currently do for 20 good repetitions) before ordering kettlebells, there is a fantastically inexpensive option: the "T-handle". Rumoured to be one of the core tools of dominant Hungarian hammer throwers, this simple device is also known as the Hungarian Core Blaster (HCB).

I have 20 kettlebells of various sizes but still prize my T-handle, as it can be disassembled for travel and packed flat at a weight of less than 2.3kg (5lb). In addition to swings, it can be used for deadlifts, two-arm bent rows, curls reverse curls, and more. For $10 (£6.20), five minutes of shopping and less than five minutes of assembly, you have an entire gym. Here's what it looks like:

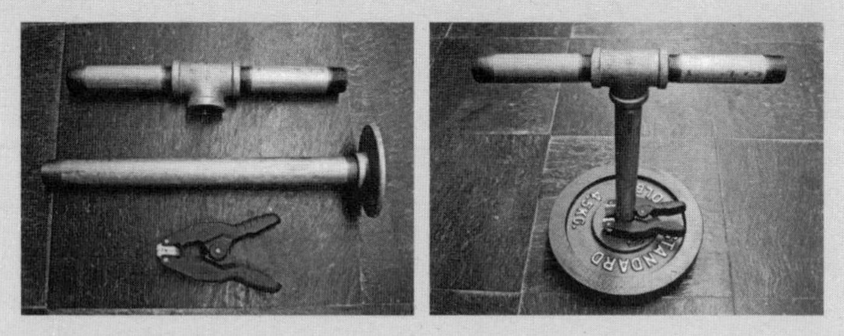

Just head to any hardware store or Home Depot and head to the plumbing aisle:

- One 8mm (¾in) diameter × 30cm (12in) long pipe nipple for the vertical shaft. A "pipe nipple" is, somewhat paradoxically, a short pipe threaded on both ends with male pipe thread.[7]
- Two 8mm (¾in) diameter × 10cm (4in) long pipe nipples for the handles. Electrical or duct tape can later be used to cover the outside threads, but I just wear leather gloves when training with the T-handle.
- One 8mm (¾in) diameter pipe "T" fitting to connect the above items.
- One 8mm (¾in) floor flange to keep the plates from falling off as you swing.

An optional but suggested addition:

- One spring clamp (I use an Irwin Quick-Grip 2.5cm/1in) to keep plates from drifting up at the top of the swing. Do not swing the weights above sternum height.

Last but not least, replace the T-handle every six months. Tossing a bunch of plates on your cat or through a wall won't win you IQ points when both are preventable for the cost of a T-shirt. Special thanks to Dave Draper for introducing me to this beautifully simple device.

7. If you are shorter than 165cm (5ft 5in), a 4cm (10in) or even 3cm (8in) pipe nipple can be used to avoid dangerous brushing of the ground.

THE MATHS OF BEAUTY: 0.7 AND BEYOND

What do Marilyn Monroe, Sophia Loren and Elle Macpherson have in common? The number 0.7 and the letters WHR.

If you measured the waist and hip circumference of these three women, you'd find that their waists are 7/10 the size of their hips. This makes their waist-to-hip ratio (WHR) 0.7, and this ratio in females appears to be hardwired into the male brain as a sign of fertility and therefore attractiveness. The wider your waist is, the higher this ratio goes towards the apple-shaped 1.0, which correlates in scientific studies with decreased oestrogen levels, increased disease risk, increased birth complications and lower fertility rates.

Professor Devendra Singh at the University of Texas–Austin has studied the pear-shaped 0.7 body and found it popping up in 2,500-year-old stone Venus sculptures across Europe and Asia, in all Miss America winners from 1923 to 1987 (0.69 to 0.72), in *Playboy* centrefolds from 1955 to 1965 and 1976 to 1990 (0.68 to 0.71), and across different cultures—from Indonesians and Indian labourers to African Americans and Caucasians.

The good news? If you were born with wide hips, no worries.

Working towards a more slender waist has been shown to have a greater effect on attractiveness than reducing hip size. If your WHR is high, dropping it even a little bit will increase your power (health and hotness) to attract a male partner.

For men, your magic numbers are 0.8–0.9 for WHR and 0.6 for the waist-to-shoulder ratio (WSR). Broad shoulders can be built.

Perhaps the simplest tool for fine-tuning WHR in both sexes? No surprise: the kettlebell swing.

SIX-MINUTE ABS

Two Exercises That Actually Work

"7-Minute Abs. And we guarantee just as good a workout as the 8-minute folk. . . . If you're not happy with the first 7 minutes, we're gonna send you the extra minute free!"

"That's good. Unless, of course, somebody comes up with 6-Minute Abs. Then you're in trouble, huh?"

"No! No, no . . . not 6! I said 7. Nobody's comin' up with 6. Who works out in 6 minutes?! You won't even get your heart goin', not even a mouse on a wheel. . . . It's like you're dreamin' about Gorgonzola cheese when it's clearly Brie time, baby."

—*There's Something About Mary*

HOTEL BEDROOM, NAPA, CALIFORNIA, MAY 2009

"You look like a cat about to vomit."

My girlfriend had come out of the shower to find me perched on the bed on all fours, stomach heaving.

Taking a huge inhale, I looked up and gave an awkward smile: "Thirty more seconds. . . ."

She tilted her head like a Labrador retriever, observing the oddness for a few seconds, then walked back in the bathroom to dry her hair and brush her teeth. She needed to get ready for my friend's wedding, and my groaning on all fours was far from the strangest thing she'd seen from me.

I continued my routine with a degree of glee.

For the first time in my life, I had reliable six-pack abs.

Cat vomiting rocked.

Single White Male Seeking Abdominals: Exploring the Path Less Travelled

I've never had visible abs.

Even when my body fat was low enough to show

veins everywhere else, my frontal six-pack—the rectus abdominus—showed almost no separation. Damnation.

Low body fat was necessary but not enough.

I performed conventional ab exercises for more than a decade with no discernible benefit, somehow convinced it was just a matter of time. Albert Einstein would call this insanity: doing the same thing over and over again and expecting different results.

Things changed only when I began testing basic assumptions in 2009. It took a week to arrive at a reductionist programme of two exercises. I performed these exercises just twice a week on Mondays and Fridays after kettlebell swings. In a matter of three weeks, I had my six-pack.

There is just one more prerequisite for visible abs: follow a diet that allows sustained low body fat of 12% or less. I suggest the Slow-carb Diet, as it has the highest compliance rate I've ever observed, but other viable options include a ketogenic diet (especially the Cyclical Ketogenic Diet) and intermittent fasting (IF). The latter will be covered in later chapters.

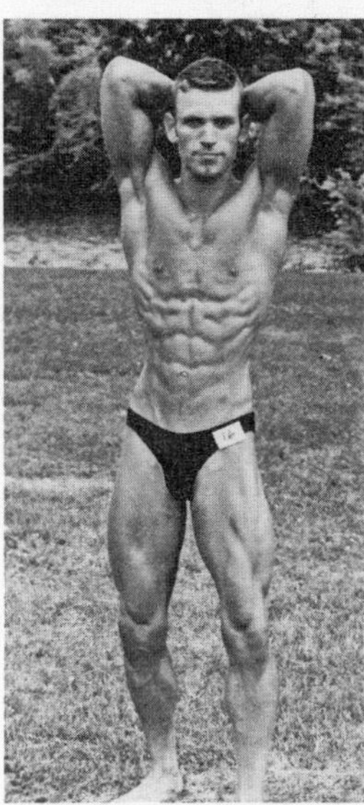

Drew Baye after more than six months of no direct abdominal exercises. It goes to show how diet is often a determining factor. (Photo: Mike Moran)

Movement #1: The Myotatic Crunch

I began my analysis by looking for common attributes in exercises that hadn't worked. The shared feature of all the dominant exercises, in particular the floor crunch, is that they used no more than half of the full range of motion (ROM) of the abdominals. If you were to imagine yourself sitting in a chair, the prescribed exercises all took you towards your knees (crunch, floor sit-up) or brought your knees towards your chest with a straight back (roman chair, reverse crunch). I decided to ignore that foetal range of motion altogether for eight weeks and focus on the stretched position achieved with full back extension.

The result was the myotatic crunch, so named because it leverages the fully stretched position and the resultant reflex (myotatic reflex or stretch reflex) for a stronger contraction than I had been able to achieve otherwise.

It didn't take eight weeks to see a difference. It took three.

Since this exercise is also effective for recruiting the transverse abdominis (explained next), if you have to choose one exercise, choose this one. If a BOSU ball is not available, use a small Swiss ball (45–55cm/17.7–21.7in in diameter) or a pile of firm cushions.

Using a BOSU or Swiss ball, ensure your bottom is close to the floor, usually no more than 15cm (6in) off the ground. Then follow these steps:

1. Start with arms stretched overhead as high as possible (I overlap my extended hands as if in a diving position). Keep your arms behind or next to your ears for the entire exercise.
2. Lower under control for 4 seconds until your fingers touch the floor, the entire time attempting to extend your hands further away from the ball.

THE MYOTATIC CRUNCH

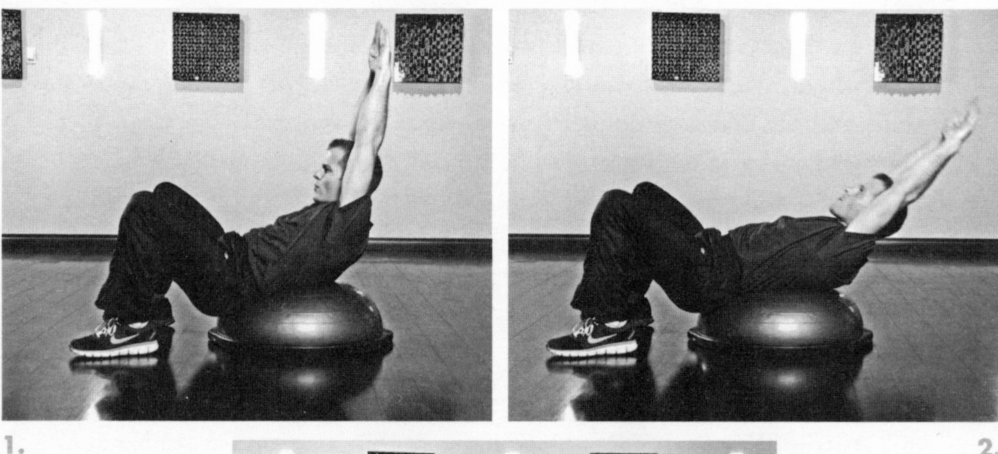

1. 2.

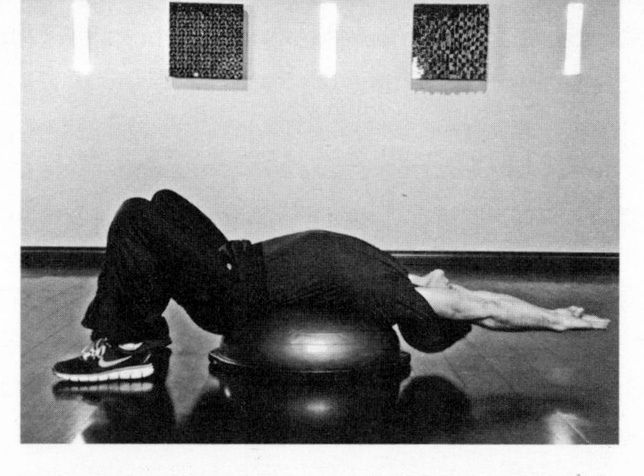

3.

3. Pause at the bottom for 2 seconds, aiming for maximum elongation (picture 3).
4. Rise under control and pause in the upper, fully contracted position for 2 seconds. The arms should *not* pass perpendicular with the ground.
5. Repeat for a total of 10 repetitions. Once you can complete 10 repetitions, add weight to your hands. I tend to use books of different sizes. If female, I don't suggest exceeding 4.5kg (10lb) in added weight (see "Hourglass" sidebar on page 179).

Movement #2: The Cat Vomit Exercise

This exercise is dedicated to my ex-girlfriend. I want only the best for you, Angelina Jolie.

Unless you purchase a corset at the same time, doing crunches will not pull your abdomen in. The muscle fibres of the six-pack (rectus abdominis) run vertically. The muscle you want to target instead is called the transverse abdominis (TVA), the deepest of the six main abdominal muscles, which is composed of fibres that run horizontally like a belt. The TVA is nicknamed the "corset muscle", and if your abs have ever ached from laughing or coughing, you've felt it working.

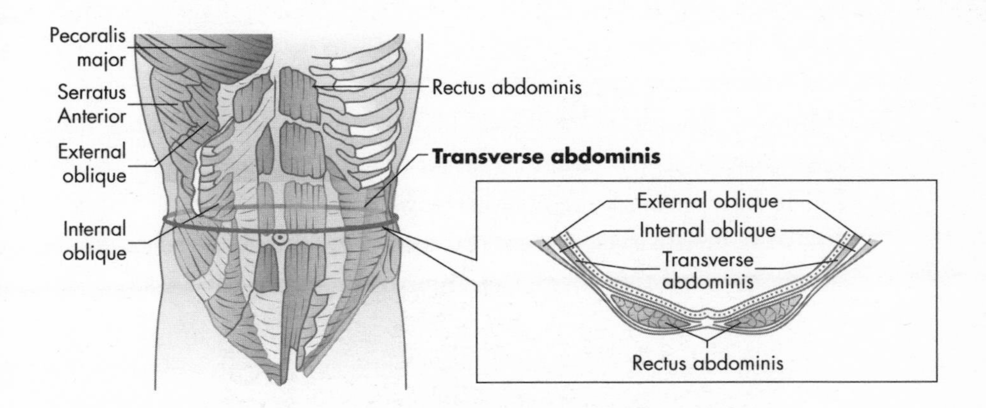

CAT VOMIT

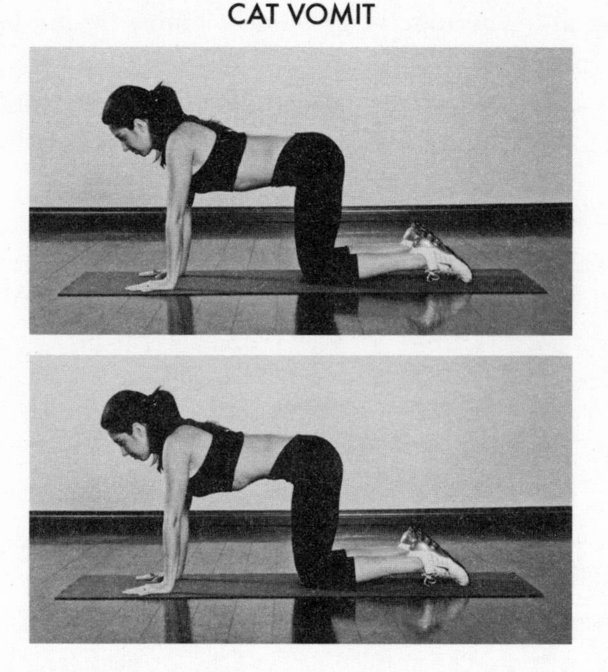

Unfortunately, laughing repeatedly in the gym will get you a strait-jacket or a plate to the head, so here is the alternative:

1. Get on all fours and keep your gaze focused either directly under your head or slightly in front of you. Don't arch your back or strain your neck.
2. Forcefully exhale from your mouth until all air is fully expelled. Your abs should be contracted from this forceful exhale. Full exhalation is necessary to contract the transverse abdominals, and you'll use gravity to provide resistance.
3. Hold your breath and pull your belly button upward towards your spine as hard as you can for a target of 8–12 seconds.
4. Inhale fully through the nose after the 8–12 second hold.
5. Take one breath cycle of rest (exhale slowly out the mouth, inhale slowly through the nose), then repeat the above for a total of 10 repetitions.

There you have it: the myotatic crunch and the cat vomit exercise. Heave, groan and be merry.

SQUARE IS NOT FEMININE: PRESERVING THE HOURGLASS

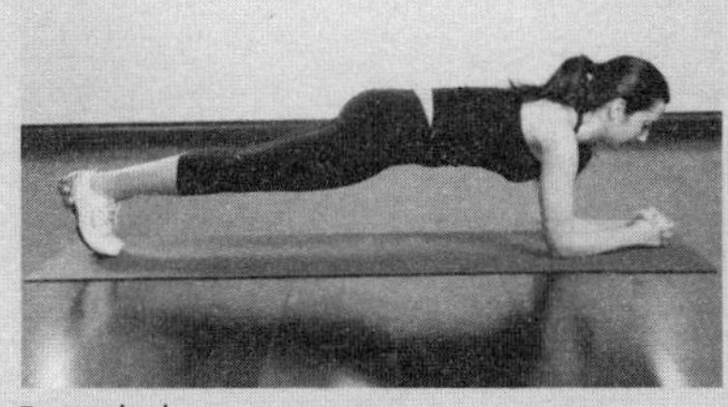

Front plank

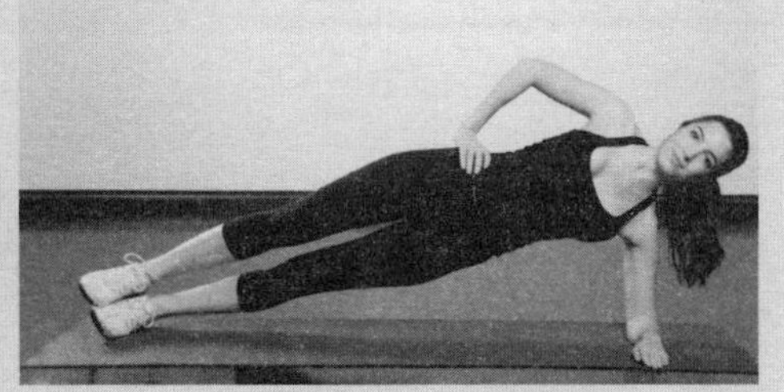

Side plank

Square obliques are unattractive on women, and using common progressive resistance exercises can create them. Fortunately, the myotatic crunch and cat vomit exercises, as described, are not such exercises.

Loss of the feminine hourglass shape is sad and leaves some women looking bloated under clothing, even when they have low body fat. Not good.

If you want additional abdominal exercises as a woman, stick with timed planks instead, which also strengthen the gluteus medius on the hip. Just as The Kiwi in the last chapter prescribed, start with 30 seconds on the front, then 30 seconds on each side, working up to 90 seconds maximum per set. One set per angle per workout is all that's needed.

Last but not least, to avoid the small potbelly look so common among women, even fitness competitors, fix your pelvic tilt with hip flexor stretches. The following can be performed once a day for 30 seconds on each side. Before kettlebells is perfect, as it will also help with hip extension.

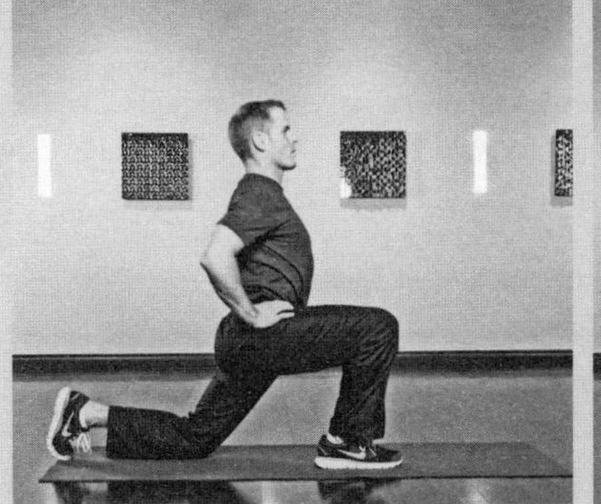

Hip flexor stretch (illustrated for left side)

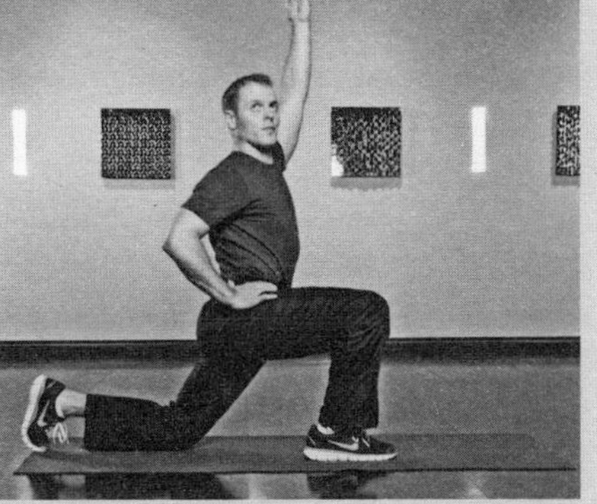

Hold in this position for 30 seconds.

MEASURING AB ACTIVATION WITH EMG: COMPARING THE USUAL SUSPECTS

Even if you ignore the two exercises in this chapter, don't rely on the plain-vanilla crunch. It's utterly ineffective.

Here's how it stacks up against other exercises when rectus abdominis activation is measured with electrodes and an EMG (electromyography machine). Google each exercise if curious. The traditional crunch is given a value of 100%.

Exercise	Activation
Bicycle crunch	248%
Captain's chair	212%
Exercise ball	139%
Vertical leg crunch	129%
Torso track	127%
Long arm crunch	119%
Reverse crunch	109%
Crunch with heel push	107%
Ab roller	105%
Hover	100%
Traditional crunch	100%
Exercise tubing pull	92%
Ab rocker	21%

TIPS AND TRICKS

BOSU Balance Trainer (www.fourhourbody.com/bosu) The BOSU looks like half of a Swiss ball with a flat plastic base attached to the underside. I use it for myotatic crunches and the torture twists featured in "Effortless Superhuman".

GoFit Stability Ball (www.fourhourbody.com/stability) If preferred to the BOSU, this 55cm/21.7in "stability" ball (usually referred to as a "Swiss" ball) can be used. It's less than half the cost of a BOSU, but I found such balls hard to store in the home and less versatile.

Crazy Hitchhiker from *There's Something About Mary* (www.fourhourbody.com/hitchhiker) The classic scene that inspired the title of this chapter. "It's Brie time, baby"!

FROM GEEK TO FREAK

How to Gain 2.4st (15.4kg) in 28 Days

Somewhere along the line, we seem to have confused comfort with happiness.

—Dean Karnazes, ultramarathoner who, in 2006, ran 50 marathons in all 50 U.S. states in 50 consecutive days, finishing with a 3 hour and 30 second time at the New York City Marathon

Often the less there is to justify a traditional custom, the harder it is to get rid of it.

—Mark Twain

On 6 July, 65-year-old John's biceps measured 37cm (14½in) in circumference. Six weeks later, his biceps measured a full 2cm (¾in) larger at 39cm (15¼in).

It seems like magic, but it wasn't.

He reduced his workouts from three per week to two per week. It was all planned. Progressive reduction.

You see, most of the conventional wisdom about muscular growth is just dead wrong.

Prelude: On Being Genetically Screwed

I come from a family of lightly muscled males. The only exception is a dramatic bubble bum on my mum's side. Not a bad look if you're a Brazilian woman.

In August 2009, to confirm the obvious, I mailed DNA samples to the Gist Sports Profile laboratory in Australia for testing of the ACTN3 gene, which codes proteins for fast-twitch muscle fibre. Fast-twitch muscle fibres have the greatest potential for growth, whereas slow-twitch fibres have the least potential.

GA Just a smidge of helpful science: muscle fibres are composed of myofibrils, which are in turn composed of two filaments—actin (thin filaments) and myosin (thick filaments)—that slide over each other to cause muscles to contract, a literal shortening of the muscle. Actin filaments, which are necessary to this process, are stabilized by actin-binding proteins. One actin-binding protein called alpha-actinin 3 (ACTN3) is expressed only in fast-twitch muscle fibre, the crown jewel of shot-putters and bodybuilders worldwide.

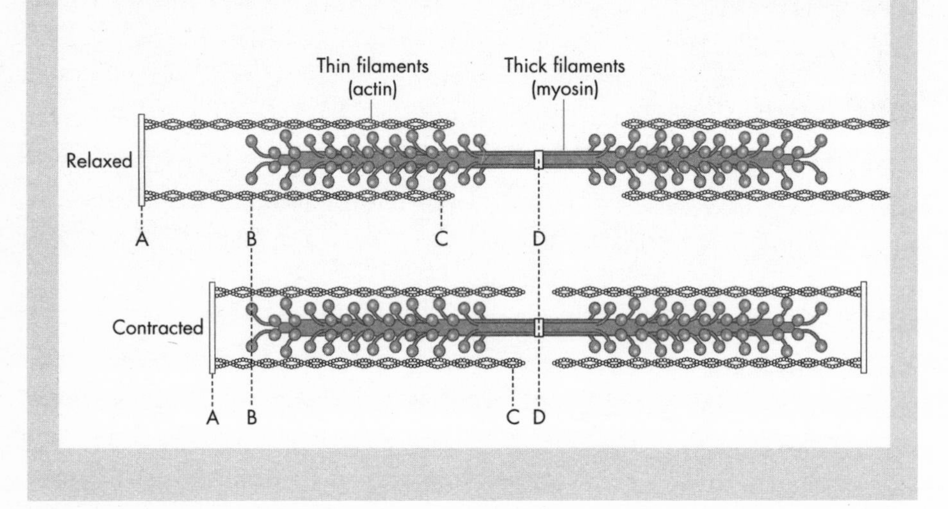

It turns out that both of my chromosomes (one from Mammy and one from Pappy Ferriss) contain the R577X variant of the ACTN3 gene, a mutation that results in a complete deficiency of our most desired ACTN3. This variant, amusingly called a "nonsense allele", is found in more than a billion humans worldwide.

Sad Christmas.

The cover letter from Gist Sports began with the following headline, which, in good humour, lacks an exclamation point:

> Congratulations Tim Ferriss. Your Genetic Advantage: Endurance Sports.

This is a diplomatic way of telling me (1) I'm not likely to win an Olympic gold medal in sprinting, and (2) I am not genetically pre-programmed to gain a lot of muscular mass.

I hadn't won the fast-twitch lottery for bodybuilding,[8] and chances are that you haven't either. Looking at family photos, this result wasn't surprising. What is surprising is how well you can override genetics.

I have gained more than 9kg (20lb) of fat-free mass within four weeks on at least four occasions, the most recent in 2005. Two of these experiments were done in 1995 and 1996 at Princeton University, where Matt Brzycki, then Coordinator of Health Fitness, Strength and Conditioning, nicknamed me "Growth".

This chapter details the exact methods I used in 2005 to gain 15.4kg (34lb) of fat-free mass in 28 days.

For the ladies not interested in becoming the Hulk, if you follow a Slow-carb Diet and reduce rest periods between exercises to 30 seconds, this exact workout protocol can help you lose 4.5–9kg (10–20lb) of fat in the same 28-day time span.

Before-and-After

I weighed 10.9st (69kg) throughout high school, but after training in tango in Buenos Aires in 2005, I had withered to 10.4st (66.2kg). I remedied the situation with a 28-day schedule based primarily on the work of Arthur Jones, Mike Mentzer and Ken Hutchins.

Before-and-after measurements, including underwater hydrostatic weighings, were taken by Dr. Peggy Plato at the Human Performance Laboratory at San Jose State University. Though this ridiculous experiment might seem unhealthy, I tracked blood variables and dropped my total cholesterol count from 222 to 147 without the use of statins[9] (see pre-bed supplementation).

Here are the results:

8. I've since confirmed this finding with three separate genetic profiles through 23andMe (two tests with different names to ensure consistent results) and Navigenics, two genetic testing companies in California, U.S..
9. I've since learned to worry less about cholesterol if HDL is high enough and triglycerides are low enough.

Age: 27 (in 2005)
Weight before: 10.4st (66.2kg)
Weight after: 12.6st (80kg) (13st ≠ 83kg three days later)
Body fat percentage before: 16.72%
Body fat percentage after: 12.23%
Total muscle gained: 34lb (15.4kg)
Total fat loss: 3lb (1.4kg)
Time elapsed: 4 weeks

To put 15.4kg (34lb) in perspective, to the right is exactly 450g (1lb) of lean grass-fed beef sirloin next to my fist.

Imagine 34 of those placed on you. It's no small addition.

Here are some select stats on the four-week change (21 September to 23 October), using combined measurements from Dr. Plato and Brooks Brothers:[10]

- Suit size: 40 (50) short to 44 (54) regular (measured at Brooks Brothers at Santana Row in San Jose)
- Neck: 40cm to 46cm (15.8in to 18in)
- Chest: 95cm to 109cm (37.5in to 43in)

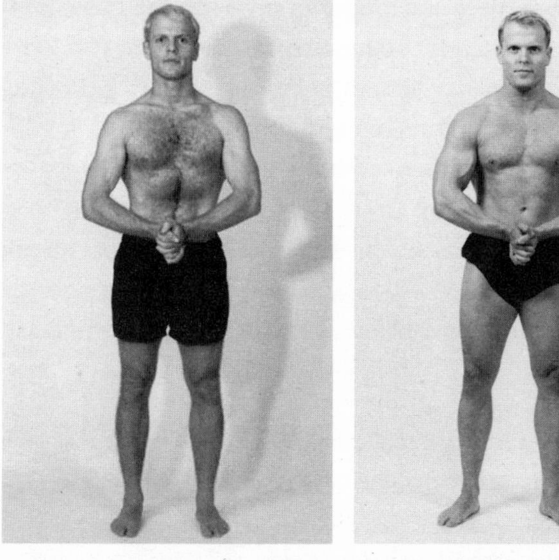

Anti-gravity shorts for dramatic effect.

10. Compiled with a combination of the lowest and highest measurements from both locations.

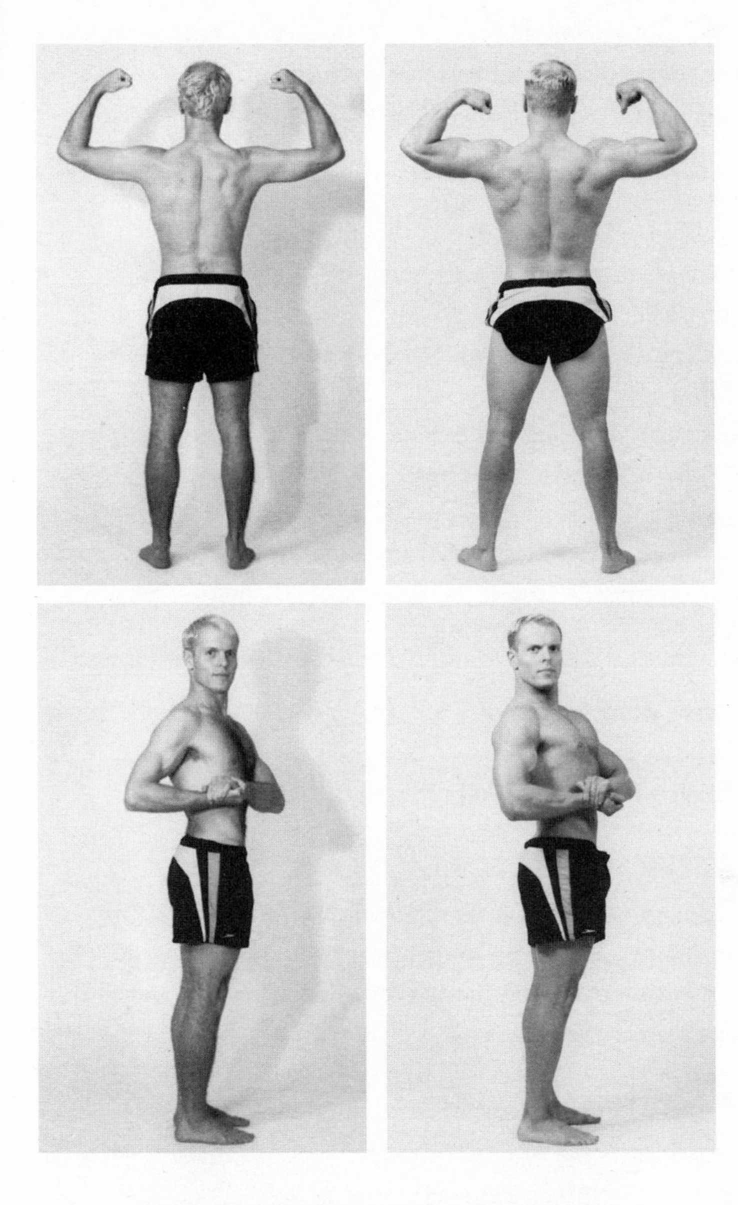

- Shoulders: 109cm (43in) to 132cm (52in)
- Thigh: 55cm (21.5in) to 65cm (25.5in)
- Calf: 34cm (13.5in) to 38cm (14.9in)
- Upper arm: 30cm (12in) to 37cm (14.6in)
- Forearm: 27.4cm (10.8in) to 30cm (12in)
- Waist: 75cm (29.5in) to 84cm (33.1in)
- Hips (bottom at widest): 86cm (34in) to 97.1cm (38.23in) (J. Lo, eat your heart out)

Oh, and I forgot to mention, all of this was done with two 30-minute workouts per week, for **a total of 4 hours of gym time**.

How Did I Do It?

First, I followed a simple supplement regimen:

Morning: NO-Xplode[11] (2 scoops), Slo-Niacin (or timed-release niacinamide, 500 mg)
Each meal: ChromeMate (chromium polynicotinate, *not* picolinate, 200 mcg), alpha-lipoic acid (200 mg)
Pre-workout: BodyQUICK (2 capsules 30 mins. prior)
Post-workout: Micellean (30 g micellar casein protein)
Prior to bed: policosanol (23 mg), ChromeMate (200 mcg), alpha-lipoic acid (200 mg), Slo-Niacin (500 mg)

No anabolics were used.

From a training standpoint, there were four basic principles that made it happen, all of which will be expanded upon in the next chapter:

1. PERFORM ONE-SET-TO-FAILURE FOR EACH EXERCISE.

Follow Arthur Jones's general recommendation of one-set-to-failure (i.e., reaching the point where you can no longer move the weight) for 80–120 seconds of total time under tension per exercise. Take at least three minutes of rest between exercises.

2. USE A 5/5 REP CADENCE.

Perform every repetition with a 5/5 cadence (five seconds up, five seconds down) to eliminate momentum and ensure constant load.

11. To give my adrenal glands and adrenergic receptors a rest, I didn't consume NO-Xplode on Sundays.

3. FOCUS ON 2–10 EXERCISES PER WORKOUT, NO MORE.

Focus on 2–10 exercises per workout (including at least one multi-joint exercise for pressing, pulling and leg movements). I chose to exercise my entire body each workout to elicit a heightened hormonal response (testosterone, growth hormone, IGF-1, etc.).

Here is the sequence I used during this experiment ("+" = superset, which means no rest between exercises):

- Pullover + Yates's bent row
- Shoulder-width leg press[12]
- Pec-deck + weighted dips
- Leg curl
- Reverse thick-bar curl (purchase cut 5cm/2in piping from a DIY store if needed, which you can then slide plates onto)
- Seated calf raises
- Manual neck resistance
- Machine crunches

All of these exercises can be found at www.fourhourbody.com/geek-to-freak.

4. INCREASE RECOVERY TIME ALONG WITH SIZE.

This is described at length in the next chapter, which describes the most reductionist and refined approach to overriding stubborn genetics: Occam's Protocol.

Occam's Protocol is what I suggest almost all trainees start with for mass gains.

12. I recommend the squat for those who have access to a Safety Bar, which provides a yolk-like shoulder harness.

THE COLORADO EXPERIMENT: 4.5ST (28.6KG) IN 28 DAYS?

Think gaining 2.4st (15.4kg) in 28 days is impossible? I might have, too, if it weren't for bumping into the curious case of Casey Viator.

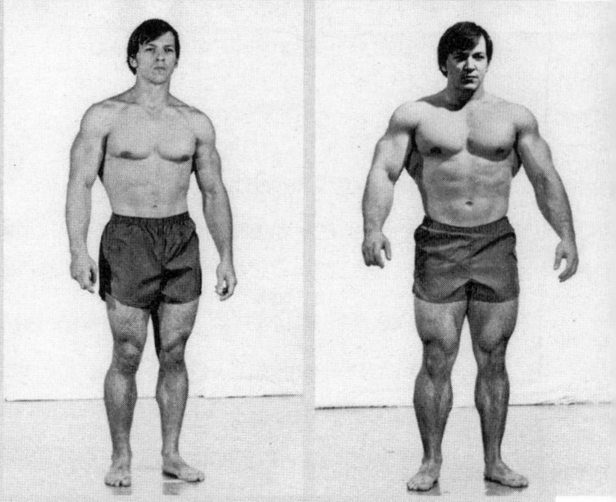

The "Colorado Experiment" was conducted in May 1973 at Colorado State University in Fort Collins, Colorado. It was designed by Arthur Jones and supervised by Dr. Elliott Plese, Director of the Exercise Physiology Lab in the Department of Physical Education. It was intended to be a brutal example of minimalist training.

Casey Viator's results, produced from three workouts per week, were otherworldly:

Photos by Inge Cook, provided courtesy of Ellington Darden PhD

Increase in bodyweight: 3st (20.5kg)
Loss of body fat: 17.93lb (8.1kg)
Muscular gain: 63.21lb (28.7kg)

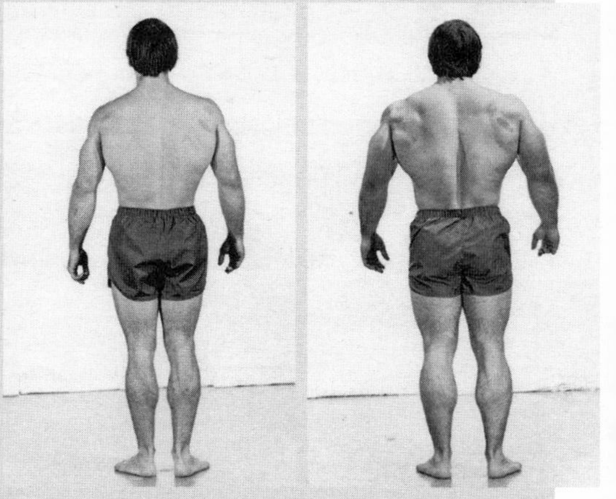

That same month, Arthur Jones followed in Viator's footsteps and gained just over 1st (68kg) in 22 days. How did they do it in workouts that averaged just 33.6 minutes each?

First, negative-only sets were often used, wherein the weight was raised with the legs using a lever and then lowered with the target muscle, allowing heavier weights than could otherwise be lifted. Second, exercises were paired into supersets to prefatigue a muscle (e.g., quadriceps with leg extension) prior to taking it to failure with a compound movement (e.g., squats). Third, Casey ate 6–8 meals per day like it was his job. That's not a metaphor. He had a cash incentive per kilogram (pound) of muscle gained. It *was* his job.

Here is one of Casey's actual workouts. Keep in mind that, unless rest is indicated, there is no rest between exercises:

1. Leg press 750 for 20 reps
2. Leg extension 225 for 20 reps
3. Squat 502 for 13 reps
4. Leg curl 175 for 12 reps
5. One-legged calf raise with 18kg (40lb) in one hand for 15 reps (Two-minute rest)
6. Pullover 290 for 11 reps
7. Behind-the-neck lat isolation 200 for 10 reps
8. Row machine 200 for 10 reps
9. Behind-the-neck lat pull-downs 210 for 10 reps (Two-minute rest)
10. Straight-armed lateral raise with dumbbells 18kg (40lb) for 9 reps
11. Behind-the-neck shoulder press 185 for 10 reps
12. Bicep curl plate loaded 110 for 8 reps
13. Chin-ups bodyweight for 12 reps
14. Tricep extension 125 for 9 reps
15. Parallel dip bodyweight for 22 reps

If you're a normal human, you would finish this workout by retching into a garbage can or dying. Both the Denver Broncos and Dick Butkus of the Chicago Bears visited Fort Collins to observe the fast-paced training, which is hard to appreciate unless you attempt it.

Though far from easy, the basic workout template is simple. The following was sent to me by Casey Viator himself:

Leg press × 20 reps
Leg extension × 20 reps
Squats × 20 reps (increase weight 9kg/20lb once you hit 20, then work back up to 20)
(Two-minute rest)
Leg curl × 12 reps
Calf raises 3 × 15
Behind-neck pull-down × 10
Row × 10
Behind-neck pull-down × 10
(Two-minute rest)
Lateral raise × 8
Press behind-the-neck × 10
(Two-minute rest)
Curl × 8
Underhand chin plus weight for reps
(Two-minute rest)
Tricep extension × 22
Dips × 22[13]

13. Most mortals will need to work up to 22.

o Experiment has, no surprise, faced incredible criticism. For start- vas neither published nor repeated. Casey has been accused of ng weight he'd lost following a car accident. Not one to speculate, I / directly about all of this and more.

swer: he dieted down for two months as instructed pre-experiment (this had alw.ys been transparent) and lost approximately 9kg (20lb) of muscle mass. Casey has no financial interest in the Colorado Experiment more than 20 years later, so I assume this to be the truth. Ditto with his response to questions about anabolic steroid use:

> *There has been a lot of questions regarding steroid use. Many people claimed that I loaded up for this experiment. I can honestly say that there was no use of steroids during this study, which is a very important point. I was closely monitored in a closed-door environment. Believe me, I would have done anything to have gained that weight, but I knew my rebound potential and I also knew I would make remarkable gains even before the study began.*

The equation is undeniable: 4.5st (28.7kg) – 1.4st (9kg) still = 3st (19.6kg) gained in 28 days above baseline. Even if drugs were used, these gains reflect a phenomenal training effect. If you believe that steroids guarantee a gain of 2.14+st (13.6+kg) in four weeks, you should look at clinical studies and real-world users. It just isn't the case.

The real significance of the Colorado Experiment is two-fold, despite the fact that Casey is clearly a genetic mutant.

First, it is physiologically possible to synthesize enough protein to produce 28.7kg (63.21lb) of lean mass in 28 days. This shows that one counter-argument ("you'd have to eat 20,000 calories a day"!) is flawed.[14] This is true even if drugs were involved.

There are mechanisms involved that the simplistic caloric argument doesn't account for.

Second, the workout logs show that the amount of stimulus needed to produce these gains (remember that Arthur also gained just over 1st/6.8kg in 3 weeks) was less than two hours per week.

To quote Casey:

"I was very proud of the results that took place in Colorado and feel that this study has contributed to the awareness of how much time is wasted in most individuals' workouts."

More than four hours per month of gym time is not necessary to reach your target weight in record time. Flip the growth switch and go home.

What to do with your new-found time? That's easy. Focus on eating.

14. Using popular caloric models from published studies, Casey would actually have had to eat approximately 39,000 calories per day to gain this muscular mass. That's 89 McDonald's double cheeseburgers or 97 chicken breasts per day. Even with chicken breasts, poor Casey would have also gained an unfortunate 189 pounds of fat at the same time, according to the same maths, leaving him looking like Cartman on "Weight Gain 4000".

THE MYTH OF 30 GRAMS

How much protein should you eat per meal?

There's a popular (mis)belief that the human body can't absorb more than 30 grams of protein per meal. The science refutes this.

Researchers in France have found that eating protein all at once can be just as well absorbed as spreading it out over your day. A group of 26-year-old women were given either 80% of their protein for the day at one meal or spread over multiple meals. After two weeks, there was no difference between the subject and control groups in terms of nitrogen balance, whole-body protein turnover, whole-body protein synthesis or protein breakdown.

In both subjects and controls, the amount of protein given was 1.7 grams of protein per kilogram of fat-free mass per day. This means that, for a 26-year-old, 8.9st (56.7kg) woman, eating 77 g[15] of protein in one meal had the same effects as spreading it out.

The experiment was then repeated in older subjects, with whom, it turns out, eating protein all at once can actually lead to better protein retention. Giving elderly women 80% of their protein for the day at one meal over a period of two weeks led to almost 20% more synthesis and retention of protein compared to dividing it into smaller doses.

So it appears that daily total protein is more important than per-meal protein.

It's also important to remember that food weight does not equal protein weight. For example, if you weigh near-fat-free chicken breasts on a food scale and the total is 140 grams, it does not mean you're getting even close to 140 grams of protein. In fact, 140 grams contains about 43 grams of protein, less than one-third the total weight. People forget the heaviest piece: water.

A good rule of thumb for daily intake, and a safe range based on the literature, is 0.8–2.5 grams of protein per kilogram of bodyweight. For muscular gain, I suggest at least 1.25 grams per kilogram (pound) of current lean bodyweight, which means you subtract your body fat first. Here are a few examples:

45.4kg (100lb) of **lean** mass = 125 grams of protein
50kg (110lb) = 137.5 g
54.4kg (120lb) = 150 g
59kg (130lb) = 162.5 g
63.5kg (140lb) = 175 g
68kg (150lb) = 187.5 g
72.6kg (160lb) = 200 g
77.1kg (170lb) = 212.5 g
81.6kg (180lb) = 225 g
86.1kg (190lb) = 237.5 g
90.7kg (200lb) = 250 g

Not gaining muscle? Track your protein over one day. Then eat more.

15. 1.7 g/kg * 56.7 kg * 80%.

TOOLS AND TRICKS

***The Concise Book of Muscles* by Chris Jarmey (www.fourhourbody.com/muscles)** World-class strength coach Charles Poliquin introduced me to this outstanding book. It is the best anatomy book for non-medical students that I've ever seen, and I've looked at them all. Get it.

"Strength Training Methods and the Work of Arthur Jones", D. Smith, S. Bruce-Low and J. E. Ponline, *Journal of Exercise Physiology* (www.fourhourbody.com/comparison) This research review compares single-set and multiple-set strength gains. The authors incorporate 112 sources to answer the question: are multiple sets really better than single sets? For muscular growth, it's hard to beat the economy of single sets. For pure strength with little weight gain (see "Effortless Superhuman"), different approaches are more effective.

"Cartman and Weight Gain 4000" (www.fourhourbody.com/cartman) Inspirational weight gain video from our friends at *South Park*. Good pre-dinner motivation for overfeeding.

Arthur Jones Collection (www.fourhourbody.com/jones) This site, compiled by Brian Johnston, is a collection of the writing and photographs of the legendary Arthur Jones, including the original Nautilus Bulletins, "The Future of Exercise", and unpublished works.

OCCAM'S PROTOCOL I

A Minimalist Approach to Mass

It is vain to do with more what can be done with less.

—William of Occam (c. 1288–1348), "Occam's Razor"

30M (100 FT) OFFSHORE, MALIBU, CALIFORNIA

I was sitting on my surfboard 6m (20ft) to the side of Neil Strauss, bestselling author of *The Game.*

The afternoon sun was shimmering off the rolling sets of blue water, and he was catching wave after wave. Me, not so much. In between bouts of falling into whitewash like an injured seal, I mentioned that my next book was a hacker's guide to the human body. Might he be interested in gaining 5 or more kg (10 or more lb) of muscle in four weeks?

He stopped catching waves and turned to look at me:

"Count me in. I'm so in." Neil weighed 8.8st (56.2kg).

The work started four months later. I was now watching Neil take 45 minutes to eat a small seafood entree at the Hawaiian-themed Paradise Cove restaurant. His fork would pause a few centimetres in front of his mouth as thoughts occurred to him, and there it would remain for minutes at a time. It drove me nuts.

This glacial pace was apparently a vast improvement. To prove this, he had e-mailed me an excerpt of an interview he did with Julian Casablancas of the rock band The Strokes:

> JULIAN: You're a very slow eater. You have had a ham sandwich in your hand for like 45 minutes.
>
> NEIL: That's true. I know.
>
> JULIAN: You just have a little bite. I don't know if you're just chewing it, or does the food dissolve in your mouth?

Given no choice, I resorted to feeding Neil spoonfuls of brown rice in between sentences. Neighbouring tables looked on in confusion. The enormous colourful umbrellas sticking out of our coconut-shell "Cocoladas" made the scene even more questionable. It was very bromantic.

Neil had been punished as a kid for taking "Neil bites" and keeping his parents waiting at the dinner table. Not eager to be sent to his room, he developed the habit of stuffing all of the food in his mouth, which often backfired with projectile vomiting across the table.

Gross.

Pausing to sip his Cocolada, Neil said he felt sick. I told him to keep eating. He looked down at his plate and repeated:

"Dude, I really feel sick."

So I once again repeated:

"No, you just don't want to eat. Take bigger bites. You'll adapt." Then, just to be safe, I inched out of vomit range.

Despite the bickering couple routine, I had complete faith: we were, after all, only 48 hours into the protocol.

Then things began to work as planned. Five days later, I received the following text message from Neil:

> Gotta tell you: you're turning me into a ravenous food-devouring machine. And, mentally and physically, between the healthy food, exercise, and Malibu air and surf, I feel frigging great.

The text was prompted by a turning point. He had demolished an entire plate of steak in half the time as his girlfriend's entire family, proceeded to eat what remained of her food, and then continued to vacuum up the steak leftovers. Tapeworm? No, his digestive enzymes and other internal flora had just adapted to the increased food intake, and now he was primed for processing.

Ten days into the protocol, Neil's sex drive was so high that it was almost a problem. His girlfriend had to push him away as if he were a single-minded 19-year-old. High sex drive is, of course, a quality problem, and it's a by-product of vastly increased protein synthesis.

In just over four weeks, Neil, who'd never been able to gain weight, gained 10lb (4.5kg) of muscle and grew from 8.9 to 9.6st (56.7 to 61.2kg), a near 10% increase in total body mass.

The Bike-Shed Effect

The goal of this chapter is to reduce everything to the absolute minimum. Before we get started, we need to discuss the "bike-shed" effect, originally described by C. Northcote Parkinson.

To illustrate this phenomenon, let's compare a conversation about building a nuclear power plant with building a bike shed. Most people rightly assume that they know nothing about something as complex as a nuclear power plant and so won't voice an opinion. Most people wrongly assume, however, that they know something about building a bike shed and will argue until the cows come home about every detail down to paint colour.

Everyone you meet (every male, at least) will have a strong opinion about how you should train and eat. For the next two to four weeks, cultivate selective ignorance and refuse to have bike-shed discussions with others. Friends, foes, colleagues and well-intentioned folks of all stripes will offer distracting and counterproductive additions and alternatives.

Nod, thank them kindly, and step away to do what you've planned. Nothing more and nothing different.

Complicate to Profit, Minimize to Grow

To earn a fortune in the diet and exercise industries, there is a dictum: complicate to profit. To grow, however, you need to simplify.

The objective of the minimalist routine I'll describe is:

1. Not to make you a professional athlete.
2. Not to make you as strong as possible, though strength will increase and the gains will surpass most protocols. Strength is the sole focus of "Effortless Superhuman".

Here is our singular objective: to apply the MED necessary to trigger muscular growth mechanisms, and then channel food preferentially into muscle tissue during overfeeding. There is one condition: we must do both *as safely as possible.*

The safety issue is particularly important to understand when considering exercises. Don't get me wrong; all movements are safe when performed properly.

This includes backflips on one leg, break-dancing headspins and the much-vaunted snatch.[16] The problem with such movements, and dozens of others, is that a minor mistake can cause serious, often permanent, injuries. These injuries are underreported because: (1) those affected don't want to be ostracized from communities that view the moves as gospel, and (2) cognitive dissonance prevents them from condemning a move they've advocated for a long time. So what is used to explain the injury? "I/he/she just didn't do it right." There is underreporting of diet failures (raw food as one example) for similar reasons. In fairness, can you learn to do snatches safely? Sure. But if there are safer substitutes that provide 80% or more of the benefits, I will suggest those substitutes instead.

In more than 15 years of resistance training, I have never been injured following the protocols I will describe here. I suggest adopting one rule of Dr. Ken Leistner, an NFL strength consultant I had the painful pleasure of training with in 1996: the goal of strength training is to reduce injury potential first, and to increase performance second.

16. Yes, in case you missed it earlier, this is a weight lifting manoeuvre.

Occam's Protocol

Recall that coach Matt Brzycki at Princeton nicknamed me "Growth". He has written more than 400 articles on strength and conditioning and dealt with everyone from SWAT teams to NFL teams. What made me different from trainees who didn't grow?

I used hyper-abbreviated training to compensate for mediocre recuperative abilities. It was the self-control to do less.

"Occam's Protocol" is a variation of the consolidation routine used by the late Mike Mentzer, who won the heavyweight class of the Mr. Olympia competition in 1979.

It is possible to get huge with less than 30 minutes of gym time per week. **The following A and B workouts are alternated, whether you choose the machine or free weight option.**

The exercises should be performed for one set each and no more. The objective is to fail, to reach the point where you can no longer move the weight, at seven or more repetitions at a 5/5 cadence (five seconds up and five seconds down). The leg press is to be performed for 10 or more repetitions at the same cadence. The only exceptions to the cadence rule are the abdominal exercises and kettlebell swing, which are described in earlier chapters.

The mechanisms of growth we want to stimulate are both local (muscular, neural) and systemic (hormonal). The longer time under tension (TUT) for the lower body will elicit a greater full-body growth hormone response while also stimulating the formation of new capillaries, which will improve nutrient delivery.

Each workout consists of just two primary lifts.

WORKOUT A: THE MACHINE OPTION

1. Close-grip supinated[17] (palms facing you) pull-down × 7 reps (5/5 count)
2. Machine shoulder press × 7 reps (5/5 count)
   (Optional: Abdominal exercises from "Six-Minute Abs")

17. Med school mnemonic for "supinated": imagine eating "soup" out of a cupped hand.

Pull-down

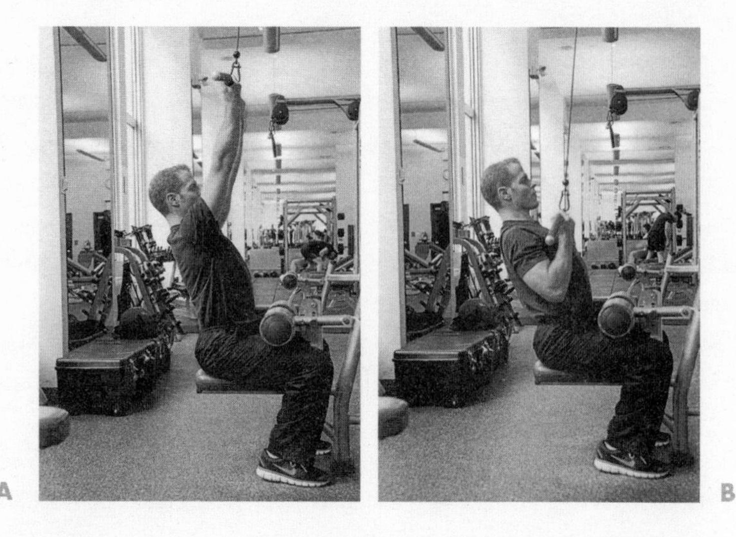

It is critical to record seating settings on all machine exercises. If there are four holes showing in the sliding seat adjustment, for example, note this in your notebook or iPhone. Even 2.5–5cm (1–2in) of difference in starting position can change the leverage and create the illusion of strength gain or loss, especially with pressing movements. Record it all and standardize the movement.

Machine Shoulder Press

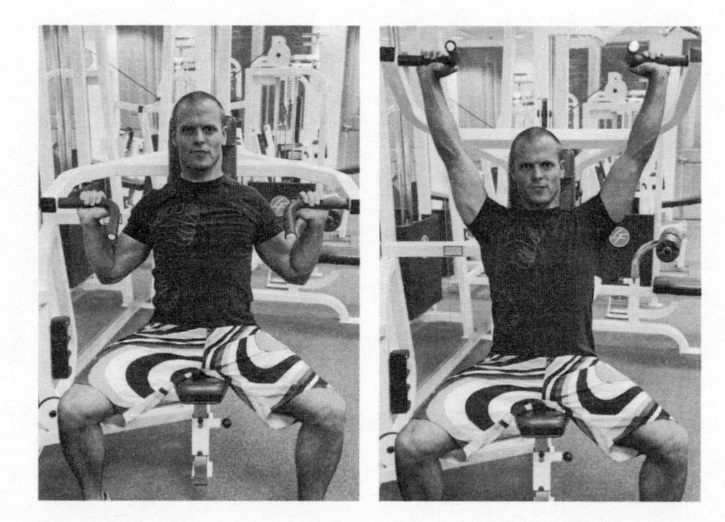

THE LOCKED POSITION

There are a million and one ways to perform exercises.

To keep things simple—and to keep you safe—I will make one recommendation: use the "locked position" to protect your shoulders in all weight-bearing exercises, whether the kettlebell swing, the bench press, the deadlift or other.

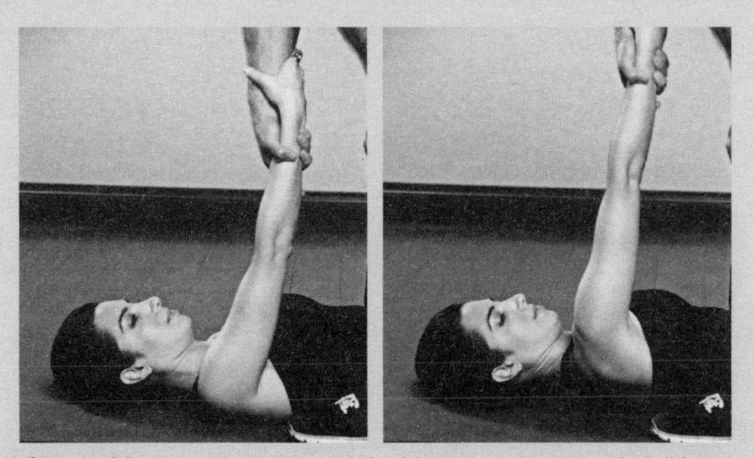

Asking for trouble. From Marie's normal shoulder position, I can easily pull her shoulder forward like a dislocation. Her entire upper body is unstable in both pictures.

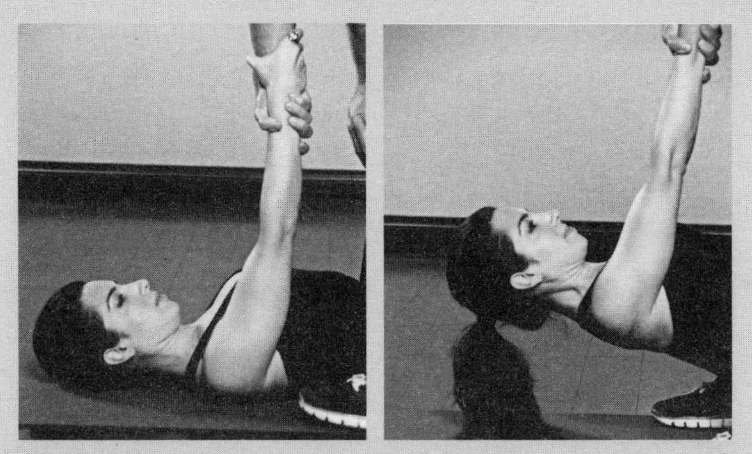

The "locked position." Marie has pulled her shoulder blades back and pushed them down toward her hips 2.5–5cm (1–2in). Notice how you can see her shoulder strap in these photos but not in the first set. There is a slight arch in the back, and if you extend your arms in front of you, the elbows should be closer to nipple height than collarbone height. Marie is now stable, and I can even lift her off of the ground with one arm.

WORKOUT B: THE MACHINE OPTION

1. Slight incline/decline bench press × 7 (5/5 count)
2. Leg press × 10 (5/5 count)
   (Optional: Kettlebell or T-bar swings from "Building the Perfect Posterior" × 50)
3. Stationary bike × 3 minutes at 85+ rpm (to minimize subsequent leg soreness)

Slight Incline/Decline Bench Press (Shown Here: Hammer Machine) If you'll injure your shoulders on any exercise, it will be the flat bench press. For this reason, I suggest a slight (less than 20-degree) incline or decline when possible. For stubborn chest development, Dorian Yates suggests the slight decline. If only flat machines are available, a phone book or thick rolled towel behind the lower back will create a slight decline angle.

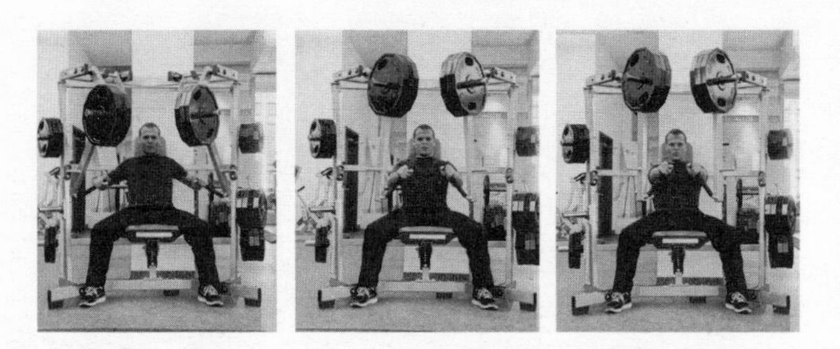

To prevent unnecessary shoulder strain, set the pins in the machine (or seat adjustment) so that your knuckles are one fist width above your chest at the bottom of the movement. I also suggest a one-second pause at the bottom of the movement without touching the weight stack, which will aid in chest development and further reduce risk.

Leg Press

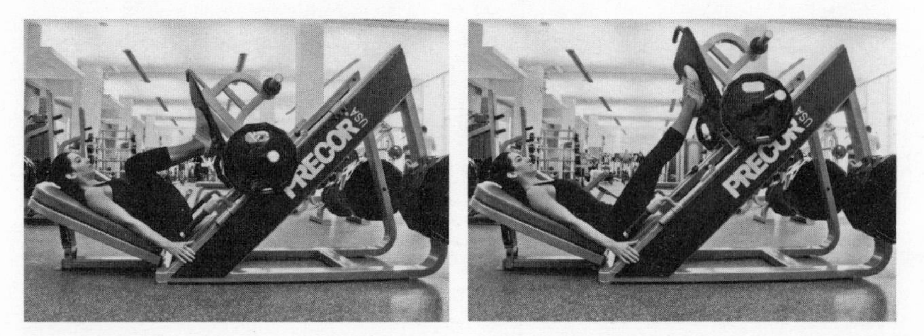

For most trainees, I suggest the above routine incorporating machines.

WORKOUT A: FREE WEIGHT OPTION

Free weights can be used if you prefer them, or if you travel often and need standardized equipment that is the same around the world:

1. Yates row with EZ bar (ideal) or barbell × 7 (5/5 count) (see pictures in the sidebar later this chapter)
2. Shoulder-width barbell overhead press × 7 repetitions (5/5 cadence) (Optional: Abdominal exercises from "Six-Minute Abs")

Barbell Overhead Press The elbows are kept in front of the shoulders and do not flare outward. The bar travels in front of the face, but the head and upper torso move forward to be under the bar once it passes the head. The split stance prevents excessive arching of the back, but a shoulder-width parallel stance can also be used.

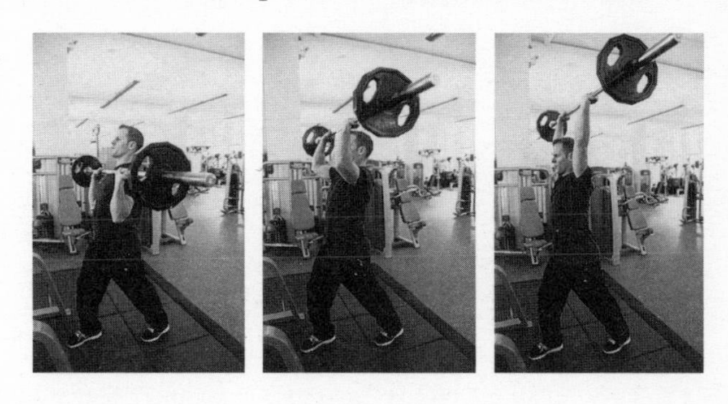

WORKOUT B: FREE WEIGHT OPTION

1. Slight incline bench press with shoulder-width grip × 7 (5/5 count) (If no Power Rack[18] is available, use dumbbells, but you'll often run into problems with adding weight in small increments.)
2. Squat × 10 (5/5 count)
   (Optional: Kettlebell or T-bar swings from "Building the Perfect Posterior" × 50)
3. Stationary bike × 3 minutes (to minimize subsequent leg soreness)

Squat (Shown on the Next Page with Smith Machine) The feet, slightly wider than shoulder width, are placed a foot ahead of your hips. Initiate the

18. These are rectangular frames with pins that can be set at various heights to catch weights if dropped. I train solo and do almost all of my barbell exercises in a Power Rack.

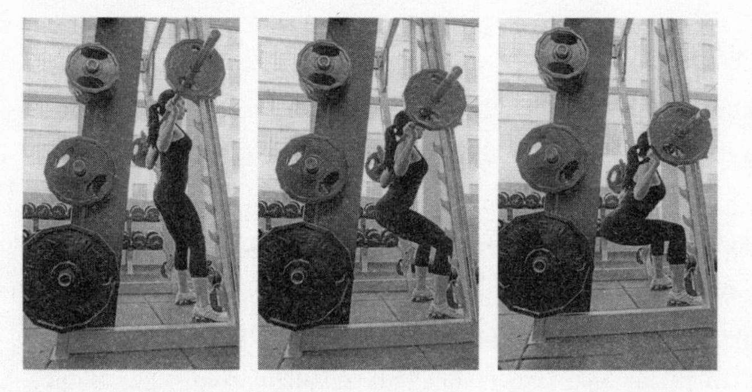

movement by breaking at the hips (imagine pouring water out the front of your pelvis) and sitting backwards, descending to where your thighs are parallel with the ground. Look up at approximately 45 degrees throughout the movement and do not pause at the top or the bottom.

Rules to Lift By

1. If you complete the minimal target number of reps for all exercises (excluding abs and kettlebell swing), increase the weight the next workout at least 4.5kg (10lb) for that exercise. If the additional 4.5kg feels easy after two to three reps, stop, wait five minutes, increase the weight an additional 2.2 to 4.5kg (5 to 10lb), then do your single set to failure.
2. Do not just drop the weight when you hit failure. Attempt to move it, millimeter by millimeter, and then hold it at the limit for five seconds. Only after that should you slowly (take five to ten seconds) lower the weight. The biggest mistake novice trainees make is underestimating the severity of complete failure. "Failure" is not dropping the weight after your last moderately strenuous rep. It is pushing like you have a gun to your head. To quote the ever poetic Arthur Jones: "If you've never vomited from doing a set of barbell curls, then you've never experienced outright hard work." If you feel like you could do another set of the same exercise a minute later, you didn't reach failure as we are defining it. Remember that the last repetition, the point of failure, is the rep that matters. The rest of the repetitions are just a warm-up for that moment.
3. Do not pause at the top or bottom of any movements (except the bench press, as noted), and take three minutes of rest between all

exercises. Time three minutes exactly with a wall clock or a stopwatch. Keep rest periods standardized so you don't mistake rest changes for strength changes.

4. The weight and repetitions used will change as you progress, but all other variables need to be identical from one workout to the next: rep speed, exercise form and rest intervals. This is a laboratory experiment. To accurately gauge progress and tweak as needed, you must ensure that you control your variables.

That's it.

The temptation to add exercises will be enormous. Don't do it. If anything, if you've never been able to gain mass, you might choose to do less. That's what we did with Neil. His programme and progress over four weeks looked like this:

WORKOUT A

Pull-down: 8 reps × 36kg (80lb) → 8 reps × 50kg (110lb)
Machine shoulder press: 8 reps × 14kg (30lb) → 5 reps × 27kg (60lb)

WORKOUT B

Seated dips: 6 reps × 63.5kg (140lb) → 6 reps × 77kg (170lb)
Seated leg press: 11 reps × 63.5kg (140lb) → 12 reps × 86kg (190lb)

Occam's Protocol is enough to stimulate a massive growth response.

Remember our tanning analogy in the beginning of this book? Forget working harder for a minute and realize that biology isn't about blunt force.

Don't add a damn thing.

Occam's Frequency

> Michael, I did nothing. I did absolutely nothing, and it was everything that I thought it could be.
>
> —*Peter Gibbons,* Office Space

The frequency of the A and B Occam workouts is based on a simple premise: you must increase recovery time along with size.

You will exercise less frequently as you increase strength and size, as you can often increase muscle mass well over 100% before reaching a genetic ceiling, but your recovery abilities might only improve 20–30% through enzymatic and immune system upregulation (increased plasma glutamine production, etc.).

Put in simple terms: it takes non-growing repair systems longer to repair a 9kg (20lb) muscle than its 4.5kg (10lb) predecessor. The bigger and stronger you get, the less often you will go to the gym.

Looking at the hypothetical two months below printed from freeprintablecalendar.net, we see that sessions are not scheduled on set days (e.g., Monday and Friday), but are instead spaced apart by set numbers of rest days, which increase over time.

In 1996, while at the Capital University of Business and Economics in Beijing, I grew to 14st (89kg) and was easily the strongest I've ever been. No supplements whatsoever were used, as none could be found. I hit a whole-food ceiling at 6,000 calories per day, as more made me ill, but I was able to resolve all progress plateaus with additional rest days, eventually ending the bulking cycle after four months at 12 days between identical workouts.

< December — January 2011 — February >

Sunday	Monday	Tuesday	Wednesday	Thursday	Friday	Saturday
26	27	28	29	30	31	1 New Year's Day
2 A	3	4	5 B	6	7	8 A
9	10	11 B	12	13	14	15 A
16	17 Martin Luther King Jr. Day	18	19 B	20	21	22
23 A	24	25	26	27 B	28	29
30	31 A	1	2 Groundhog Day	3	4	5

< January — February 2011 — March >

Sunday	Monday	Tuesday	Wednesday	Thursday	Friday	Saturday
30	31 (A)	1	2 Groundhog Day	3	4 B*	5
6	7	8	9 A	10	11	12 Lincoln's Birthday
13	14 St. Valentine's Day B	15	16	17	18	19 A
20	21 Presidents Day	22 Washington's Birthday	23	24 B	25	26
27	28	1 A	2	3	4	5

Two sample months

GETTING STARTED

Step 1: Take at least seven days off of all training that causes significant muscular damage. No bodyweight resistance training or weight training allowed.

Step 2: Begin Occam's Protocol with two days between A and B workouts. After two of both the A and B workouts, increase the rest days between workouts to three days. As soon as you have a workout where more than one exercise has stalled (indicated in our hypothetical calendars with the B*), but not before, increase to four days between workouts.

Continue adding rest as needed to resolve plateaus until you hit your target weight or end your bulking cycle.

Important caveat: this spacing assumes you are consuming enough food to support rapid growth. Of the trainees who fail to gain significant muscular weight (significant = at least 1.1kg/2.5lb per week) on Occam's Protocol, 95%+ of them fail due to insufficient caloric/nutrient intake. The remaining 5% have nutrient absorption issues such as leaky gut syndrome, impaired stomach acid production, excessive fat excretion, insufficient bile, etc., or other conditions requiring medical attention before the protocol can do its job.

I've encountered only one such clinical case in the 5% group. He was 8.8st (56.2kg) at 185cm (6ft 1in), and even when he attempted to gain weight by eating bag after bag of doughnuts in 24-hour periods, he could not gain a single kilogram.

Don't assume you are in this unlikely minority. The most common problem is insufficient food intake.

That leads us to the real challenge of Occam's Protocol.

Eating.

Occam's Feeding

In the 1995 gaining experiment, I set an alarm to wake me four hours into sleep so that I could consume five hard-boiled eggs as an additional meal. It helped, to be sure, but it was also uber-inconvenient. Inconvenient eating schedules, no matter how effective, have a high abandonment rate after initial enthusiasm wanes. I prefer low-friction approaches that are less disruptive, even if it takes a few more weeks to reach my goals. Taking two to four more weeks to reach a mass goal is much better than constant irritability or quitting a program altogether.

Some athletes eat 10 times per day to break up caloric load and avoid excessive fat gain. I find this unnecessarily inconvenient, particularly when you are on a regimen of supplements that increases insulin sensitivity and GLUT-4 activity (see "Damage Control"). I eat four main meals per day for both fat loss and muscular gain.

MY STANDARD NIGHT-OWL SCHEDULE

10:00 A.M.—Wake up, immediately breakfast + ½ shake (details later in this chapter)
2:00 P.M.—Lunch
6:00 P.M.—First dinner

7:30 P.M.—Training, if scheduled (I sip low-fat protein just before and throughout. Neil used Isopure®.)
8:30 P.M. (30 minutes post-training)—Dinner
15 minutes before bed—Second half of morning shake

The meal composition is nearly identical to the Slow-carb Diet, as are the tenets, though we now add a starch such as brown rice or quinoa to the non-shake meals. There is no need to mimic my hours, of course. Just look at my meal spacing as one option that has worked.

Neil was different. He was prone to skipping breakfast and had little appetite. It was impossible for him to consume large meals from the get-go. The solution was to prescribe a calorie-dense shake for breakfast and increase the number of meals to achieve a proper food volume, even with smaller portions.

NEIL'S FOOD SCHEDULE

9:00 A.M.—Protein shake (see below)
11:00 A.M.—Protein bar (Pro Muscle Protein Bar)
1:00 P.M.—High-protein/-carb lunch (usually chicken breast with potatoes)
3:00 P.M.—Protein bar
5:00 P.M.—High-protein/-carb dinner (usually sushi/sashimi with extra rice)
7:00 P.M.—Protein bar
9:00 P.M.—Protein snack with carbs (chicken or eggs or tuna)
11:00 P.M.—Protein shake

The choice is yours: eat big or eat often. Fat gain will be slightly more with the former, and inconvenience will be much greater with the latter.

Pick one and make it your religion for four weeks. It's easy to lose a little extra fat later.

A NOTE ON SKIPPING BREAKFAST

If you skip breakfast even once a week, or opt for a non-breakfast like coffee and toast even once a week, make the blender your first stop after getting out of bed.

The following recipe can also be used as a meal replacement or pre-bed snack:

750ml (24 fl oz) 2% (semi-skimmed) or whole organic milk
30g (1oz) whey protein isolate (chocolate tends to work best)
1 banana
3 heaped tbsp almond butter with no added sugar, maltodextrin or syrups
5 ice cubes

Caloric and protein profile with 2% (semi-skimmed) milk (approximate): 970 cal, 75 g protein

The Fixer: GOMAD

> Everyone on these heavy squat programs who drank enough of it [milk] gained weight. Yes, ***everyone*** we've ever heard of.
> —*Dr. Randall J. Strossen*

If the preceding diet and high-protein snacks don't elicit at least 1.1kg (2 ½lb) per week of gain, add in one litre of 2% organic milk between meals, up to 4l (135 fl oz) per day. Four litres = roughly one gallon. This is the simple and rightly venerated GOMAD (Gallon Of Milk A Day) approach to mass gain, which—along with squats—has produced monsters for more than 75 years, including the incredible Paul Anderson and some of the greatest lifters the world has ever seen.

I suggest adding 1l (32 fl oz) per day each week (often in the aforementioned shake) and keeping a close monitor on fat gain, which can accelerate. Fat gain is not inevitable, but it needs to be monitored. Navel circumference measurements are a good estimation if you don't have access to other body composition devices.

Reader Matt gained 6lb (2.7kg) per week for three weeks (18lb/8kg total) using GOMAD as his only means of increasing calories during his "Geek to Freak" (G2F) trial, and his abdominal skinfold (5cm/2in to the side of the navel) remained 4mm (⅛in) throughout.

If you're eating enough at your main meals, you shouldn't need more than 1l (32 fl oz) per day to accelerate growth. Lactose-intolerant? Try incorporating one glass of organic whole milk per day into your diet. Don't be surprised if you can comfortably consume milk after 1–2 weeks.

For many people, GOMAD or LOMAD (Litre Of Milk A Day) will be the only dietary change required to stimulate growth.

If simple does the job, keep it simple.

Occam's Prescriptions

This protocol works without any supplementation whatsoever.

There are, however, four supplements that I would suggest to those with the budget. The first two minimize fat gain and are covered in "Damage Control" and "The Four Horsemen": **1.** Cissus quadrangularis (2,400 mg, three times per day) **2.** Alpha-lipoic acid (300 mg, 30 minutes before each whole-food meal). Here are the other two:

3. L-GLUTAMINE

L-glutamine is an amino acid commonly used as a post-workout supplement for tissue repair. In our case, I suggest it for an alternative use from strength coach Charles Poliquin: intestinal repair.

The food you ingest does no good if it isn't absorbed. It's like panning for gold with a chain-link fence. The anatomical equivalent of this porous chain-link fence is an assortment of digestive conditions, including leaky gut syndrome, for which L-glutamine has been shown to be a promising treatment.

Rather than risk suboptimal food absorption, consume 80 grams of L-glutamine during the first five days of Occam's Protocol.

I recommend 10 grams at a time every two hours on the dot until the daily 80-gram quota is reached. Powder mixed in water is easiest to consume, but capsules are more convenient for travel. After the initial five-day loading period, if you wish to consume 10–30 grams post-workout, it will speed repair and help prevent soreness.

4. CREATINE MONOHYDRATE

Creatine increases both maximal force production and protein synthesis. Doses of 5–20 grams per day have been demonstrated as safe and largely devoid of side effects, though people with preexisting kidney conditions should use creatine under medical supervision. Athletes generally use a "loading phase" of five to seven days at 10–30 grams per day, but this can cause severe intestinal discomfort. You can achieve the same muscular saturation with lower doses for a longer period of time.

Take 3.5 grams upon waking and before bed for the entire 28-day duration. If you use powder, mix in 5–6 grams total, as losing one to two grams in solution is hard to avoid.

MY FAVOURITE AND EASIEST-TO-CONSUME HIGH-CALORIE MEAL

My single favourite meal for mass is macaroni (preferably durum whole wheat), water-packed canned tuna and fat-free turkey/bean chilli. Use a little whole milk or Irish butter with the macaroni, add only one-third of the orange-flavoured cancer powder and prepare this in bulk.

Mix the macaroni with a can of tuna and as much chilli as you like, microwave it for one minute on high, and have it for breakfast in a bowl. I sometimes ate this meal two or three times per day, as prep time was less than three minutes if I made the macaroni in advance. For a higher-protein change of pace, feel free to substitute quinoa for the macaroni.

It might sound funky, but trust me: this mess tastes delicious.

Lessons From Neil

Neil gained significant muscle for the first time in his life using Occam's Protocol.

Not only did he add 4.5kg (10lb) to his frame in four weeks, he also improved his strength 22.7kg (50lb) on some lifts and doubled others. His minimum improvement was 21.4%. He used machines exclusively and used a dip machine in place of the incline bench press, as the former had less traffic:

WORKOUT A

Pull-down: 8 × 80 to 8 × 110 (+37.5%)
Overhead shoulder press: 8 × 30 to 5 × 60 (+100%)

WORKOUT B

Seated dips: 6 × 140 to 6 × 170 (+21.4%)
Seated leg press: 11 × 140 to 12 × 190 (+35.7%)

There is no need to reinvent the wheel or face challenges alone. Here are some of Neil's notes, in his words, on what to expect and what to do:

"An unexpected side effect of the experiment is how, after the first few days and the initial shock of having to stuff my gullet to the point of feeling ill actually passed, I began to feel incredibly happy and content.

"Like everything, there's a pain period when you step out of your comfort zone. And just when it seems toughest, and you most want to give up (because it's too much time/work/energy, because you don't understand it, because you don't trust it), if you push through that moment, immediately afterward you break free and it becomes a habit that you feel you've been doing all your life (and know you should have been doing all your life).

"The workouts are the least challenging part of it. Going to the gym so rarely and for so short a time left me wanting more. I think the key is, like you told me in the gym, to know that you only grow in those last reps when your muscles want to give up. To really focus and keep pushing to complete failure is an internal battle, so one has to really have the mental strength to keep going when the body wants to quit, rush or use bad form in those last reps.

"My main advice would be to: write out a meal/supplement plan and keep it with you at all times. Have a workout buddy in the gym to push you and help spot. Do this at a time when you aren't travelling and can have a pretty routine schedule. And carry a pack with supplements and protein bars in your car or with you at all times, in case your schedule changes during the day. Interestingly, it was only the first few days when the creatine made me piss like a racehorse; after four days, my body began absorbing it like it should.

"I think my biggest worry was that all the food would just create a tyre around my abdomen, but like you said, it all went to the right places and people noticed . . . there was no downside and no reason not to do this."

TOOLS AND TRICKS

Free Printable Calendar (www.freeprintablecalendar.net) Use this free custom calendar maker to schedule your workouts and rest spacing for each month.

YouBar Custom Protein Bars (www.fourhourbody.com/youbar) Custom design your own protein bars with Pro Muscle Protein Bars, which allows you to choose protein type and dozens of add-ons like cashew butter, chia seeds, goji berries and much more. Anyone can have their own branded (you choose the label type) protein-on-the-go for a minimum of 12 bars. For my preferred mix, search for the "Training 33" bar.

***Parkinson's Law* by Cyril Northcote Parkinson (www.fourhourbody.com/parkinsons)** This is the seminal book on Parkinson's Law, written by Parkinson himself. Everyone you meet will want to tell you how to train and eat. Read this hysterical book to cultivate your selective ignorance of these "bike shed" discussions, which will derail more than help.

FOR MEN: THREE EXERCISES FOR DEVELOPED BICEPS

Biceps are a male obsession. This usually leads to throwing everything and the kitchen sink at them.

In reality, to build large and vascular biceps, there is no need to do isolated arm work.

All you need are two compound exercises (one high-rep and high-speed, and the other low-rep and low-speed) and, if you absolutely must do curls, include one lesser-known version called the "reverse drag curl".

The First Compound Exercise: The Two-Handed Kettlebell Swing
We covered this exercise in detail in "Building the Perfect Posterior". Reps are 50+.

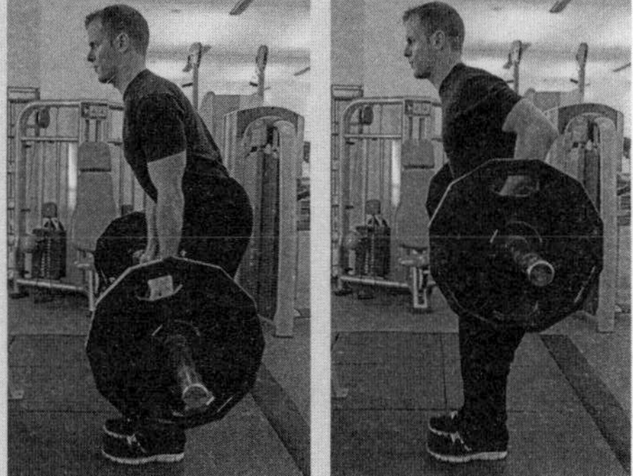

The Second Compound Exercise: The "Yates" Bent Row
Named after six-time Mr. Olympia Dorian Yates, who used it as a staple of his back routine, this exercise is a palms-up bent row performed with a slight 20–30-degree bend at the waist from standing. The bar will generally be at the top of the kneecaps in the bottom hang position. To minimize wrist pain, perform with an EZ bar if possible (here demonstrated with a standard Olympic barbell) and pause for a second at your hip crease, where the bar should make contact.

The Reverse Drag Curl
This exercise, ideally performed with a thick bar, develops the brachialis on the side of the upper arm and provides more constant tension than traditional curls.

Traditional curls often place the elbow under the weight at the top of the moment, minimizing resistance:

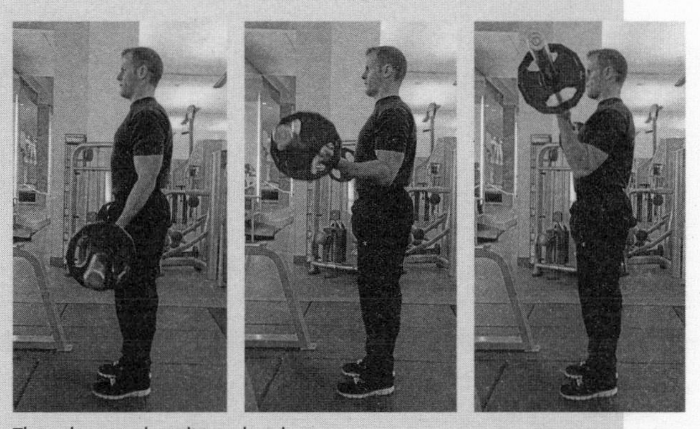

The suboptimal traditional curl

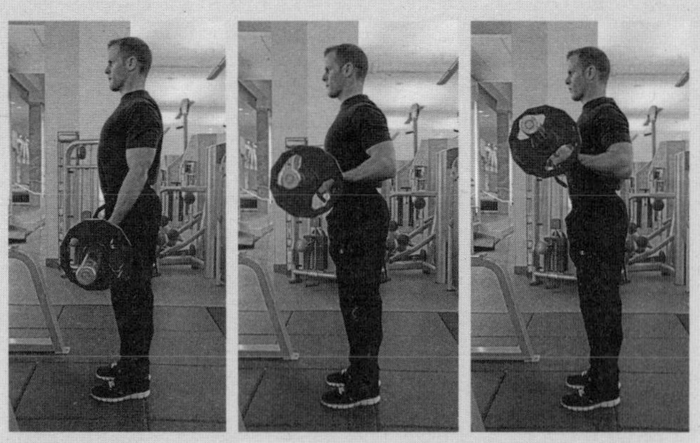
The "drag curl"

The drag curl, in contrast, raises the bar straight up rather than in a circular motion, grazing the front of the body and maintaining tension throughout.

The above photos show a standard drag curl with palms up. To reverse it, as suggested, ensure your palms are shoulder width apart and facing down.

Tempo and reps on both the row and the drag curl are the same as in Occam's Protocol, 5 up and 5 down.

DAVE "JUMBO" PALUMBO—FROM 10 TO 22.6ST (63.5–144KG)

Dave Palumbo was going to become a doctor.

Then, somewhere between running track in college and his third and final year in medical school, he became fascinated by muscular growth. That marked a fork in the path, and he opted to step outside of the laboratory and make himself a real-life experiment.

He weighed less than 10st (63.5kg) when he started in 1986. By 1997, he was 22.6st (144kg) at less than 10% body fat.

In 2008 alone, in addition to training professional athletes and celebrities like WWE star Triple H, he trained more than 150 bodybuilders and physique competitors. Getting to 3.5% body fat or doubling your body mass isn't normal, but that is precisely Dave's forte: creating freaks of nature.

This brings us to the kitchen in 1997, just before his apex of mass proportions.

Dave was standing completely still, braced with his hands on the sink.

He hadn't been gaining weight. Despite consuming six to eight Met-Rx meal replacement packets and four to five whole-food meals per day, the scale wasn't budging. He needed to eat more, but he couldn't chew and digest more solids without regurgitating. It was impossible. He'd reached his solid food limit, so he had to augment with liquid.

His Jewish grandmother harassed him about consuming raw eggs and the risk of salmonella poisoning, so he compromised: 12 eggs mixed in a blender and then microwaved for one minute. That formed the base. The full recipe was four ingredients:

12 warm blended eggs
225ml (8fl oz) apple juice
85g (3oz) uncooked porridge oats
2 scoops whey protein powder

Blending the concoction created a cement-like substance, which he then had to pour down his throat while stationed at the kitchen sink. He'd conditioned himself to inhibit the gag reflex, which was critical, as the sludge moved at a glacial pace down his oesophagus to his stomach.

Just another day at the office.

Then he waited.

Dave had learned from experience—and three times daily cement feedings—that he had to remain perfectly still for 15 minutes, no less, breathing slowly and allowing things to settle. Even shifting on his feet could trigger immediate retching. Stillness was important.

There were times, of course, when the world didn't cooperate.

He had once been late for a training appointment, so he force-fed himself, threw the blender in the sink and jumped in his car to beat the clock. Keep in mind that, at 178cm (5ft 10in) and more than 21.4st (136kg), his legs were only a few centimetres from his stomach when seated. He had outgrown his car.

In minutes, as he rushed through traffic, his mouth began to produce copious amounts of saliva, preparing his digestive tract for rejection. He did his best to achieve a Zen-like state, repeating "Please don't puke, please don't puke, please don't puke," like a mantra. He was almost there.

Dave approached a light, and the car in front of him stopped short.

He slammed on the brakes. This made his stomach slam into his thighs and he projectile-vomited onto the windshield, like Linda Blair in *The Exorcist*, for several long seconds. Not a centimetre of windshield was spared, and nothing remained in his stomach.

Towelling off just enough to see, he raced to his client's house, jumped out of the car and ran up to the front door. "What the hell happened to your car?" was all his client could say as Dave walked past him directly to the kitchen.

It was time to have another shake. The calories were not optional.

Gaining more than 81.6kg (180lb) of muscle is possible, as is squatting with fourteen 20kg (45lb) plates on the bar, but neither is common. Doing the uncommon requires uncommon behaviour. Rule #1 for Dave: eating would not always be for enjoyment.

If you're attempting to gain large amounts of muscular weight, it won't always be enjoyable for you either. This is particularly true for the first week.

Buckle up and get the job done.

OCCAM'S PROTOCOL II

The Finer Points

It's the little details that are vital. Little things make big things happen.

—John Wooden, Hall of Fame NCAA basketball coach (10 NCAA titles in 12 years)

Common Questions and Criticisms

CAN THIS FREQUENCY REALLY BE ENOUGH?

Yes. Doug McGuff MD compares burn healing to muscle tissue healing to explain:

> *Building muscle is actually a much slower process than healing a wound from a burn (which typically takes one to two weeks). A burn heals from the ectodermal germ line, where the healing rate is relatively faster, because epithelial cells turn over quickly. If you scratch your cornea, for instance, it's generally going to be healed in 8–12 hours. Muscle tissue, in contrast, heals from the mesodermal germ line, where the healing rate is typically significantly slower. All in all—when you separate all the emotion and positive feedback that people derive from the training experience—solid biological data indicate that the optimal training frequency for the vast majority of the population is no more than once a week.*

For a much more in-depth discussion of recovery intervals, especially if you're science-inclined, I suggest Dr. McGuff's book *Body by Science.*

HOW DO I DETERMINE STARTING WEIGHTS?

The first A and B workouts will be longer than subsequent workouts, as you need to use trial-and-error to determine starting weights.

Do this by performing sets of five repetitions in each exercise with one minute of rest in between. Cadence should be fast but controlled on the raising and two to three seconds on the lowering. Do not perform more than five reps per set. If you can lift more, wait a minute, increase the weight 4.5kg (10lb) or 10% (whichever is less), and attempt again. Repeat this until you complete fewer than five reps.

After you fail to complete five reps, calculate 70% of your last full five-rep set. Take a three-minute rest and perform a 5/5 cadence set-to-failure using this weight. Congratulations, you just performed your first proper set-to-failure for this exercise, and this weight will be your starting point for Occam's Protocol. For the shoulder press, use 60% of the last successful five-rep set instead of 70%.

Let's look at a hypothetical first workout A, performed on a Monday. Here is how things might look for a semi-trained 10.7st (68kg) male doing the pull-down (weights will differ from person to person of course, and that's why you budget at least an hour for these first workouts):

41kg (90lb) × 5 reps (f/2)[19]
(1-min rest)
45kg (100lb) × 5 reps (f/2)
(1-min rest)
50kg (110lb) × 5 reps (f/2)
(1-min rest)
54kg (120lb) × 5 reps (f/2)
(1-min rest)
59kg (130lb) × 4 reps (f/2) (he failed to complete 5 reps, so 54kg (120lb) was the last full 5-rep set)

19. "(f/2)" indicates "fast but controlled" on the lifting portion and a two-second lowering.

Then we do the maths: 120 × 0.7 = 84, and we round up or down to the nearest weight we can actually use on a machine or bar, which leads us to 39kg (85lb).

(3-min rest)
39kg (85lb) × 8.4 to failure (5/5)

The 8.4 just means your failure was reached at 8 + 4/10 of a repetition.

Take a five-minute rest, then repeat this process with the shoulder press. Once finished with this first workout A, record the target weights you will use for your next A. Since this A was done on a Monday, your next few workouts will look like this:

(Just finished: Monday—Workout A)
Thursday—Workout B
Sunday—Workout A
Wednesday—Workout B
Sunday—Workout A (notice the planned increase to 3 rest days preceding this workout)

HOW DO I ADD WEIGHT?

If you complete your required minimum of reps, add 4.5kg (10lb) or 10% of the total weight in the subsequent workout, whichever is greater. In the example above, we crossed our seven-rep threshold with 39kg (85lb) in the pull-down, so we will increase the weight to 43kg (95lb) for the next workout, as a 10% increase would be less at 42.4kg (93.5lb).

To maintain this rate of progress for even two months, you will need to eat like it's your job. Add shakes or milk if whole food is too difficult.

WHAT IF I MISS A WORKOUT DUE TO TRAVEL?

It is better to take an additional one to three days off than to half-ass a workout with different equipment that makes it impossible to determine progress or proper weights when you return. There is nothing to be lost by an additional one to three days of rest.

The other solution is to always use free weights with standard Olympic barbells, as these will be universal and comparable between facilities. Free-weight options are outlined in the preceding chapter.

WHAT IF I DON'T MAKE THE TARGET NUMBER OF REPETITIONS?

This means one of two things: either you didn't stimulate growth mechanisms (insufficient failure during the last workout), or you haven't recovered (insufficient rest/food).

If you miss your target by more than one repetition on the first exercise of a given workout, go home, take the next day off, then repeat the workout.

Let's say you're scheduled for workout A on a Monday. The first exercise is close-grip pull-downs, and your target number of repetitions is a minimum of seven. If you complete six good repetitions or more, complete the entire workout. If you don't complete six repetitions for pull-downs, do NOT proceed to the shoulder press.

Instead, pick up your gym bag and go home. Rest Tuesday, ensure proper nutrient intake by eating a ton and come in Wednesday prepared to crush both exercises and proceed as planned.

If you fail before the requisite number of reps, do not—as many people do—decrease the weight and do another set (called a "drop-down" or "break-down" set). Do nothing but leave. If you haven't recovered, you haven't recovered. Continuing can easily stagnate you for two weeks or more.

Cutting a workout short takes tremendous self-control and runs counter to gym culture.

Be smart and opt for a 48-hour reboot instead of a two-week or three-week reboot.

Last but not least, if you abandon a workout because you miss a set, add another recovery day between all workouts moving forward. In effect, you're just accelerating the planned decrease in frequency. There is very little downside to doing this. Twenty-four hours of additional time cannot hurt you, but underrecovering will screw up the entire process.

HOW MANY CALORIES SHOULD I CONSUME?

If you fail to gain weight after adding milk and shakes, chances are that you have a medical condition. It shouldn't be necessary to count calories, and I never have.

There is one exception.

If you believe you're doing everything right and still aren't adding kilograms, confirm that you aren't vastly overestimating your food intake and hence undereating. Count calories and weigh food for a 24-hour period.

For recording like this, I use the Escali food scale, which allows me to input the code for a food, provided in an included manual, to determine the protein, carbohydrate, and fat breakdown.

Ensure that you are eating 20 calories per kilogram of lean bodyweight *for 4.5kg (10lb) more than your current lean bodyweight.* Note that this is not necessarily your ultimate target weight (assuming you want to gain more than 4.5kg/10lb). Adjust this target number on a weekly basis.

Let's say you are 11.4st (73kg) lean bodyweight (determined by body composition testing) and want to have 81.6kg (180lb) of lean mass. You would check your diet to ensure that you are consuming 170 × 20 = 3,400 calories. This is the absolute rock-bottom minimum and also applies to non-workout days.

All that said, remember: you shouldn't have to count calories.

Keep it simple and you will gain. If the number on the scale isn't getting bigger, eat more.

BUT WHAT ABOUT CARDIO?

Think you need to hit the stationary bike or run to maintain or improve aerobic capacity? This isn't always the case. Doug McGuff MD explains:

> *If you are intent on improving your aerobic capacity, it's important to understand that your aerobic system performs at its highest when recovering from lactic acidosis. After your high-intensity workout, when your metabolism is attempting to reduce the level of pyruvate in the system, it does so through the aerobic subjugation of metabolism ... since muscle is the basic mechanical system being served by the aerobic system, as muscle strength improves, the necessary support systems (which includes the aerobic system) must follow suit.*

If you're a sprinter or marathoner, can you prepare with weight training alone? Of course not. But, if you're a non-competitive athlete looking to avoid cardiovascular disease, do you need to spend hours spinning your wheels, literally or figuratively? No. The artificial separation of aerobic and anaerobic (without oxygen) metabolism might be useful for selling *aerobics,* a marketing term popularized by Dr. Kenneth Cooper in 1968, but it's not a reflection of reality.

Occam's Protocol develops both anaerobic and aerobic systems.

WHAT IF I'M AN ATHLETE?

Though it depends on the sport, if you are a competitive athlete with frequent sports training, I would suggest a protocol designed for maximal strength gain and minimal weight gain. See "Effortless Superhuman".

WON'T THIS SPEED OF LIFTING MAKE ME SLOW?

Though this programme is not designed for athletes (again, see "Effortless Superhuman" for that), there is no evidence that a 5/5 lifting cadence will make you slow. Let's take a look at one counter-example in a sport where speed is paramount: Olympic lifting.

In 1973, an Olympic weight lifting team with no prior experience was formed at DeLand High School in Florida. Their main training protocol was slow, mostly eccentric (lowering) lifting. The team went on to amass more than 100 consecutive competitive wins and remained undefeated and untied for seven years.

Letting weight training displace skill training is what makes athletes slower. A focus on muscles shouldn't replace a focus on sport. For competitors outside of the iron game, lifting is a means to an end. It shouldn't interfere with other sport-specific training.

WHAT ABOUT WARM-UPS?

Take 60% of your work weight for each exercise in a given workout and perform three reps at a 1/2 cadence (1 second up, 2 seconds down). This is done to spot joint problems that could cause injuries at higher weights, not to "warm up" per se. Prep sets for all exercises should be performed prior to your first real set at 5/5.

In practical terms, the first few repetitions of each work set act as the warm-up. I have never had a trainee injured using this protocol.

HOW SHOULD I WORK OUT WITH A PARTNER?

If you work out with a partner, ensure that your rest intervals remain consistent. Three minutes should not bleed into three and a half because your partner is socializing or slow in changing weights. This is non-negotiable. I have always lifted alone and use training time as near-meditative "me" time, which the counting of cadence reinforces. Many people benefit tremendously from workout partners, but I don't appear to be one of them.

The exercises are chosen to be safe when performed alone. Even if you elect to train with partners, do not let partners help you. It will lead to them lifting the weight while shouting "All you!" This makes it impossible to know how much weight you actually lifted.

Feel free to lift together, but fail alone.

WHAT ABOUT DROP SETS, REST-PAUSE AND OTHERWISE EXTENDING FAILURE?

This isn't needed and screws up your ability to control variables. Keep it simple and follow the rules.

Most advanced trainers who use one-set-to-failure methodologies have observed better results from not extending failure. If you cannot move the resistance, it means you have failed. Extending it just consumes resources that could be applied to growth.

ISN'T X BETTER THAN Y? CAN I [INSERT CHANGE TO PROTOCOL]?

If you want to be a competitive powerlifter, you will need another programme.

If you want to be outstanding in other lifts, you need another programme.

For the purposes of gaining 10+lb (4.5+kg) of fat-free mass in four weeks, however, this programme does not require any modification whatsoever.

If you want something else, choose something else. Otherwise, don't change it.

CAN I JUST WORK OUT EVERY 12 OR 24 DAYS AS GURU X SUGGESTS? I'M STILL GETTING STRONGER.

There are some trainers who advocate training as infrequently as possible to produce strength gains. This can mean one workout per month in some cases.

This isn't a bad thing, but let us make an important distinction:

Doing the least *possible* to *experience* strength gains
v.
Doing the least *necessary* to *maximize* size gain

The latter is the objective of Occam's Protocol.

Tissue growth is our highest priority, even though there will be significant strength gains. Doubling and tripling of your lifts in one to two months, as Neil and other trainees have experienced, is not uncommon.

To support a high rate of fat-free growth, we need to overfeed and direct those excess calories to muscle. This is accomplished by stimulating protein synthesis and increasing the insulin sensitivity of muscle tissue itself through activation (translocation) of the GLUT-4 glucose transporters. Recall from "Damage Control" that the latter is best done through exercise, as we don't want to overdose on insulin.

If you work out just once a month, this might represent one whole-body GLUT-4 window per month for effective overfeeding. This is unacceptable for us, and we'll aim for one workout per week at a minimum.

WHAT TO DO IF YOUR GAINS SLOW WITH ONE SESSION PER WEEK?

Rather than doing one full-body workout every 10–14 days, for example, test a split routine to facilitate strength gains while increasing your GLUT-4 windows to at least two per week.

This is how you get very big, very fast without getting very fat.

I've successfully used the following three-workout split, most notably in 1997:

Session 1: Pushing exercises
Session 2: Pulling exercises
Session 3: Leg exercises

If you are unconditioned or deconditioned (atrophied), take one day between workouts (e.g., pushing, one day off, pulling, one day off, legs, one day off, ad nauseam) for the first two weeks, two days between workouts for the next three weeks, then move to three days between workouts.

The exercises I used, all performed at 5/5, were:

Push:

- Incline bench press
- Dips (add weight when possible)
- Shoulder-width grip shoulder press (never behind the neck)

Pull

- Pullover
- Bent row
- Close-grip supinated (palms facing you) pull-downs
- *Slow* shrugs with dumbbells (pause for two seconds at the top)

Legs

- Leg press with feet shoulder width (do higher reps on this; at least 120 seconds before failure)
- Adduction machine (bringing the legs together as if using the Thighmaster)
- Hamstring curl
- Leg extension
- Seated calf raises

In retrospect, I believe this volume of exercises to be excessive for most trainees. Using the first two exercises listed for each workout will produce at least 80% of the desired gains with less risk of plateauing.

UNDERSTANDING THE SARCOPLASM: ISN'T IT JUST WATER?

"It's just water weight."

This dismissive comment is common in the lifting and diet worlds.

Now, carrying so much subcutaneous water that your head looks like a Cabbage Patch Kid is bad. However, purposefully putting more fluid and substrate in specific parts of muscle tissue can be incredibly useful. There are two different types of muscular growth that you can use to your advantage with a bit of inside knowledge.

The names of both sound complicated—myofibrillar and sarcoplasmic—but the difference is really very simple.

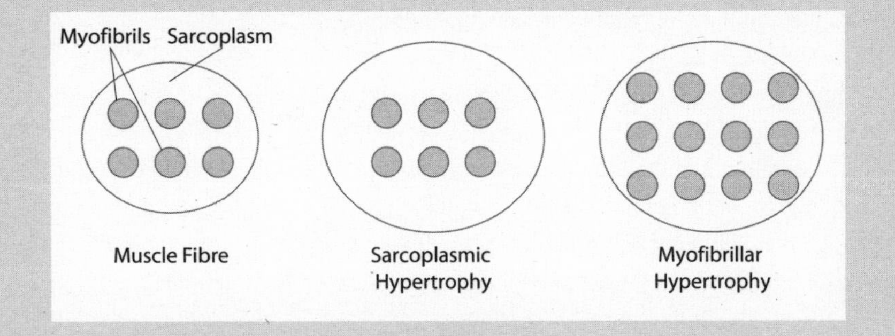

Let's start with a basic primer on muscle fibres.

Every muscle fibre has two main parts: myofibrils, which are cylinder- shaped filaments that contract to create movement, and the sarcoplasm, which is the fluid surrounding the myofibrils that contains glycogen stores and mitochondria to provide energy (ATP).

Myofibrillar hypertrophy[20] can be thought of as growth for maximal strength. The myofibrils in the muscle fibre increase in number, adding primarily strength and some size to the muscle. This kind of muscle growth is achieved by high tension—doing one to five reps at 80–90% of your one-repetition maximum, for example. The strength output is limited to brief intervals, as you're developing fast-fatiguing type 2 muscle fibres.

Sarcoplasmic hypertrophy can be thought of as growth for maximal size or anaerobic fatigue resistance. The volume of fluid in the sarcoplasm increases instead of the myofibrils, adding primarily size and some strength to the muscle. This kind of muscle growth is achieved through metabolic adaptations—doing 8–12 reps to failure at a submaximal 60–80% of your one-repetition maximum, for example.

20. Also called *sarcomeric* hypertrophy.

But which is better? Is sarcoplasmic hypertrophy useless, nothing more than water?

First things first: the claim that it's "nothing more than water" doesn't square with the science. Dehydration of even 4% bodyweight can decrease muscular endurance 15–17%. More relevant to tissue growth, researchers such as Dr. Clyde Wilson of UCSF School of Medicine believe that water effectively acts as a transcription factor—much like testosterone or growth hormone—for protein production. There is evidence that growth factors are triggered by cell volume regulating elements (CVRE) that, in effect, tell DNA to replicate when intracellular hydration is optimal. If that weren't enough, as Dr. Doug McGuff has pointed out, when the water-containing interior of the cell is maximally hydrated, receptors for hormones, "sitting as they do on the surface of the cell membrane, become maximally convexed into the environment where the hormones are circulating, thus allowing for maximal hormonal interaction with the receptor sites".

Just water. Bah.

Second: the sarcoplasmic volume increase is not just a fluid (water) increase. It also corresponds to more mitochondria, more glycogen and larger stores of both adenosine triphosphate (ATP, the energy currency of cells) and phosphocreatine (PC, a high-energy reserve). Not to mention increased capillarization from such training, which results in more efficient nutrient delivery through additional blood vessels.

This is why Neil gained an average of 48.65% strength on his exercises (100% on one) in four weeks using what would be considered a sarcoplasmic lifting protocol. These strength increases are impressive by any measure, myofibrillar or otherwise.

Will Occam's Protocol give you more strength than a protocol specifically designed for maximal strength? No, that's what the chapter "Effortless Superhuman" is for. But can Occam's make you much, much stronger and allow you to surpass most people in the gym? Yes.

The conclusion: to decide on the best programme for you, you need to know your objective.

As usual, the more specific your goal and the more precise your training, the better your results will be.

IMPROVING SEX

THE 15-MINUTE FEMALE ORGASM

Part Un

The pleasure of living and the pleasure of the orgasm are identical. Extreme orgasm anxiety forms the basis of the general fear of life.

—Wilhelm Reich, Austrian psychologist (1897–1957)

An orgasm a day keeps the doctor away.

—Mae West, American actress and sex symbol (1892–1980)

9:00 P.M., OSHA THAI RESTAURANT, SAN FRANCISCO

My Thai food hovered between my plate and my mouth, broccoli dangling off the fork. Then it fell. I was focused more on the conversation than the eating.

"For almost all women, the most sensitive part of the clit will be the upper-left-hand quadrant from their perspective, around one o'clock from the man's perspective."

Tallulah Sulis, a specialist in female ejaculation, paused to take a sip of water and raised her eyes to meet mine:

"Sometime you should really try and meet Nicole Daedone."

Tallulah was an old friend, and had now become my first orgasm consigliere. I wrote the name down on a note, and we meandered from our love-life catch-up to other topics.

Two hours later, we settled the bill and I walked her to her car. As we ambled over the pedestrian crossing, I turned to her and joked:

"Now all I need to do is find a beautiful single girl who's never had an orgasm."

It was a funny ending to a funny night.

Little did I realize how important the note in my pocket would become.

The Quest

Exactly 24 hours later, serendipity entered stage left.

I was enjoying French food and a bottle of Bordeaux with a 25-year-old female yoga instructor new to San Francisco, fresh from the Midwest. Talk drifted to the singles scene and then to her culture shock in places like the Castro, where drag queens and transsexuals have dinner next to dot-com millionaires. Nothing is taboo, and she was just getting acclimatized. SF is, after all, the world's capital city of sexual exploration.

Several glasses further into the evening, she casually admitted that she'd never experienced an orgasm. How we got to that topic, I don't remember, but I looked around to see if God was playing a trick on me. I've never won the Powerball lottery, but I felt like I had.

My daydream was interrupted when her follow-up comment slapped me back to reality:

"It's fine, though. I've realized that sex just isn't that important."

Time-out.

"What?!" I blurted, a little too loudly. (Thank you, wine.)

This gorgeous woman in her prime, let's call her Giselle, had compartmentalized sex as an unimportant and uninteresting activity. As the drinks flowed and we continued to talk, it became clear that this rationalization was a direct product of her inability to fully enjoy it.

And so it came to be that I made her a drunken promise: I would fix her inability to orgasm. Not that night, not necessarily through me,[1] but somehow.

In retrospect, it was a foolish and overconfident promise. But with

1. C'mon, people. I'm a *professional*.

alcohol-induced optimism on my side, I viewed it as a watershed moment, an opportunity to harness my OCD for the greater good.

Most men assume they kinda-sorta understand female anatomy, but—the upper-left quadrant at one o'clock? That was a new one.

Tallulah had given me a glimpse of a different world altogether.

Later that evening, somewhere between Wikipedia and PornHub, I realized Giselle wasn't alone. Sex researcher Shere Hite had long ago concluded that 70% of U.S. women couldn't experience orgasm from intercourse, and Alfred Kinsey's data suggested that up to 50% of U.S. women weren't able to achieve orgasm at all.

My quest for the elusive female "O" had begun.

The outcome, four weeks later, was better than I ever could have imagined.

I was able to facilitate orgasms (the word *facilitate* will be explained later) in every woman who acted as a test subject.[2]

The results: those who'd never experienced manual-only orgasm were able to do so, and those who'd never experienced penetration-only orgasm were also able to do so. The success rate was 100%.

Here is what I learnt.

The Process

The morning after wine with Giselle, I wrote down a number of questions that seemed like good starting points. Several of them related to extending male endurance, if that were to prove a limiting factor. I figured I might need to train men to become Energizer bunnies.

Some of the assumptions, reflected in the wording, turned out to be totally wrong, but here are my original questions:

1. How do you tweak the most common sexual positions to make it more likely that the woman will orgasm?
2. How can you reduce the refractory periods (the erection-impossible period after ejaculation) for men? This would allow more sessions per night.

2. How do you legally get eager test subjects? That's a topic for another book.

3. Is it possible for men to have multiple orgasms without ejaculating?[3]
4. How do you keep *it*—the hoo-ha, that is—from stretching out over time? (A female friend insisted I throw this one in.)[4]

Once I had questions, I needed some answers. For that I would need two things: experts and lots of practice.

First things first: experts.

There is no shortage of how-to sexual information. From Chigong Penis (competes with the Iron Penis Kung-Fu school, not kidding) to orgasm training on elaborate vibrator-saddle machines like the Sybian, it's a paradox-of-choice problem. Considering the options, I started to think that I might be re-enacting *The Snow Leopard* by Peter Matthiessen.

In 1973, Peter travelled with zoologist George Schaller 423km (250 miles) into Himalayan no-man's-land in search of the near-mythical snow leopard. Not to be a spoiler, but he didn't find the goddamn cat. He saw rare mountain sheep, foxes, wolves—even signs of the snow leopard itself—but it was never found.

Fortunately, Peter's experience led to a Buddhist-like search for meaning and a beautiful classic in nature writing. I doubted I could pull the same beauty out of Iron Penis Kung-Fu. My quest was all-or-nothing, and it needed a happy ending in all senses.

I had no choice but to narrow down the field, to find someone who'd already tried everything.

There was only one place to look.

Nina and 400 Hollywood Nights

Nina Hartley became a registered nurse in 1985 after graduating magna cum laude from San Francisco State University.

She also started stripping during her sophomore year, which led to experimenting in adult films. It was not a college phase. Nina has since

3. Short answer: yes. But if you don't have a stamina problem, this often aggravates the woman and robs her of the psychic payoff of bringing you to orgasm. Not a fan. If you want to extend your stamina, I recommend breathing and better positioning.
4. Ladies, this is answered in the sidebar and resources of the next chapter.

starred or featured in more than 650 porn films and is one of the most recognized and respected names in the business. Lexington Steele, the only person ever to win the AVN (the Oscars of porn) Male Performer of the Year Award three times (three times!), has publicly stated "without hesitation" that the single greatest sexual experience of his life was with Nina.

My friend Sylvester Norwood[5] later told me the same thing.

But . . . WTF?

His confession confused me. Not because I doubted Nina had the skills. But how the hell did Sylvester enter the picture? The same well-behaved Jewish boy too shy to talk to girls?

[Shimmer and fade to re-enactment] Straight out of *Ripley's Believe It or Not*: Sylvester's mum attended a group dinner in Berkeley, California, that Nina also happened to be attending, and the two ended up seated next to each other. Mrs. Norwood came home and said to then-22-year-old Sylvester, "Guess who I was at dinner with? A famous porn star: Nina Hartley. Have you ever heard of her?"

Sylvester nearly choked. In his secret double life, he had a huge collection of videos featuring Nina, his personal snow leopard.

"Mum, I have to meet her. If I never do anything again in this life, I MUST meet Nina Hartley."

Three days of insistent begging and nagging later, Sylvester's mom raised a hand and picked up the phone.

"Hi, Nina, it's Mrs. Norwood. I had such a wonderful time meeting you at the party. Listen, I have a question for you. Do you ever make love to younger men?"

Nina's answer: "Why, yes! I love breaking in younger men . . . but only once."

And so it happened.

Summary: Coolest. . . mum. . . ever.

A decade later, Sylvester is still friends with Nina, and he introduced us via e-mail. The two-hour phone call that followed was a master's degree in all things sexual, but the most actionable highlights related to (1) the single most important precondition for female orgasm and (2) technical modifications of positions.

5. Not his real name. I've immortalized his cat's name in the tradition of porn name creation: childhood pet's name + the street you grew up on.

THE PRECONDITION: WOMEN NEED TO STEP UP TO THE STARTING LINE FIRST

"No man can *give* you an orgasm. He can only help you do it yourself."

This is why I used the word *facilitate* earlier. First and foremost, Nina emphasized, a woman has to be comfortable masturbating. "If she doesn't masturbate regularly, she'll be more trouble, baggage-wise, than it's worth, unless you get off on being the fixer. She has to at least come up to the starting line and be comfortable conversing with her own orgasmic potential." For years, Nina herself was too embarrassed to show her "O face"—her face during orgasm—to partners, thinking it was ugly or unattractive, not realizing that men go nuts for it. "The woman needs to know how beautiful and exciting she is in that state."

Truer words never spoken.

To those women who don't masturbate, Nina recommends starting in small increments, five minutes a night before bed or immediately after waking up, and listening to self-talk. What is your head telling you? Unwarranted guilt and shame? Both will pass with practice, and you must be comfortable solo before it's possible with someone else.

Thirty minutes after the interview with Nina, I called Giselle.[6] The verdict: she never masturbated.

She was the eldest daughter in her family, an unexpected recurring theme I found among inorgasmic women, and had been raised Catholic. Her mother used scare tactics with religious overtones, repeating phrases like, "I hope your decision to abstain includes remembering your faith." This fuelled a feeling of obligation to be a role model for her younger sisters, and the end product was predictable: she disallowed herself pleasure, viewing it as a hazard, and was now well on the path to asexuality.

Step 1: I gave Giselle, who'd agreed to play along, the book *Sex for One* by Betty Dodson,[7] along with a homework assignment to masturbate prior to bed for five minutes each night.

Then I crossed my fingers.

The next few weeks would show if her discomfort and disinterest could be fixed through simple conditioning.

6. Giselle is a composite of several subjects from here forward.

7. Recommended by Nina and dozens of other sex educators. Giselle found this book a bit too over-the-top due to rather creepy illustrations and a group sex description in the beginning. She preferred *I Love Female Orgasm: An Extraordinary Orgasm Guide* by Dorian Solot, later given to her by an enthusiastically orgasmic female friend.

In boxing, there is an expression: "Everyone has a plan until they get hit." For Giselle and other women I later interviewed, it seemed that they often had Rocky-like sexual confidence until game time with a partner, when all the buried insecurities surfaced despite (or perhaps because of) their best efforts to suppress them. It was practice facing these demons that they needed, not better self-talk. Masturbation it was.

I hoped five minutes of nightly homework would be enough.

THE POSITIONS: PRECISION AND PRESSURE

Nina emphasized two slight modifications to most positions:

1. **Changing the angle** of penetration so that the head of the penis makes more contact with the female g-spot, which is generally about a quarter (or 10 pence) in size and 2.5–5cm (1–2in) inside the vagina on the top side. If the male inserts an index finger up to the second knuckle (palm up), and makes a come-hither motion, the fingertip should touch a sponge-like tissue or be within an inch of it. This is the g-spot.
2. **Changing the pressure** of the position so that the man's pelvic bone is in direct contact with the clitoris.

The descriptions that follow are based on Nina's suggestions, as well as my [cough] research testing. The three positions described were chosen because the woman need not necessarily stimulate herself, as would be the case in doggy style.

Improved-angle Missionary

On the facing page, notice that the woman's hips are elevated on a pillow to tilt her hips towards her head. Nina suggests buckwheat hull pillows, which are firm and, unlike foam or feather pillows, don't collapse. I fell in love with them in Japan, as the hulls conform to your head and neck to offer the perfect night's sleep. They conform equally well to female buttocks, while keeping them a perfect 15cm or so (6in or so) off the bed.

The man then moves his hips as close as possible to the woman's hips while keeping his heels under his buttocks. He should be sitting Japanese-style, sitting on heels with knees spread as wide as is comfort-

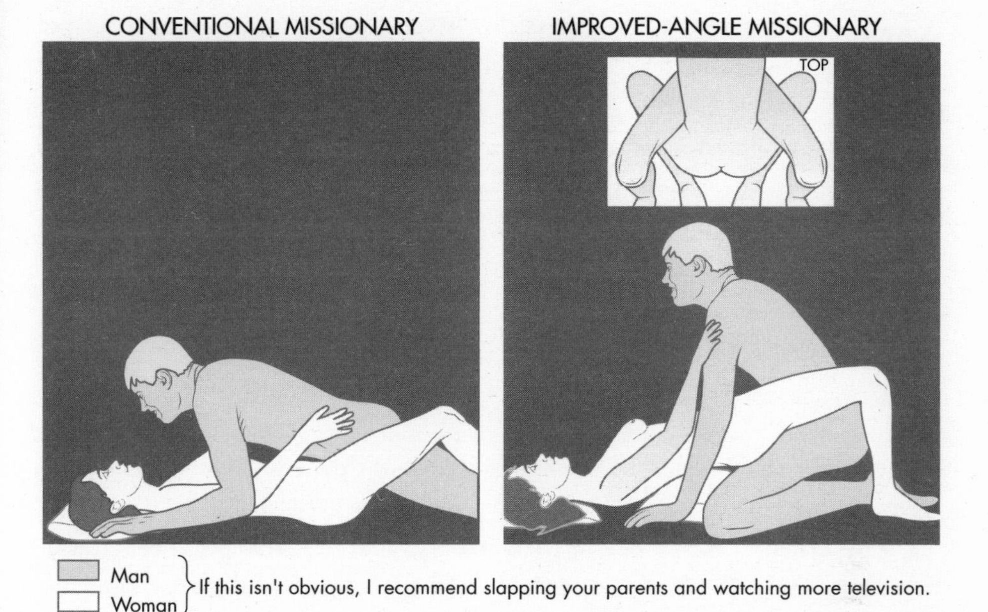

able. The lower he keeps his hips, the better the angle to hit the g-spot.[8] Experiment with different depths of penetration. Using a rhythm of nine shorter half-length penetrations with one long is particularly effective. Use the bottom of the opening of her vagina as a fulcrum for the penis, which will act as a lever.

The woman should test (a) pulling her knees towards her chest to tilt her hips towards her, and (b) placing her feet flat on the bed to elevate her hips. One will usually feel awesome, while the other will feel awkward.

Note for the big gents on long strokes: if your penis is apt to hit her cervix in this position, which is not pleasant for women, "open up" one hip, as they say in the adult film business. Putting her bellybutton at twelve noon, aim your penis at ten or two o'clock. This works for all positions where deep penetration is possible (doggy style, knees on shoulders, etc.). Pain isn't sexy unless the woman tells you it is.

Improved-pressure Missionary

To accomplish this position, the male must shift his weight forward a few centimetres. First, he must straighten his legs (bringing them closer to-

8. In doggy style, if you wish to expand your repetoire later, the woman would want to keep her hips as low as possible.

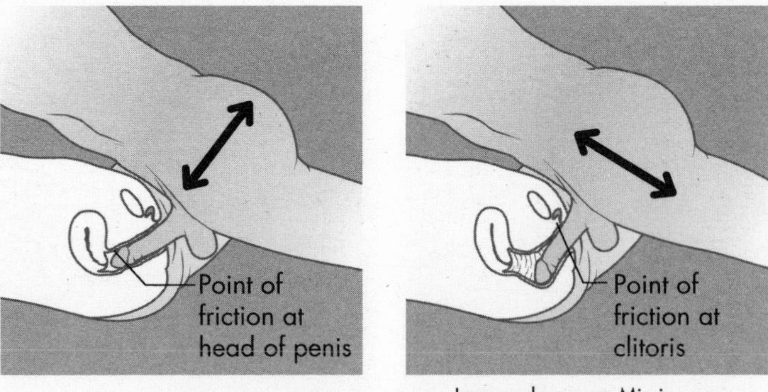

Improved-pressure Missionary

gether makes this easier) so the knees are off of the bed. Then he'll support more weight on her pelvis (the entire purpose) and his arms.

This changes the angle of penetration so that the focal point of friction is no longer the head of the penis against the vaginal wall, but rather the man's pelvic bone on the woman's clitoris. This kills two birds with one stone: the man can last far longer, and the woman receives direct clitoral stimulation.

This modification was recommended by Nina, but she is not alone.

Tallulah was emphatic: "The number-one move I would offer to men is the targeted pelvic grinding in this position, either moving the hips in small circles or slowly side to side."

I later found bracing the abdomen muscles, even extending them a bit, and rocking the hips back and forth in a short 2.5–5cm (1–2in) motion to be most effective. Imagine that, from just below your navel to the base of your penis, you are connected to the woman—never lose contact with the clitoris. If you do this right, expect to feel like you did 1,000 sit-ups the next day.

Just as one friend said to me as I ground the gears of my car on a steep hill in San Francisco:

"If you can't find it, grind it."

Bad advice in cars, good advice in girls.

Conventional Cowgirl Position v. Improved-pressure Cowgirl Position

Improved-pressure cowgirl puts the woman on top and re-creates the same penile position as in improved-pressure missionary.

CONVENTIONAL COWGIRL

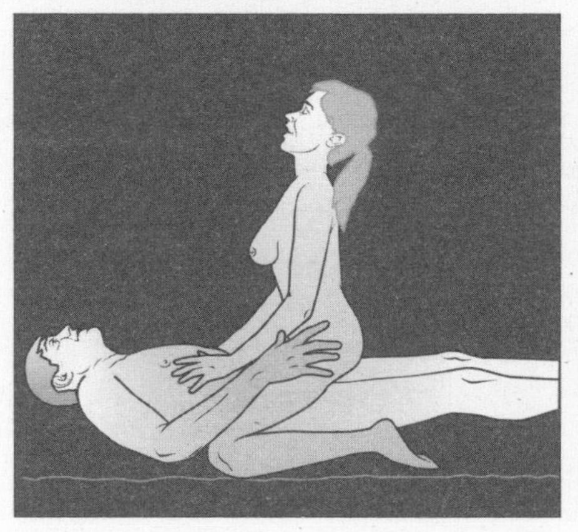

IMPROVED-PRESSURE COWGIRL

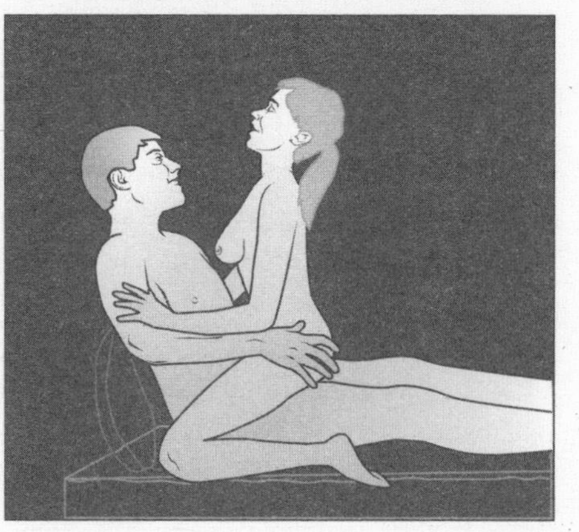

The man should not be flat on his back, nor should he be sitting straight up. He should be leaning back about 20 degrees. This can be accomplished with pillows on a bed or, ideally, on an armless chair with a back that the woman can hold on to. The advantage of this position is simple: the woman can control the motion.

Professor Nina offers the following advice for all intercourse: "When in doubt, you supply the pressure and she provides the movement."

The male can hold a vibrator to the clit in this position, but I opted not to because of the risk of distraction on both sides. As Nina-san sayeth: "A vibrator can be a girl's best friend, or it can be as annoying as a mosquito."

I could always bring in the heavy artillery after the fact, but I wanted to be ready for empty-handed encounters. I wanted to deconstruct the orgasm, and create it at will, without any tools.

That's when the note in my pocket became the keys to the kingdom, which we explore in the next chapter. That's also where we'll learn what happened with Giselle.

TOOLS AND TRICKS

Buckwheat Hull Pillows (www.fourhourbody.com/buckwheat) Bucky manufactures comfy pillows filled with natural buckwheat hulls. Buckwheat hulls are lightweight, durable, and fit the contours of your body without getting flattened like normal pillows. The hulls are hypo-allergenic and allow constant air circulation through the pillow, keeping you cool. Perfect for better sleep and better sex.

Liberator Bedroom Adventure Gear (www.liberator.com) Spice up your bedroom with all the Liberator sex gear you can afford. The website is explicit, and I want to hire their photographer (or maybe it's just the female models?). If nothing else, the "wedge" is a must-purchase item (www.fourhourbody.com/wedge). Enough said.

Beautiful Agony (www.beautifulagony.com) Beautiful Agony is a bizarre but oddly hypnotic experiment. The site features videos that users submit of their "O" faces. It may be the most erotic thing you've ever seen, yet the only nudity it contains is from the neck up. Perhaps it's just me, but I wish they had a "Would you like to see men or women?" landing page.

SexWise with Nina Hartley (www.sexwise.me) This is where Nina explores and explains it all. Based on the belief that most sexual "problems" are conflicts between true sexual nature and what you've been taught to believe is acceptable, nothing adult, legal and consensual is taboo on this site.

Tallulah Sulis (www.tallulahsulis.com) Tallulah is a female ejaculation expert. She was the first to introduce me to the missile coordinates that form the basis for the next chapter.

***I Love Female Orgasm: An Extraordinary Orgasm Guide* (www.fourhourbody.com/loveorgasm)** This book, given to Giselle by a female friend, was so good that she suggested I make it my default recommended reading. It uses levity and humour to explain how to have an orgasm during intercourse (and why most women don't), detailed advice on how to have your first orgasm, and advice for better oral sex, among other things. Anecdotes from real-world couples create an experimental eagerness around topics that might otherwise be intimidating. It's a great book.

THE 15-MINUTE FEMALE ORGASM

Part Deux

Parental Guidance Suggested: If graphic illustrations of female anatomy bother you, you might want to skip this chapter. For real. It's vajayjay galore.

There's very little advice in men's magazines, because men think, "I know what I'm doing. Just show me somebody naked."

—Jerry Seinfeld

Stupid Animals

Below is a composite scene that repeats itself millions of times per night around the world:

Man finally gets to go downtown and fumbles to get his hand where it counts.
Man starts random up-and-down or circular motion, hoping to God he can hit the spot and not act surprised.
Woman moans and man thinks he's doing well.
Woman stops moaning.
Man shifts technique or goes into hyperdrive, and woman asks him to slow down a bit.
Man slows down, and exactly five seconds of mild positive response later, nothing.
Man feels like a dog trying to open a door with no thumbs.
If he's out to beat the clitoris, dead or alive, as most men are, woman gently stops his increasingly erratic attack after 10 minutes.
Best case, they move on to something the man can understand, like penis in vagina.
He's a stupid animal, folks. Have mercy.

Clitoral Confusion

The clitoris looks something like an Imperial Guard from Star Wars.

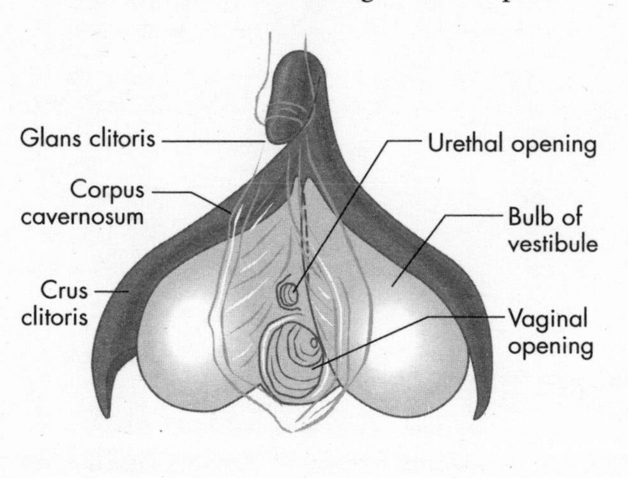

It's also much larger than most people realize. The clitoral glans, what most refer to as the "clit", extends back and splits into an upside-down V. Those legs, the clitoral crura, are concealed behind the labia minora. Some researchers believe that "g-spot" stimulation is actually stimulation of the crura and that all orgasms originate from stimulation of the clitoris.

Other researchers, mostly male, disagree.

This is nothing new. Men have been arguing about the clitoris for 2,500 years.

It all (seemingly) started in 1559. Realdo Colombo of the University of Padua in Italy announced the discovery of the clitoris and planted his flag: "Since no one has discerned these projections and their workings, if it is permissible to give names to things discovered by me, it should be called the love or sweetness of Venus." Gabriele Falloppio, Realdo's successor and later of Fallopian tube fame, refuted his claim, as did Italians, Danes and every Y chromosome in between.

Hippocrates actually had Realdo beat by more than 1,300 years, but the clitoris seems to periodically go into hiding, often for decades at a time. Is it real? Is it an illusion? Is it alive? Is it dead? No one knew until it made a sudden reappearance, like Osama bin Laden on CNN.

It's not hard to understand why men pretend it doesn't exist. If it doesn't exist, or if it's unpredictable, men can write it off as a female problem. If it's purely a female problem, men can't have their egos crushed like a grape between Serena Williams's buttocks.

Clitoral Confidence

Leaving dinner with Tallulah, I became fixated on the idea of a hypersensitive upper-left quadrant on the clitoris. Could it really be that straightforward?

I walked home from the restaurant that evening and jumped on my laptop to begin researching the one method Tallulah had mentioned by name: the Doing Method.

Seventy-two hours later, I tested the upper-quadrant technique on a willing test subject who'd never experienced an orgasm from finger-only stimulation. Two strong peaking orgasms and an extended 15-minute continuous orgasm later, I was shocked speechless.

It worked on the first shot.

But it was still guesswork, and I needed to make the technique bulletproof. To do that, I would need to meet not just *a* master but *the* master.

Luckily, I had her name on a little scrap of paper: Nicole Daedone.

Origins: More University

Lafayette Morehouse was established by Dr. Victor Baranco in 1968 on Purson Lane in Lafayette, California.

Operating as More University from 1977 to 1997, it was a commune founded on the ideal of "responsible hedonism". The residents painted the buildings and automobiles on the property purple, and their newsletter explained the rationale:

> *We tell people that all the houses here are purple so that there is no mistake that one has changed realities should they wander onto our property.*

If people missed the purple, there were other warning signs for wanderers.

In the 1960s, Baranco and his wife, Suzie, began researching how to improve their sex lives. Both believed that the amount of sensual pleasure available to an individual far exceeded the expectations commonly held in society.

In 1976, after more than a decade of experimentation, they blew the floodgates open by giving the first public demonstration of female orgasm. It lasted *three hours.* That's a genital *Dances with Wolves.* The female student who demonstrated the orgasm, Diana, recalled the result it had on the wall-to-wall audience:

> *When that demonstration was over, people RAN to every available space on the property so that they could get off, too . . . get the women off! It was really the women.*

Not surprisingly, students flocked to Morehouse.

Two students of the Morehouse methods for extending orgasm were Drs. Steve and Vera Bodansky, founders of the Doing Method I had taken for a test drive.

Another was Ray Vetterlein, who took his first class at Morehouse in 1968, eight years before the public demo. He earned its highest private qualification in 1989 and has been refining his methods ever since. . . for more than 40 years.

8,000 Nerve Endings and Two Sheets of Paper

Less than a month after dinner with Tallulah, I was witnessing some of Ray's findings first hand.

"You want to use about two sheets of paper worth of pressure," explained my chaperone Aiko,[9] who had organized the visit and was sitting to my right.

Roger that.

"Go by how it feels, not by how it sounds."

I scribbled down notes as four OneTaste practitioners, two seated next to me and two on the floor, demonstrated and explained the fine-tuning I needed. OneTaste was founded in 2001 by Nicole Daedone, a student of Morehouse and Vetterlein, to give women a clean and brightly lit place to learn about orgasm from another woman. I'd met with Nicole the afternoon before, and our conversation had started at neuroscience and ended with me recounting my trial run of the Doing Method. One thing was clear to her: there was much room for improvement.

9. Not her real name.

Now I found myself at OneTaste's coaching location in the SOMA district of San Francisco.

Their expansion in both New York City and California has been funded largely by Reese Jones, who sold his software company Netopia to Motorola for $208 million (£130 million). The "slow-sex" movement thus began and Nicole was its default leader.

In San Francisco, I was playing Larry King: "So, can I ask exactly where you are touching the clit now? It's still an upward motion?"

I was positioned on an office chair with my elbows on my knees, looking down at the woman's vulva from about 1.5m (5ft) away, where she and her male partner were positioned on pillows and throw rugs.

"You can get closer," said Aiko.

"Sure. Get as close as you need to," added the woman on her back.

So I did. I watched from a distance of about 60cm (2ft), sometimes closer, as the woman's entire physiology changed over 15 minutes, asking questions and watching the man's technique.

Then it was my turn.

"Are you ready?" Aiko asked.

"Ah . . . sure." Personal clitoral coaching was the last thing I thought I'd be doing at 10:00 A.M. on a weekday, but I already had four pages of detailed notes. If I didn't put theory into practice, none of it would make sense later. So on went the latex gloves.

My research partner arrived, and we repeated what I'd just seen. The two coaches who'd been sitting next to me earlier were now seated in front of me, kneeling about 91cm (3ft) from the woman's clitoris. They reached in occasionally to correct my hand position and offered intermittent suggestions ("Ensure your forearm is parallel to her body") or encouragement ("Good stroke!").

It was like playing for the coolest Little League team in the world. Go, Timmy, go!

My partner experienced all of the involuntary muscle contraction I had hoped for, and the group coaching, though a little weird, wasn't uncomfortable in the least.

Aiko asked me if I had any feedback after the session ended.

I did.

"This should be required education for every man on the planet."

A MORE USEFUL DEFINITION OF ORGASM

Orgasm, as defined by most women, is not gratifying. It's an all-or-nothing pressure that prevents the very phenomenon we're after. For purposes of practising what's in this chapter, the following definition of orgasm is the most useful composite I found:

> *Orgasm is when there is no resistance—no physical or emotional blocking—to a single point of contact between one finger and the clitoris.*
>
> *This state naturally leads to the involuntary contractions and flushing that most associate with the word* orgasm.

Diana, the original Morehouse demo subject, concurs:

> *I think, for men and for women, it's true that when you feel "this is it from the first stroke", that it really gets better from there.*

The Practice and How-to: The 15-minute Orgasm

I believe the two principal reasons the OneTaste method works so well is that (1) it is presented as a goalless practice, and (2) it decouples orgasm from sex.

Kissing, fondling, disrobing, whispering and requesting are all fun and wonderful parts of sex. Unfortunately, multi-tasking these actions often fractures the attention a woman needs to reach orgasm. We'll develop singular focus through isolated practice, and it can later be brought into sex.

The technique requires 15 minutes of 100% concentration on approximately three square millimetres of contact. Nothing more.

Test this and practise it. The payoff will alter your sexual experiences forever.

I'll explain this from the standpoint of a man, as that's what I am, meng.

1. EXPLAIN TO YOUR PARTNER THAT IT IS A GOALLESS PRACTICE.

This is 100% critical. There is no objective, just a focus on a single point of contact. The phrasing should emphasize this and remove all expectations and pressure:

"I'm going to touch you for 15 minutes. You don't need to do anything, and you don't have to do anything afterwards. There is nowhere to get to, nothing to make happen. Just focus on the single point of contact. It's an exercise."

The only focus should be on the short stroke—one stroke, one stroke—just as the emphasis would be on the breath—one breath, one breath—in most forms of meditation. View it as an exercise in mindful awareness. There is no goal.

2. GET INTO POSITION.

First, the woman disrobes from the waist down and lies on her back using a pillow for neck support. Her legs are bent and spread, feet together in butterfly position. If this makes her hips uncomfortable on one or both sides, pillows can be put underneath her knees.

Based on the premise that it is easier to achieve the proper angle of contact with the left hand, the man should sit to her right side on top of at least two pillows and straddle his bent left leg perpendicularly across her torso, foot flat on the opposite side. Add as many pillows as necessary to relieve any pressure from his left leg on her abdomen. Too many is better than too few. His right leg is straight or relaxed in butterfly position.

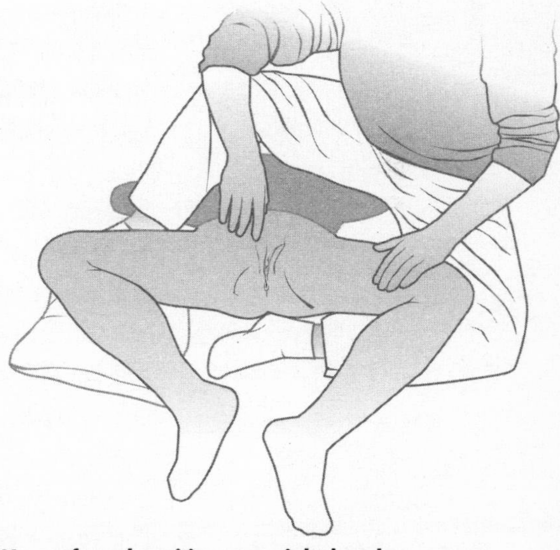

My preferred position as a right-hander

Despite the left-handed positioning, which is ideal, I'm right-handed and impatient with poor fine motor control. I had more consistent luck sitting on the woman's left side and using my right hand. If you choose to do the same, it's important to tilt your right wrist towards you slightly as if you were looking at a watch. This creates a better finger angle.

Since I had the most success with this right-handed position, and since most of the world is right-handed, all illustrations are from this position, man seated on the left side of the woman.

3. SET THE TIMER FOR 15 MINUTES, FIND THE UPPER-QUADRANT POINT OF GREATEST SENSATION AND STROKE.

Limit the session to exactly 15 minutes. I used a kitchen timer. This removes performance pressure and creates a safe start-and-end container for the woman. Look at it as you would a yoga routine or deep breathing sequence. It is an exercise in *focused repetition*, not a goal.

Finding the upper quadrant and anchoring (illustrated on the next page with the right hand):

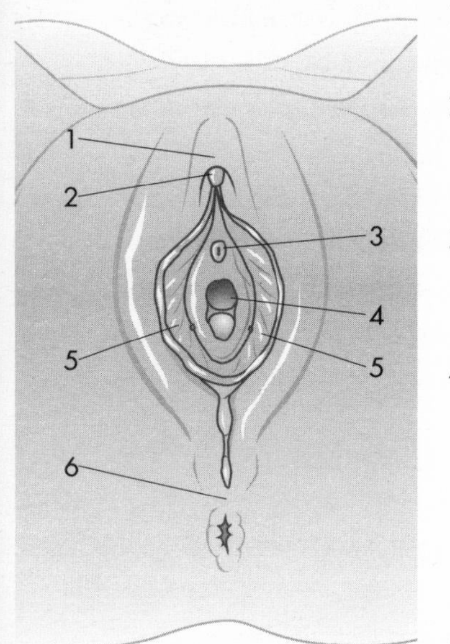

1. Clitoral hood; **2. clitoral glans (the point of contact)**; 3. urethral orifice; 4. vaginal opening (introitus); 5. labia minora; 6. perineum.

1. Separate the labia.
2. Retract the clitoral hood upwards with the heel of the palm.
3. Anchor the clitoris with the right thumb by holding the hood back.
4. Put your left hand under her buttocks, two fingers under each cheek, with the thumb resting on (not in) the base of the entrance to the vagina (ring of introitus). This will act as an anchor and help the woman to relax.
5. Imagine you are looking directly at the clitoris from between her legs, with the top of the clitoris as 12 o'clock on a clock face. Find 1:00 P.M.—ideally a small indentation or pocket between the hood and her clitoris—with your right hand's index finger and begin stroking using the lightest touch possible and only 1.5mm ($^1/_{16}$in) or so of movement. The tip of the finger is better than the pad, so cut your nails beforehand.

Nicole emphasizes the start: "If I can suggest one thing to the guys: take the time to find the spot. Once you find it, she won't be able to take more than a very light touch, like brushing satin against her skin."

Stroke like a metronome at a constant speed for periods of two to three

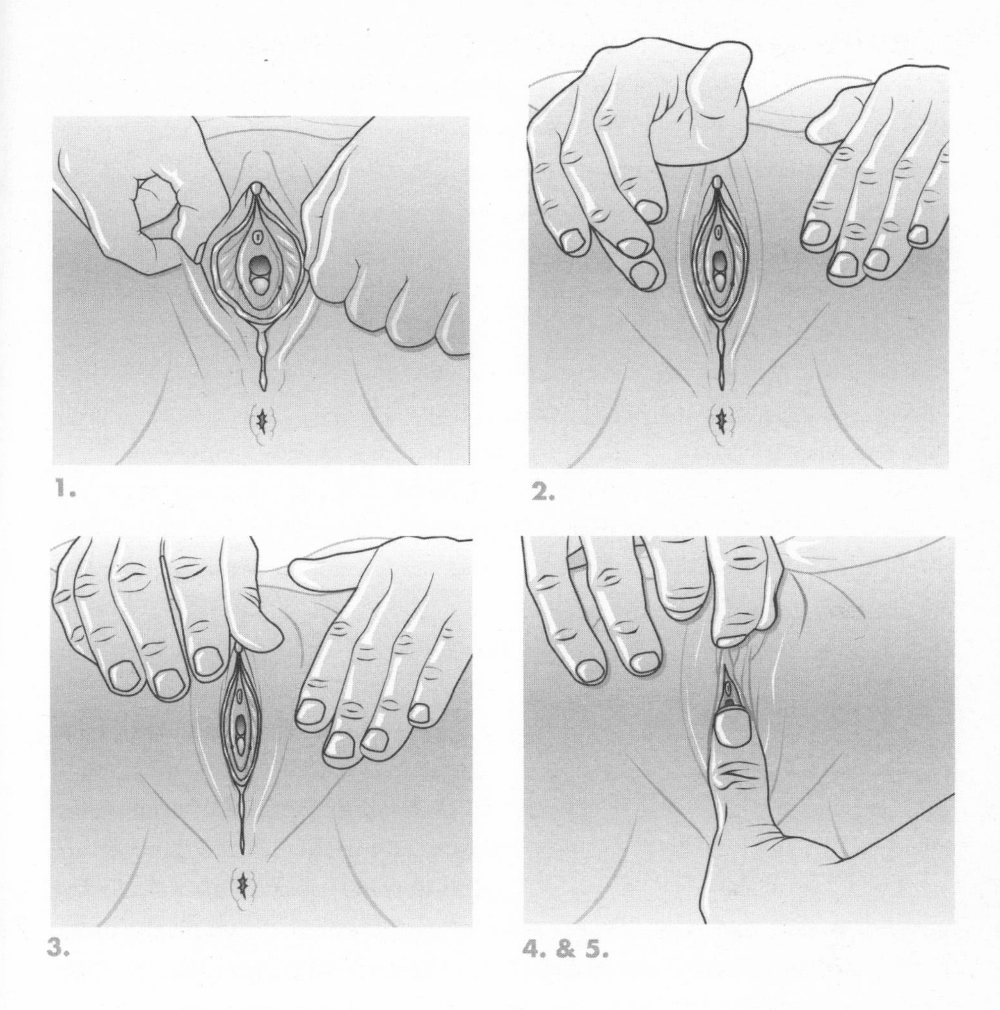

It is not uncommon for the man's lower back to tire. Fidgeting screws up everything, so I began testing an alternative elbow-brace position, seen on the next page.

You'll notice my left elbow is braced on my left shin. Since the angle no longer works for the introitus placement, I instead use my left hand to immobilize her right leg. Two women I practised this alternate position with preferred it to the textbook version.

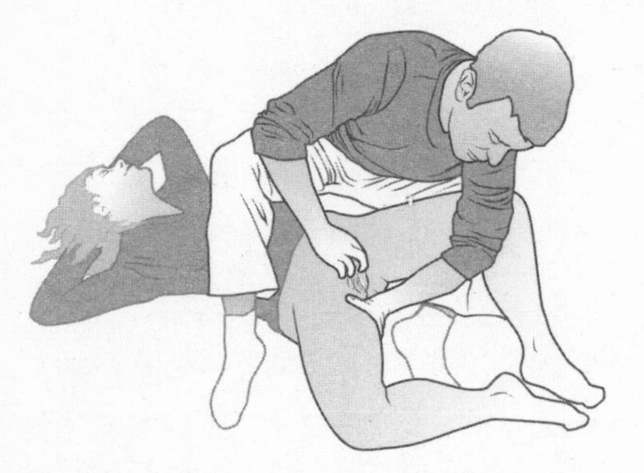

Elbow brace variation.

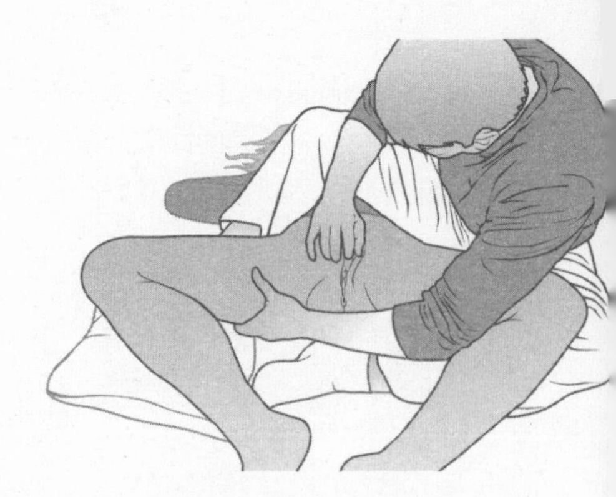

Front angle of the elbow brace variation.

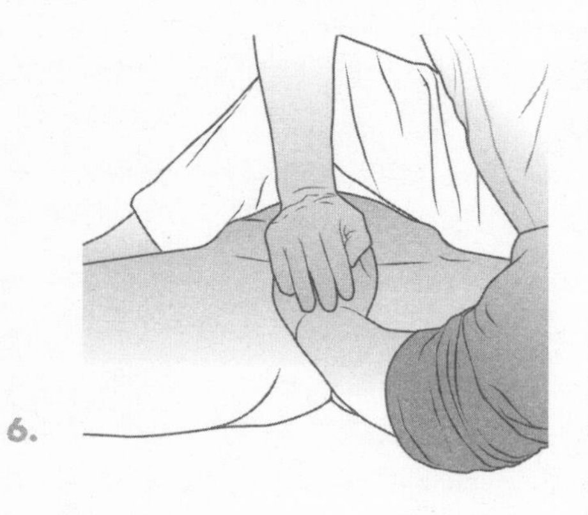

minutes, but feel free to change speed between periods.

6. "Ground" at the end.

Once the 15 minutes have elapsed, "grounding" is performed to (ostensibly) ease the woman out of the experience. Though there are sophisticated options for this closing portion, novice males can simply apply strong pressure down on the pubic bone and up towards the woman's head, using overlapping hands as indicated. Let her dictate the pressure. Most women, in my experience, find the strongest possible pressure the most pleasurable for ending a session.

I initially thought this closing portion was a waste of time. "Grounding"? It sounded like a bunch of New Age nonsense.

Now I believe that grounding is important not as some type of energetic witchcraft, but rather for closure. It consummates a complete experience with beginning (setup), middle (stroking) and end (grounding). This format gives both parties a sense of accomplishment that artfully helps avoid fixation on a full-blown orgasm as closure. Remember that it's the goalless nature of the practice that allows the relaxation that produces the orgasm. This guaranteed outcome (grounding) is smart and—I now believe—critical to include.

Suggestions for a Successful Beginner's Session

Based on coaching and practice, here are some helpful guidelines:

- Light contact. Remember: two pages of paper as depth of pressure. No more. It takes a lot of strength and concentration to stroke lightly.
- It isn't building towards anything. Keep the practice goalless and remember the intention: singularly focused repetition for 15 minutes.
- Consider using a blindfold or airline eye mask on the woman. I've found it makes them less self-conscious and increases tactile sensitivity.
- Have her "turn off the show". She doesn't need to please you. Make this clear. She doesn't need to moan and groan. It's about subtle sensation and nothing extra.
- Make it fun and even call it an "experiment". Serious = tension. Keep it light.
- Related to the above: *no* idle chatter. Some women will talk to distract themselves and prevent orgasm, or to prevent facial expressions of pleasure. This is an exercise in overcoming embarrassment, so the talking crutch should be removed. Using an eye mask helps minimize the talking impulse.
- Reinforce relaxation gently if the woman seems tense or anxious: "I notice you're tensed. Try and relax a little bit." If she's experiencing strong contractions which will clearly exhaust her before 15 minutes are up, encourage her to breathe and push out slightly as if she were going to pee. She won't pee, and it will help her extend the plateau and minimize fatigue.

Most common mistakes:

- Being goal-oriented. This includes women who will ask for insertion or penetration. Do not oblige them until the 15 minutes are up. Sex is fine afterwards, but not until the session is finished. Don't give in. She might beg in the moment, but she will thank you later for holding off. Once you've completed five 15-minute sessions without caving in, feel free to break the rules and go nuts before 15 minutes are up. But *not* until you've followed the rules for five sessions.

- Asking "non-winning" questions of the woman such as "Does it feel good?" or "Are you enjoying this?" almost guarantees lying. Asking questions is encouraged, but use directional questions instead: "Would you like a lighter or stronger stroke?" "More to your left or right?" "Higher or lower?"
- Once again: using too much pressure. I consciously focused on a light touch when practising the Doing Method for the first time, and I assumed it was light enough. It wasn't. I was using at least three times too much pressure. Imagine tickling a sleeping friend's nose just enough to make him scratch his own nose, but not enough to wake up.

Once you're comfortable with the basic practice (five stroke-only sessions), but *not* before, try these:

1. Insert the middle finger of the non-stroking hand, palm up, and use a come-hither motion to stimulate the g-spot. After five minutes, add in the index finger for a total of two fingers and continue the come-hither motion.
2. Place a buckwheat pillow[10] under her hips for the same angle as the improved-angle missionary, and use your left thumb to anchor the clitoris while you perform cunnilingus at the one o'clock upper quadrant of the clit. Do this as lightly as you would perform the stroke for at least five minutes, without finger insertion, and then add in #1 above with the right hand. Build a strong neck so she doesn't pop your head off.

Afterword: The Snow Leopard Cometh

So did Giselle get to the finish line? Yes. And she ended up getting much more.

It started with her masturbation homework assignments.

10. Or normal pillow folded in half.

"I'm similar to my closest friends in most ways, so I'd assumed this would also be the case. It wasn't. I was the only one [who didn't masturbate]." Once she started talking to her girlfriends about it, the entire subject became less taboo and became "normal". Suddenly sex wasn't something to be avoided. Now, it was something fun to talk about over a glass of wine.

She also realized that she'd been suppressing a critical part of herself, and that without a developed sexuality, she wasn't a fully developed person. It took discipline to overcome old habits and subconscious sabotage:

"It was really tempting to come home from work and say, 'Oh, I'm tired,' and go to bed without doing it. I really had to view it as practice, just like yoga. Practice is something you do even when you don't want to."

Rediscovering her sensual self went far beyond the bedroom. Giselle started taking salsa lessons and was finally comfortable as a sensual being. Comfortable in her own skin, she finally felt free to express herself. Not in a haphazard manner, but free from unwarranted guilt or shame. The mind can rationalize terrible voids, and there is no need for it.

Life is short, and sex should be a wonderful part of it. It's a fundamental part of our natural hardwiring.

Isn't it time you let your hair down and had some real fun with it?

All it takes is 15 minutes.

VIOLET BLUE: THE JOY OF CAFFEINE AND SELF-DISCOVERY

It's no secret that I'm fascinated by pharmaceuticals.

I was buzzing on one of my favourites, caffeine, as I listened to my friend Violet Blue wax poetic about drugs at a pavement café:

"Antihistamines can make you taste bitter, but it's simple to fix. Just add cucumber, mango, pineapple, papaya or citrus to your diet." Benadryl was now on my blacklist. Cucumber was on the shopping list.

The week prior, Violet, one of *Wired* magazine's "Faces of Innovation" and sex columnist for the *San Francisco Chronicle*, had kept Oprah rapt onstage for more than an hour. I wasn't surprised. Self-proclaimed sex educators often fall in the extremes, whether involving sex parties or worshipping the sex goddess Ix Chel. Violet was a different breed. Between lecturing to MDs at UCSF and speaking about sex to Google executives at their world headquarters, she had a simple person-to-person mission: to teach people how to safely get what they want in sex.

"Stimulants like caffeine also make it harder to come," she added.

I looked down at my coffee, and I looked down at my twins. Something else to experiment with. I'd come to our lunch date armed with a list of must-answer questions, and she had already knocked most of them off like a major leaguer at a Little League game.

But there was one question, *the* question, remaining:

What would you recommend, step by step, to a woman who wants to have her first orgasm?

Violet bounced a little in her chair and smiled, and I prepped my wrist for note-taking. She first brought up the cornerstones, erotica and self-exploration, and then added the details:

1. First, ask yourself a few simple questions: Have you ever felt anything close? Were you previously interested in sex but now you're not? Are you even interested in having an orgasm? Then watch Mary Roach's TED presentation entitled "10 Things You Didn't Know About Orgasm".
2. If embarrassment is an issue, get a copy of *When the Earth Moves: Women and Orgasm*.
3. Know thyself. Learn as much as possible about what turns you on. Give yourself permission to explore *all* fantasies. After all, they're just fantasies. Read some quality erotica written and curated by women. Violet has edited hundreds of erotica stories, and her top two picks were *The Best Women's Erotica 2009*, which she edited, and *60-Second Erotica* by Alison Tyler.
4. Get a variable-speed vibrator. Violet recommends a simple egg vibrator with a cord for starters, such as Smoothies or Bullet Vibes. If money is no object, get a Jimmyjane Little Chroma ($125/£78) or Little Something ($195–2,750 /£121–1,716[!]). Practise masturbating with your hands as well, inserting the vibrator just prior to orgasm or when you're close. Be playful and try it all. Her favourite supplier for all such goodies is the women-run BabeLand.
5. If you want to take it to the next level, strengthen your pubococcygeus (PC) muscle, which will create an "active" vagina (and pelvic floor) that can contract from the entrance to the cervix. Insert either a "vaginal barbell" or LELO Luna Balls—Violet prefers the latter—into the vagina and contract against it as you attempt to remove it. This can produce results with as little as five minutes, three times a week. The LELO Luna Balls arrive in two sets so you can use progressive resistance as you get stronger. In tug-of-war with the PC, everyone wins. Your man, in particular, will thank you.

TOOLS AND TRICKS

***The Illustrated Guide to Extended Massive Orgasm* by Steve and Vera Bodansky (www.fourhourbody.com/doingmethod)** This is a comprehensive illustrated how-to manual for the Doing Method, which I used for my first successful test-drive of the basic upper-quadrant technique discussed in this chapter. This book also describes the female technique for use on men.

OneTaste (http://onetaste.us) OneTaste was founded by Nicole Daedone to give women a place to learn about sex and orgasm from other women. In addition to events and classes at the New York City and San Francisco locations, private coaching is available in person and by phone.

San Francisco Sex Information (http://sfsi.org/wiki/Main_Page) Have a question about any aspect of sex? Confidentially and anonymously contact SFSI, which provides free and non-judgmental information about sex and reproductive health. The telephone hotline is available in the United States (or from anywhere if you use Skype), and the "Ask Us" e-mail service is available to English and Spanish speakers.

"TED Talk—Mary Roach: Ten Things You Didn't Know About Orgasm" (www.fourhourbody.com/roach) Sexual physiology has been studied for centuries, behind the closed doors of laboratories, brothels, Alfred Kinsey's attic and, more recently, MRI centres, pig farms and sex-toy R&D labs. Mary Roach spent two years wheedling and conniving her way behind those doors to bring you the answers to the questions Dr. Ruth never asked. In this popular TED presentation, she delves into obscure scientific research to make 10 surprising claims about sexual climax, ranging from the bizarre to the hilarious.

Violet Blue's Website (www.tinynibbles.com) Violet Blue is a sex-positive pundit and educator whose audiences range from medical doctors to the viewers of the *Oprah Winfrey Show.* She is also regarded as the foremost expert in the field of sex and technology. If you want to improve your time between the sheets, her site offers dozens of articles as jumping-off points.

VIOLET'S RECOMMENDED READING

***Got a Minute? 60-Second Erotica* by Alison Tyler and Thomas Roche (www.fourhourbody.com/60second)**

***Best Women's Erotica 2009* by Violet Blue (www.fourhourbody.com/erotica)**

***When the Earth Moves: Women and Orgasm* by Mikaya Heart (www.fourhourbody.com/earth)**

VIOLET'S RECOMMENDED TOOLS

BabeLand (www.babeland.com) Babeland was originally opened in response to the lack of women-friendly sex shops in Seattle. Now it is a one-stop nationwide shop for women who want to explore their sexuality.

Vibrator MVPs
Bullet vibes (www.fourhourbody.com/bullet)
Smoothie (www.fourhourbody.com/smoothie)
Jimmyjane Little Chroma (www.fourhourbody.com/chroma)
Little Something (www.fourhourbody.com/something)

LELO Luna Balls System (www.fourhourbody.com/luna) LELO Luna Balls are the answer to the "How do you prevent your 'hoo-ha' from loosening?" question. Used for five minutes, three times a week, to strengthen the PC muscle, they are also the answer to the question, "How do you make your hoo-ha tighter?" Normal Pilates exercises can be used for a complementary effect. Squeeze hard and prosper. Trust me, these are worth the investment.

The Kegelmaster (www.kegelmasters.com) Though Luna Balls have the most enthusiastic rave reviews, The Kegelmaster is a popular vaginal barbell and a less expensive alternative. Oddly enough, there is an endorsement from Teri Hatcher on the home page. Meow.

SEX MACHINE I

Adventures in Tripling Testosterone

Sex is one of the nine reasons for reincarnation. The other eight are unimportant.

—George Burns

NOONISH, ONE BEAUTIFUL SATURDAY, SAN FRANCISCO, 21 FLOORS ABOVE THE EMBARCADERO PIERS

"That's kind of creepy. They're already 75% healed." Vesper had come out of the shower and was staring at my shoulders.

"Are you kidding? It's fucking awesome! I'm becoming Wolverine." I was referring, of course, to the superhero with mutant healing powers. He also has adamantium claws, but that's where Vesper was a much better comparison.

The night before, she'd inflicted bedroom wounds on my back and arms that weren't really "scratches". The masterpiece: four 10–18cm (4–7in) gashes in my right shoulder streaming blood that made me look like Bruce Lee from *Enter the Dragon*. Bruce in dire need of Neosporin. Now, less than 10 hours later, three of the gashes had disappeared completely, and the last and deepest was barely visible.

Strange.

The strangeness started much earlier, well before the bedroom, at The Americano restaurant.

Friday at 8:00 P.M. brought the crowds, and the

alpha investment bankers were fighting the alpha lawyers for female attention everywhere inside Hotel Vitale. The pressed shirts and dresses spilled from the outdoor patio into the restaurant, where we had reservations. It took a chaperone using football-like blocking to get us to our booth in a secluded back corner.

The catch-up chat with Vesper looked like this:

Her: "How are you?"

Me: "Unbelievable. But I need to give you fair warning. My biochemistry is very different from the last time you saw me. I feel . . . well, superhuman."

Her (eyebrows raised): "Oh reeeeally? Details, please."

Yes, really. The last time we'd met, I had just taken my total testosterone from 244.8 to 653.3 ng/dL (nanograms per decilitre), while cutting my oestradiol (oestrogen) in half. The subsequent roughhousing had been a physical encounter of the first class. This time around, I'd just returned from Nicaragua, where I ate grass-fed beef three times per day for 21 days. I had protein-loaded for the last three days, eating 900–1.3kg (2–3lb) of fatty organic grass-fed beef per day, including at least 400g (14oz) just before bed. (Don't worry. I won't suggest that you do this.)

The result?

Fifteen minutes after we sat down, Vesper was in a sexually aggressive stupor. The bread hadn't arrived and she was already climbing on top of me. This is not a boast. This is not Penthouse Forum. It's a statement of pure confusion. She is a CEO, and this is not typical public CEO behaviour. I thought she was on drugs. Heavy nose breathing, interrupted occasionally with "What is going on? I don't understand what's going on . . ." The whole spectacle was surreal.

She was, literally, intoxicated on pheromones.

I excused myself to the bathroom at one point, and what came next was even more absurd. Vesper witnessed it later when we left. Both en route to the bathroom and coming back to the table, it was as if I had a 3m (10ft) radius field of hormonal impact. I received at least three times the normal eye contact from women.

The animal kingdom was alive and well in San Francisco.

Dinner ended immediately thereafter, and it was a short trip to her apartment on the 21st floor and our version of *Enter the Dragon*, complete with furniture smashing and most of the same sound effects.[11]

The next morning, after more of the same, I asked her, "Do you have a gong on the other side of your headboard?"

It turned out to be metal artwork hanging on the neighbour's wall. After her second shower, and taking another look at my shoulder, Vesper had just one thing to say:

"Whatever you're doing—keep doing it."

The Death of the Metrosexual: Reclaiming Aggression

Things hadn't always been this way. In fact, for several years, things were quite the opposite.

Somewhere between late 2007 and 2009, at 30–32 years old, I found myself in an odd place: able to perform in the bedroom as well as I had in college, but having less and less desire to do so.

Even with the most attractive of girls, after a week or two of rabbit love, sex frequency would drop to once a day. Then it would drop to a few times a week or once a week. I enjoyed sex as much as ever, once in the act, but fatigue or disinterest often led me to opt-out. "I'll get to it in the morning" became a constant self-promise.

It made no sense.

I was young, athletic and felt perfectly healthy. Then, looking under the hood, I ended up in the lower range of "normal" for total testosterone in blood testing.

What was the problem?

POSSIBLE SHORT CIRCUITS

Testosterone is a molecule of many dependencies.

The **hypothalamus** releases gonadotropin-releasing hormone (GnRH), which tells the **pituitary** (anterior pituitary) gland to release luteinizing hormone (LH) and follicle-stimulating hormone (FSH). LH then stimulates the Leydig cells in the testicles to produce—ta-da—**testosterone**.

11. Check out the original at www.fourhourbody.com/enter-dragon. My massage therapist later asked me: "Have you been crawling through barbed wire?"

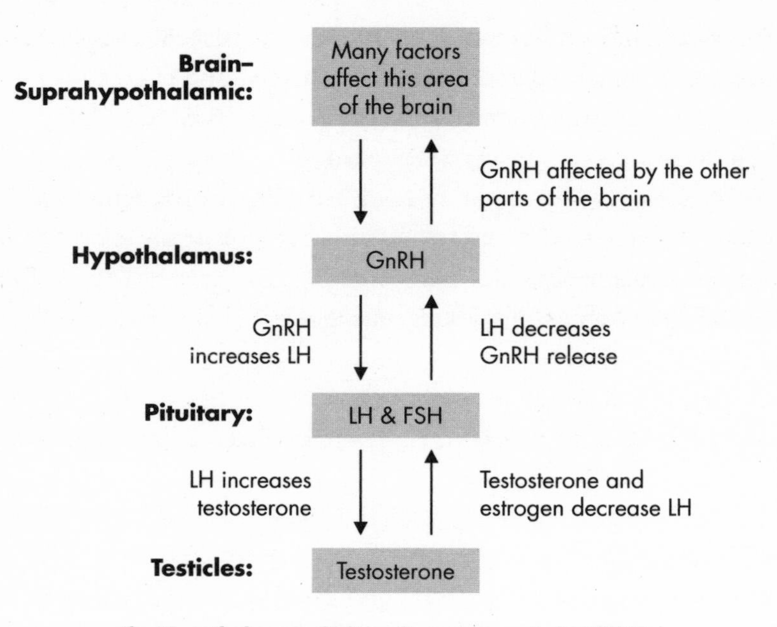

The Hypothalamus-pituitary-Testosterone Axis (HPTA)

It is a major but rampant mistake to treat low testosterone with external testosterone in the form of a gel or injection[12] without troubleshooting the upstream parts of the axis first.

It's also a mistake to think of low libido as strictly a low-testosterone problem.

In 2004, I experimented with a hormone and drug called human chorionic gonadotropin, commonly known as "hCG", which effectively acts as a form of luteinizing hormone. Injected once per week, it immediately had the effect of more than tripling seminal volume and requiring—*requiring*—ejaculation three to four times per day just to think straight. If you want to kill productivity, look no further than hCG. This inconvenience was compensated for by sex with my girlfriend, which jumped from a few times a week to a few times a day. Happy days.

So just inject hCG and problem solved, right?

Not quite. Here's the catch: repeated use of hCG can desensitize the testes to real luteinizing hormone.[13] Then the testes can't receive the signal to produce testosterone naturally. Big trouble.

12. Called "exogenous" testosterone (created outside the body), as opposed to "endogenous" (created inside the body). Think of "external" to remember the difference.
13. hCG can also inhibit GnRH at the hypothalamus. It's a serious drug and shouldn't be taken lightly.

This disqualifies hCG as a permanent solution, but it suggests that increasing luteinizing hormone (LH) increases sex drive.

GA

But, you might ask, couldn't the sex drive be due to more testosterone, since luteinizing hormone (and therefore hCG) stimulates its release in the flow chart? This is true, but I'd also used straight testosterone injections earlier in 2004 (as detailed in "The Last Mile"), which more than doubled testosterone levels but didn't improve libido at all.

LH seems to do more.

LH also correlates perfectly with the heightened sex drive experienced by women just prior to ovulation.[14]

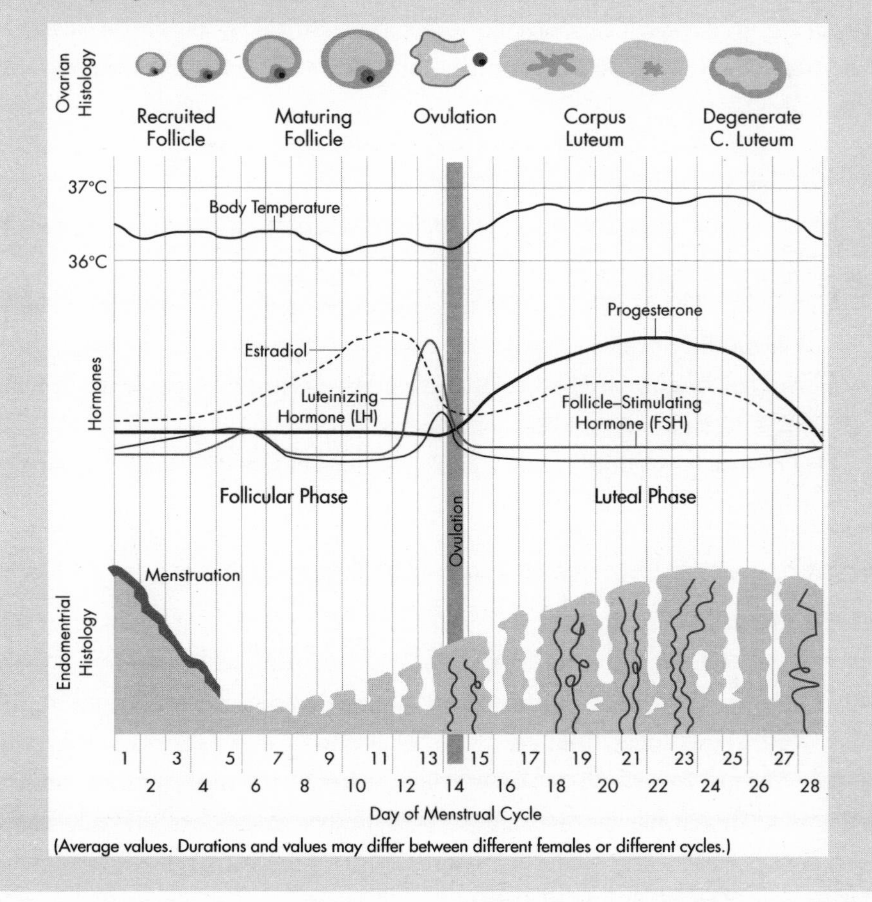

14. Though other hormones like FSH also correlate to the increased sex drive, LH shows the most pronounced jump.

My Solution: Two Protocols

I didn't consume much red meat for my first increase from 244.8 to 653.3 ng/dL, and I believe this type of jump can be achieved without eating red meat at all. The meat marathon was actually for tracking changes in food allergies.

I now use two protocols that I believe are effective for increasing both testosterone and LH, based on repeated blood test results. Neither requires needles or prescription meds.

The first is for long-term maintenance and general wellbeing. The second is for short-term "nitro" boosts of sex drive and testosterone. Sheer fun, in other words. The detailed rationales behind each can be found in "Sex Machine II" in the Appendices, but let's start with the nutshell version.

PROTOCOL #1: LONG-TERM AND SUSTAINED

Fermented cod liver oil + vitamin-rich butter fat—2 capsules upon waking and before bed

Vitamin D3—3,000–5,000 IU upon waking and before bed (6,000–10,000 IU per day), until you reach blood levels of 55 ng/mL

Short ice baths and/or cold showers—10 minutes each, upon waking and right before bed

Brazil nuts—3 nuts upon waking, 3 nuts before bed (see important footnote).[15]

PROTOCOL #2: SHORT-TERM AND FUN "NITRO BOOST"

20–24 Hours Prior to Sex

Eat at least 800 milligrams of cholesterol (example: four or more large whole eggs or egg yolks) within three hours of bedtime, the night *before* you want to have incredible sex. The Wolverine intro to this chapter was partially thanks to two 350g (12oz) rib-eye steaks the night before, but it's easier to stomach hard-boiled eggs. Why before bed? Testosterone is derived from cholesterol, which is primarily produced at night during sleep (between midnight and 4:00–6:00 A.M.).

15. This is personal, and I don't suggest the same unless you're deficient in selenium. See SpectraCell in the resources, as well as the explanation in "Sex Machine II".

Four Hours Prior to Sex

4 Brazil nuts
20 raw almonds
2 capsules of the above-mentioned fermented cod/butter combination

SHBG—THE PARTY SPOILER

Sex-hormone binding globulin (SHBG) is the party spoiler.

SHBG binds to testosterone[16] and renders it inert for our purposes, and "total testosterone" in blood tests can therefore be misleading. Some vegans have been shown to have higher testosterone levels than both meat-eaters and vegetarians, for example, but higher levels of SHBG cancel out this advantage. In other studies, consumption of cholesterol has been shown to be inversely correlated with SHBG. In other words, the more cholesterol you eat, the less SHBG you have.

From Carruthers's *Androgen Deficiency in the Adult Male: Causes, Diagnosis, and Treatment:*

> *Strict low cholesterol diets have been shown to lower total and free testosterone levels by 14%. Vegetarian diets, especially if low in protein, can increase SHBG, further reducing FT [free testosterone]. However, men put on a low-fat, high-fibre, vegetarian diet have a 18% reduction in both total testosterone and FT, which is reversed when they go back on a normal diet. . . . Conversely, high-protein, low-carbohydrate diets, such as the fashionable weight-reduction Atkins diet, may partly exert their slimming action by raising total testosterone and lowering SHBG.*

SHBG isn't evil, and we don't want to eliminate it, but a little less SHBG equals a little more free testosterone. This isn't evil either. It actually makes life much more interesting. This is the reason for our cholesterol-loading in Protocol 2.

How Well Can It Work?

Here is a sample of before-and-after sex hormone results from my first experiment (protocol 1), excluding Brazil nuts, which were added later:

16. Albumin also does this to a lesser extent.

3 APRIL 2009 (BEFORE) TO 20 AUGUST 2009 (AFTER)

Total testosterone: 244.8 to 653.3 (normal: 170–780; it would later jump to **835,** more than tripling my original value, with the addition of Brazil nuts)
Free testosterone: 56 to 118 (normal: 47–244)
Percentage free testosterone: 2.3% to 1.8%
Bio-available testosterone: 150 to 294 (normal: 128–430)
Albumin: 5 to 4.6 (normal: 3.5–4.8)
DHEA-S: 170.5 to 201.8
FSH: 6 to 8.5 (normal: 1.27–19.26)
Oestradiol: 39 to <20 (normal in males: <47)

Eager to give it a shot?

This chapter is enough to get started, but the real magic happens when we finesse the details. Be sure to read "Sex Machine II: Details and Dangers" in the Appendices if you're serious about kicking testosterone and sex drive into overdrive.

TOOLS AND TRICKS

SpectraCell Laboratories (www.fourhourbody.com/spectra) SpectraCell is the micronutrient testing lab allegedly used by Lance Armstrong. I uncovered my selenium deficiency through SpectraCell and used Brazil nuts, among other things, to correct it. To find local SpectraCell clinicians, go to: www.fourhourbody.com/spectra. More on this in "Sex Machine II".

Blue Ice™ Butter Oil/Fermented Cod Liver Oil Blend (www.fourhourbody.com/butterblend) This is the cod/butter combination I used. Blue Ice™ is from a small manufacturer and production is limited.

Carlson Super 1000mg Cod Liver Oil (www.fourhourworkweek.com/cod) A decent substitute if the above is sold-out, but consume at the same time as the below.

Vitamin-Rich Butter Fat: Kerrygold Irish butter (www.kerrygold.com/usa/locator.php) This site helps you find local stores where you can buy Kerrygold Irish butter. If you'd prefer to order online, check www.foodireland.com and click "Deli Counter" at the top of the screen.

ZRT At-Home Vitamin D Test Kits (www.fourhourbody.com/testd) If you spend a lot of your time indoors, there's a good chance that you are deficient in vitamin D. Don't just guess what amount of vitamin D you need, as overdosing will produce side effects.

SpectraCell is a more reliable blood-based test, but ZRT's saliva mail-in kit can give you an inexpensive estimate of your vitamin D levels. Once you've established your baseline, you can use sunlight, supplementation, and UV-B lamps to increase levels, following eight weeks of which you can perform an "after" test to track changes.

Vitamin D3

NOW Liquid Vitamin D3, 60ml/2 fl oz (www.fourhourbody.com/vitamin-d)

UV-B/F Lamps

Sperti Ultraviolet Systems (www.sperti.com)

The KBD D/UV-F fluorescent lamp was developed in 2010 for individuals who can't tolerate direct sunlight exposure or oral Vitamin D supplements.

21 DAYS OF MEAT AND NUTS—AM I NUTS?

Let's take a closer look at what happened to my blood and cholesterol after those 21 days in Nicaragua, 21 days of consuming at least 30% of my calories as beef fat and 200–300 grams of protein and 40–70 almonds per day. I expected the worst. Here is the real impact on two common concerns: cholesterol levels and kidney function.

BEFORE (20 AUGUST 2009) v. **AFTER (25 SEPTEMBER 2009)**

Cholesterol

Total cholesterol: 200 (borderline out-of-range) v. **190**
HDL: 57 v. **57**
LDL: 133 (out-of-range) v. **108**
VLDL: 10 v. **25**
Cholesterol/HDL ratio: 3.5 v. **3.3**
Triglycerides: 48 v. **124** (normal: <150)

Kidney function

BUN: 17 v. **18** (normal: 7–25)
Creatinine: 1.0 v. **1.1** (normal: 0.7–1.2)
BUN/creatinine ratio: 16.4–**17** (normal: 10–20)

Even I was stunned.

I took no cholesterol-lowering (or HDL-raising) drugs or supplements, and a 21-day marathon of red meat actually improved my cholesterol/HDL ratio, which most doctors view as an indication of cardiac health. I also lowered both total and LDL ("bad") cholesterol. I ended up within the "low-risk" range for triglycerides, according to the American Heart Association, but there was an elevation. I expected the increase for three reasons:

1. Triglycerides transport dietary fat, and I had been consuming massive quantities of fat.
2. Fat loss can produce transient elevated triglycerides (as it did with my dad, who lost 32+kg/70+lb) of fat), and I had lost substantial body fat in the preceding 21 days.
3. I had consumed 400ml (14 fl oz) of pulp-free orange juice the morning before the blood draw—the first time I'd done so in at least a year—to measure my blood sugar response. Fructose, the sugar in fruit, is well known for rapidly increasing both triglycerides and LDL.

All cardiac markers were brought within normal range within weeks of stopping the animal flesh binge. When I retested on 16 October (21 days later), my triglycerides had dropped from 124 to 82, and my VLDL had dropped from 25 to 16.

What of the BUN and creatinine, considered indicators of kidney stress? Both were nominally elevated but well within normal range.

I'm amazed that both weren't higher, considering that muscular damage can increase both BUN and creatinine, and I had done a squat workout 48 hours prior to the "after" blood draw on 24 September.

But isn't cholesterol bad for you?

This belief is predicated on the Lipid Hypothesis of cardiac health (cholesterol = bad), which I disagree with based on the sum total of available evidence. Between 2006 and 2009, I had obsessed over lowering my total cholesterol. The outcome? Lower testosterone and fatigue.

I'll take my egg yolks, thank you very much.

RECIPE FOR DISASTER: THE SALMONELLA SPECIAL

It appears that splitting up the 800 milligrams of cholesterol also works for the earlier "Nitro Boost" Protocol 2.

If you know your local sources and can avoid salmonella and raw milk issues, I've found the following shake to produce incredible effects when mixed with a hand blender and consumed at both 4:00 P.G. and before bed. It also helped me achieve the 45+kg (100+lb) strength gains as detailed in "Effortless Superhuman":

350ml (12 fl oz) whole raw milk
4 tbsp raw almond butter
2 raw egg yolks
3 tbsp chia seeds
1 tsp vanilla extract
½ tsp cinnamon

This is more appropriately called a "fat shake" instead of a protein shake, but I still dropped body fat while consuming it. How? The fat loss was predicated on otherwise maintaining a slow-carb diet and taking the shakes only on workout days, no more than three times a week. If you've ever wondered what anabolics feel like, one week of these shakes will give you a good idea.

Here is the nutritional yield, with all percentages of USRDA (recommended daily allowance):

Total calories = 966
Calories from fat = 627
Fat grams = 73 g (113%)
Saturated fat grams = 15 g (76%)
Cholesterol = 456 g (152%)
Protein = 34 g (69%)
Carbohydrate grams = 55 g (18%)
Dietary fibre = 20 g (81%)
Sugars = 19 g
Calcium = 93%
Glycaemic load = 15 (out of maximum 250)

Know your food sources, and the statistics on salmonella poisoning, etc., before consuming this. If raw milk scares you, and I wouldn't blame you, use organic whole milk instead.

HAPPY ENDINGS AND DOUBLING SPERM COUNT

The two canals, fashioned by the gods, in which man's power rests, in thy testicles . . . I break them with a club.

—*Atharva Veda*, sacred text of Hinduism

"Each man in this room is half the man his grandfather was."

Louis Guillette PhD, a researcher from the University of Florida, opened his discussion in front of a congressional committee without preamble. Named one of just 20 Howard Hughes Medical Institute professors nationwide, Guillette was not speaking in metaphor. He had the data to prove it.

The sperm counts of men in the United States and 20 other industrialized countries have been falling since 1942 at a rate of roughly 1% per year in *healthy* males.

The average northern European sperm count in the 1940s was more than 100 million sperm per millilitre (million/ml) of ejaculate. In 2008? "The sperm counts of the majority of 20-year-old European men are now so low that we may be close to the crucial tipping point of 40 million per milliliter spermatozoa. . . we must face the possibility of more infertile couples and lower fertility rates in the future." In Denmark, more than 40% of men have already dropped below the 40 million/ml threshold and entered "sub-fertility".

The research is, as always, controversial.

Some studies confirm the trend, while other studies contradict the findings, and we all end up more confused than before.

To sidestep the bickering, I tracked my sperm count and quality over 18 months and looked at the trends first-hand. From a selfish Darwinian standpoint, I didn't care about Henrik's balls in Copenhagen. I cared about my own.

It all started with a trip to a sperm bank in 2008 (see sidebar in this chapter), when I had no intention of trending anything.

I'd had a few too many brushes with mortality, witnessed a 30-something friend get testicular cancer, and decided it was a good idea to begin freezing my swimmies while at their healthiest. Unlike fine wine, sperm count does not improve with age. After all, what if I got married and then had an accident or needed chemotherapy? I wanted a worst-case scenario insurance policy.

Getting an accurate sperm count never occurred to me as important. My blood work was immaculate. I was a strapping 31 years young. My diet was as clean as a Mormon's breakfast, and I was hitting new personal records in the gym. Why would I bother to think about it? It was obvious that I didn't need to.

Unpleasant Surprises

Then the shocker: the lab results, which were available the afternoon after my session, put my sperm count on the low range of normal, borderline problematic. I couldn't believe it. Assuming it was a lab mistake, I repeated the drill three weeks later and came back with an even lower count. The more tests I did over the next 12 months, the lower the results.

Holy Christ. I was terrified.

But what were the possible causes?

Was it the phthalates in everything from shampoo to deodorant? Bisphenol A in everything from household electronics to plastic bottles? Tightie-whities? There was no consensus. It could have been one of a million suspects, or it could have been all of them.

No matter the causes, the real question was: could I do anything to reverse it?

To start, I attempted to remove environmental pollutants from my body using injections (IV DMPS, etc.) and dietary changes, and the changes in blood work were almost unnoticeable.

What else could I do?

Besides avoiding plastics and going organic, the sad answer seemed to be: not much. I called some of the most experienced and innovative urologists in the United States, including Dr. Dudley Danoff, founder of the Tower Urology Medical Group at Cedars-Sinai Medical Center, who served as a clinical faculty member at UCLA Medical School for 25 years. His most striking comment was a disheartening one: "Male fertility is a relatively 'infertile' field. There is so little one can do."

Then came 31 August 2009.

In preparation for an unrelated interview with famed strength coach Charles Poliquin, I had asked a friend in the fitness business for his dream list of questions. One of the side notes in his e-mail read:

> He won't use a cell phone due to radiation, states they have a high tested correlation between low T levels in athletes and cell phone carried in pocket.

"T" in this case refers to testosterone.

The interview with Charles was a fascinating romp through all things performance-related, ranging from the endocrine system to intravenous vitamin C treatment and genetics testing. In the middle, as we were shifting topics, I asked Charles if he'd observed a correlation between mobile phone use and low testosterone counts.

"It's not just something I've observed. Take a look at the studies."

So I did.

Lo and behold, jumping from article to article on MedLine, there were more than a handful of studies that showed significant decreases in serum testosterone in rats following even moderate exposure (30 minutes per day, five days a week, for four weeks) to 900 megahertz (MHz) radio frequency (RF) electro-magnetic fields (EMF), which is what most GSM mobile phones produce.

Then, the epiphany.

In the "related articles" pane next to one such study, I noticed research focusing on the effects of mobile phone radiation on sperm.

One click opened Pandora's box, but let's cover basics before we look at what I found. There are principally three things an MD will first look at when evaluating sperm:

1. **Count:** How many swimmers do we have total?
2. **Morphology:** How many swimmers have the proper tadpole-like shape?
3. **Motility:** How many of them can actually swim forward, which is the right direction?

If the sperm is misshapen or can't move, it doesn't matter how many you have. If you have great swimmers but not enough to survive the kamikaze one-way trip, you are equally screwed.

Of the dozens of studies that I found, most done in Europe, more than 70% concluded the same thing:[17] mobile phone radiation impairs sperm function. The explanation for how it does this varied, but the outcome was never good.

Here are just two abstract highlights from 2008 and 2009:

Three hundred sixty-one men undergoing infertility evaluation were divided into four groups according to their active mobile phone use: group A: no use; group B: <2 h/day [hours/day]; group C: 2–4 h/day; and group D: >4 h/day.... The laboratory values of the above four sperm parameters [mean sperm count, motility, viability, and normal morphology] decreased in all four mobile phone user groups as the duration of daily exposure to cell phones increased.

• • •

Male albino Wistar rats (10–12 weeks old) were exposed to RF-EMR [radio frequency electro-magnetic radiation] from an active GSM (0.9/1.8 GHz) mobile phone for 1 hour continuously per day for 28 days. Controls were exposed to a mobile phone without a battery for the same period.... Rats exposed to RF-EMR exhibited a significantly reduced percentage of motile sperm. CONCLUSION: Given the results of the present study, we speculate that RF-EMR from mobile phones negatively affects semen quality and may impair male fertility.

The rat balls were exposed for *one hour per day* for 28 days?!

In California, where I live, 30% of the population relies exclusively on

17. Most of the studies performed in the United States that conclude no negative effect are funded either directly or indirectly (as with many IEEE studies) by mobile phone manufacturers and carriers. Does this prove malfeasance? No, but it should raise a red flag.

mobile phones for communication. I had carried a mobile phone in my pocket an average of at least 12 hours a day for the last 10 years.

No more.

It didn't hurt me to put it somewhere else, and the evidence was strong enough to warrant a trial.

Eleven weeks later, I had my first round of results.

Happy Endings

For eleven weeks, I adopted one new rule: my phone was no longer allowed to cuddle with my testicles.

Its new home was a black InCase iPod armband intended for jogging. I could strap it to the outside of my upper arm or calf, or—if headed somewhere jogger fashion wasn't cool—I could simply turn the phone off before putting it in my pocket. In the latter case, or when running quick errands sans armband, checking messages every 30 minutes resulted in a grand total of zero problems. The front pocket of a backpack or bag also works.

I waited 11 weeks to retest for a specific reason: sperm production (spermatogenesis) takes an estimated 64 days in humans. I wanted to wait at least that long and added two weeks as an extra buffer.

I returned to the sperm bank for my deposit and testing on 19 November 2009, nervous as hell.

The anxiety wasn't necessary. I had nearly tripled my motile sperm per ejaculate. The numbers were almost unbelievable:

Ejaculate volume: 44% increase
Motile sperm per millilitre: 100% increase
Motile sperm per ejaculate: 185% increase

I let out one of the longest exhales of my life as I looked at the lab test fax. The trend had reversed.

Can I attribute these increases to removing the mobile phone and nothing else? It isn't quite that easy. I also started cold treatments and supplemental selenium (Brazil nuts), both of which could have contributed, the latter more likely than the former. Do I care about the academic purity?

No. I was more concerned with increasing sperm count than isolating variables. Even with two confounding variables, the experiment is directionally valid.

Should you wait for a scientific consensus? I don't think so. This is a case where the current literature is strong enough, and the inconvenience minimal enough, to not wait for doctor's orders.

It can't hurt you, and it might get your swim team off the bench and back in the game.

If you want kids some day, consider yourself warned.

STORING SWIMMIES—JUST IN CASE

I never thought I'd visit a sperm bank.

Perhaps it was flipping a motorcycle at 145km (90 miles) per hour on Infineon Raceway.

Perhaps it was tearing my Achilles tendon in jiu-jitsu practice, then getting thrown on my head.

Maybe having my scuba mask fill with blood at 37m (120ft) underwater in Belize?

That could have done it.

Or perhaps it was just crossing the 30-year age threshold and having friends who didn't make it. Suicide, 9/11, accidents—bad things happen to good people.

I came to realize then: it's really not that hard to die. And that's when I started thinking about storing my genetic material.

Yes, my little swimmies.

In this sidebar, I'll talk about the process, how I did it, and why it's cheap insurance in an unpredictable world. I'll also throw in some curious details (sexy time!) just for entertainment.

THE REASONS TO STORE SPERM

Doing the research, the pros far outweigh the cons:

1. **Men are becoming progressively infertile.** Go munch on some soy crisps for a mouthful of phytoestrogens, or just stick with preservatives. It's hard to avoid testicle-unfriendly food and toxins. Talk to endocrinologists

who do clinical analysis and also get your sperm count measured. It is probably less than your dad's. Real-world *Children of Men* (for men) is in full effect.

2. Many medical conditions and procedures (cancer treatment, for example) can render men infertile.
3. People who "know" they don't want kids change their minds. A lot. Just look at the number of vasectomy reversal procedures. And no, these procedures do not work well. Failure rates are high.
4. **Above all, why do it?** If you can afford it, it's a no-brainer for peace of mind. The potential downside of doing it (cost) is recoverable; the potential downside of not doing it is irreversible.

Think it's easy to get someone pregnant? Sometimes. Most of the time, after looking at the numbers, it seems surprisingly hit-or-miss.

To be clear, I think adoption is a beautiful thing. I just also want to have children who look like me, and I see no reason not to ensure both can happen. I want Mama Ferriss to be Grandmama Ferriss at some point, even if my testicles check out before I do. Call me old-fashioned.

Is this ego-driven? On some level, of course it is. But so is owning a home or having a decent car, wearing clothing besides what will keep you warm, and doing anything past the base necessities for survival. Humans are ego-driven. I'm human, ergo I'm ego-driven.

SPERM STORAGE—THE STEPS IN BRIEF

1. FIND A SPERM STORAGE FACILITY.

Google "sperm storage", "sperm bank" or "sperm donor", along with your state or city.

2. MAKE AN INITIAL APPOINTMENT AND GET TESTED FOR INFECTIOUS DISEASES.

Most reputable locations will require testing for common STDs prior to storage. I was tested for:

HIV 1 & 2
HTLV I & II
RPR (for syphilis, Al Capone's farewell song)
HCV (for hepatitis C)
HBsAG and HBcAB (for hepatitis B)

Cost of initial consult: $100–150 (£62–95)
Cost of STD lab panel: $150–200 (£95–125)

It's a romantic first date. And yes, I cleared with flying colours.

3. WARM UP YOUR WRISTS AND GET BUSY. SIX SESSIONS PER KID.
Think it's "one shot, one kill", macho man? Think again. You're no Peter North, and even if you were, 50%+ of your sperm count is annihilated by the freezing process.

You should make six sperm deposits for each child you'd like to have. It can take over eight months for a woman to get pregnant with insemination, although in vitro fertilization (IVF) ups the chances somewhat at much higher cost, generally $9,000–12,000 (£5,600–7,500) per attempt.

Oh, and forget about abstaining for long periods of time, oddly enough.

For best storage and later fertilization, abstain from ejaculation for at least 48 hours but no more than three days (72 hours) before each session. It's a tight window. More than four days and dead sperm cells begin to accumulate and cause trouble, as you need a certain ratio of live sperm to dead sperm per 1 cubic centimetre (cc) of volume. I scheduled one deposit every fourth morning: e.g., Monday, 10:00 A.G.; Friday, 10:00 A.G.; Tuesday, 10:00 A.G., etc.

Cost per sample frozen: $150–200 (£65–125) (× 6 = $900–1,200 (£560–750) per potential kid)

4. STORE ALL THE SUSPENDED SWIMMIES SOMEWHERE SAFE.
This is usually handled by the facility that did the initial freezing. This is also where the credit card comes out.

Cost per year: $300–600/£185–375 (often for all samples)

SEXY TIME DETAILS

So, cover the baby's ears. I'm going to tell you something stunning and disgusting. Something you probably don't want to hear. Ready? Most guys like pornography. And Santa Claus doesn't exist.

I'm sorry.

Here's how the storage facility website sells the "donation" process:

He [the donor/storer] is then shown to a private room where he can collect his specimen in a provided sterile cup.

About as sexy as lethal injection, right?

Well, upon arrival, there were surprises in store. I was led to a cornucopia of porn DVDs around a secret corner. Right in front of a bunch of female lab technicians looking awkward. There was something for everyone in this motley selection. Blind juggler fetish? It would've been there. No expense was spared in covering all bases.

I grabbed a few titles (I'll spare you the names) and headed to a small white room with a sliding door. I followed the lead of a quiet male Asian assistant in a white lab coat. He looked at his feet and departed with, "Please wash your hands when you finish." I didn't expect a call the next day.

The den of clinical sin was about the size of a hotel bathroom, with a paper-sheet-covered cot on the floor (yeah, baby!), a metal chair, a 33cm (13in) TV/DVD combo on a small stool, and a stack of magazines suspiciously adhered to one another.

So I sat down, still quite content and ready to do my duty. For once, I could think of solo time as a productive activity! I enthusiastically popped in the DVD, sat down to get relaxed, and then. . . my brain got sodomized.

See, I live in San Francisco, and, well, there are a lot of "alternative" sexual orientations. It also happens, sad times for Tim Ferriss, that Mr. Wash-Your-Hands was not good at matching DVDs to their cases.

Within seconds of sitting down, I'd come to the realization that this room, with paper sheets in all their glory, had been used by hundreds of other donors. That alone required me to enter a state of focus reserved for Olympians and Iron Chef competitors. Then I turn on the DVD and see two hairy boys doing something resembling wrestling. But not wrestling.

Second DVD, same story. Third time was the charm, but I was already suppressing so many images and realities that it was like bending a spoon with my mind to get done what every guy has mastered by age 12.

Ah, Mr. Wash-Your-Hands. We will meet again, and I shall give you a judo chop.

Mentally prepare, gentlemen. It won't be as easy as you think. These are tough, dangerous times. Good times to save your swimmies as cheap insurance.

And don't forget to wash your hands.

TOOLS AND TRICKS

InCase Sports Armband Pro (www.fourhourbody.com/armband) This is the neoprene armband I used for holding my mobile phone. Though designed for the iPod Touch, it's large enough to hold BlackBerries, iPhones and most other pocket microwaves.

Pong Case for iPhone (www.fourhourbody.com/pong) This is the only case that's been tested in FCC-certified laboratories and proven to reduce your iPhone's radiation to a third of what it would be without the case, all while maintaining signal strength. If you have to keep your mobile phone in your pocket, this will help minimize the damage, but I still suggest "off" around the twins.

***The Disappearing Male*, CBC Documentary (www.fourhourbody.com/disappearing)** This no-cost download of *The Disappearing Male* is about one of the most important, and least publicized, issues facing the human species: the toxic threat to the male reproductive system. Frightening and required viewing.

Sperm Bank Directories Find a bank or storage facility in your area using the below websites, or use Google to search for "sperm storage or bank or donor" in combination with your city and state names.

www.spermbankdirectory.com
www.spermcenter.com/sperm_bank_listings

Fertility Clinic Directories

Society for Assisted Reproductive Technology (www.sart.org/find_frm.html, site compatible with BlackBerries and iPhones)
"Local Doctors, Physicians, and Surgeons Directory" (www.healthgrades.com/local-doctors-directory)
Fertility Journey, "Fertility Clinic Locator" (www.fourhourbody.com/fertility)
Find a Fertility Clinic (www.findafertilityclinic.com)

"Semen Analysis", WebMD (www.fourhourbody.com/semen-analysis) Further reading on the process of semen analysis (e.g., what medications and conditions can affect your semen).

PERFECTING SLEEP

ENGINEERING THE PERFECT NIGHT'S SLEEP

Insomnia is a gross feeder. It will nourish itself on any kind of thinking, including thinking about not thinking.

—Clifton Fadiman, former chief editor, Simon & Schuster

*"God, what a beautiful beach. Calm. Translucent turquoise water. I should really go back to Thailand. I wonder what time it is in Thailand. But . . . why is there a mangy German shepherd on my beach? Orange collar. That makes no sense. Kind of looks like John's dog. Actually, I owe John a call. F*ck. Did I put his birthday party in the calendar? Birthdays and clowns. Clowns?! Why the hell am I thinking about clowns?!?"*

And so my internal monologue continues until 3:00, 4:00, or even 6:00 A.M., rotating through images, ideas, commitments, anxieties and fantasies.

This mental slide show is combined with perverse sleep yoga: sometimes the twisted-into-a-pretzel posture, sometimes lying on my back like Dracula in mock-paralysis, and always ending in the foetal position with a pillow or arm between my knees. Foetal position never works, but I continue to try it, like a full-bladdered dog scratching at a door that never opens.

I have insomnia. Horrific "onset" insomnia.

My father and my brother are the same. It's not

because we're stressed out, necessarily, it's not because we're not tired. It's because we just can't freaking fall asleep.

So, in the interest of finally getting a good night's rest and helping others with insomnia, I tried everything from folk remedies to smart drugs, from light therapy to fat loading.

Now I can say that I *had* chronic insomnia.

The Hidden Third of Life

Is good sleep a simple matter of length, the longer the better?

If you've ever needed a nap after sleeping too much, you know it isn't that simple. Let's look at the problem through an easier question: what is bad sleep?

- Taking too long to get to sleep ("onset" insomnia, my major problem)
- Waking too often throughout the night ("middle" insomnia)
- Waking too early and being unable to get back to sleep ("terminal" insomnia)

The challenge for a self-tracker is measuring things when drooling into a pillow. I could record the times when I got into bed and when I woke up, but I couldn't pinpoint when I fell asleep, much less what happened while asleep.

Taking courses like "Biology of Sleep" at Stanford University didn't fix my insomnia, but the academic searching did help me formulate more specific questions, including:

- For memory consolidation: how much REM sleep am I experiencing?
- For tissue repair: how much delta-wave sleep am I experiencing?
- For both of the above: am I experiencing sleep apnoea?

The problem with testing these in a proper sleep lab (the test is called a polysomnogram) is that you generally have at least 22 wires attached to you to measure brain activity (EEG), eye movements (EOG), skeletal muscle activation (EMG), heart rhythm (ECG), respiration and sometimes peripheral pulse oximetry.

Guess what? No one can sleep in a weird lab with 22 wires attached to them on the first night. So the data are terrible. But let's assume you try. The second night, you come in after an all-nighter and crash within minutes like a post-sugar-high two-year-old. Double-bad data.

To really test and tweak things under realistic sleeping conditions, I would need a pocket-sized sleep lab.

That didn't happen until 2009.

My First F*cking Sleep Lab

JULY 2009

"You should try what Brad Feld used. He has some gadget to measure your sleep," offered one of my friends.

This caught my attention. I had been bitching about my insomnia after another horrible night's sleep, and I'd also been meaning to reach out to Brad.

Based in beautiful Boulder, Colorado, Brad is a venture capitalist and angel investor famous for (1) his incredible track record and (2) dropping F-bombs on business panels.[1] Exhibit A: He was one of the few initial backers of Harmonix Music Systems, which he helped raise $500,000 (£312,000) in financing. They bled money for almost 11 years. A fool's errand! Then, in 2005, it had a small (sarcasm) video game success called "Guitar Hero". It sold in 2006 to Viacom/MTV for $175 million (£109 million).

Brad's contrarian decisions often follow an elegant logic that others only pick up on well after the fact.

If he had found a tool for sleep analysis, I wanted to know all about it.

Of Motion and Waves: The Tools

Brad's obsession ended up being the Zeo. It would be my first legitimate, next-generation sleep gadget.

Then I added more gadgets.

In the subsequent four months of testing, I also used heart-rate monitors, thermometers, continuous glucose monitors, two movement-detection

1. Not to be remiss, investor Dave McClure gives Brad a run for his money.

devices (FitBit and WakeMate) and video recording of sleep movement. Often all simultaneously.

I looked like a comatose Robocop.

Both WakeMate and FitBit, worn on your wrist during sleep, use motion-sensing technology (accelerometry) similar to what's found in a Nintendo Wii controller. The data are interpreted using actigraphy algorithms, which are used to determine whether someone is awake or in one of the various stages of sleep. WakeMate features an alarm clock that can be set to wake you during specific "arousal points" in REM sleep (ostensibly to minimize grogginess) up to 30 minutes before a chosen wake time.

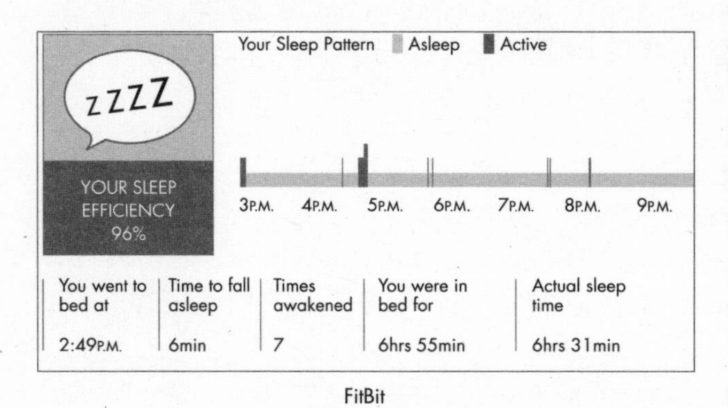

FitBit

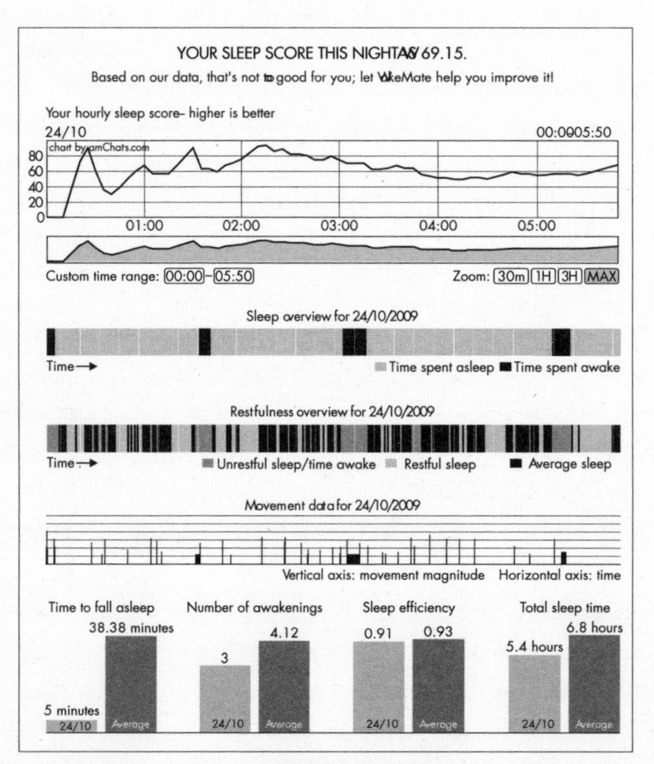

WakeMate

The Zeo, in contrast, uses a headband that measures electrical patterns generated in the brain. It also has an alarm clock intended to wake you during periods of most elevated brain activity to minimize grogginess.

The first attempts to track and fix things were not encouraging.

For both accelerometer devices, time to fall asleep—the critical problem of "onset" insomnia—did not appear

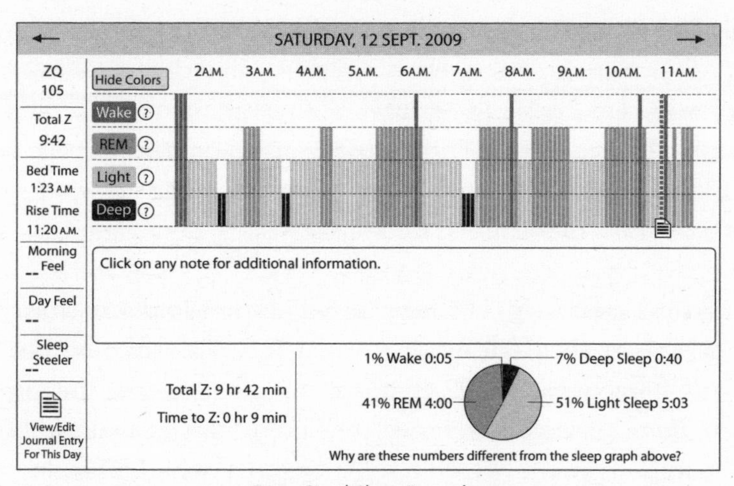

Zeo—Good Sleep Example

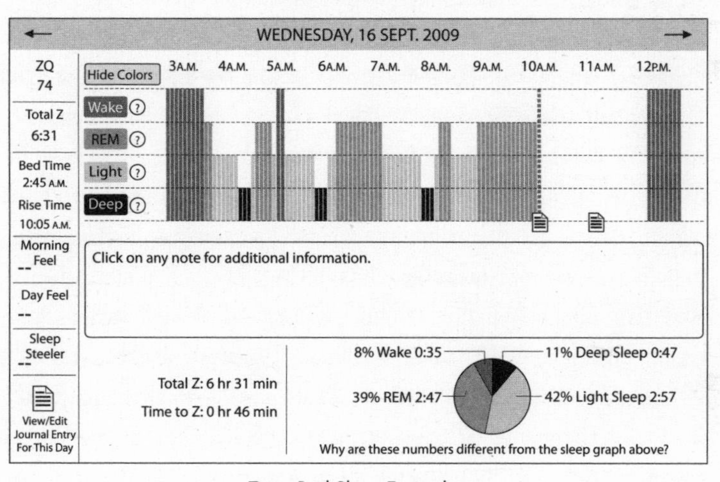

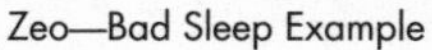
Zeo—Bad Sleep Example

accurate. Despite claims to the contrary, it didn't appear that the accelerometers could distinguish between simple lack of movement and sleeping. I tested this by watching television for 30 minutes, remaining as perfectly still as possible before attempting to sleep. My "sleep" started roughly when I started watching TV.

The first good news came a week later: the intelligent alarms, Zeo and WakeMate, seemed to reduce grogginess. I was less bastardly in the morning and could think without two cups of coffee. Placebo or true cause and effect, the "smart alarms" seemed to help. This was an improvement, but I needed better sleep, not just better wake times.

This is where the Zeo really became valuable.

I began with a trial period of answering a subjective question each morning and assigning a number: do I feel like shit (1–3) or do I feel awesome (8–10)? Nebulous answers between 4 and 7 that would skew interpretation were logged but ignored. In both extreme ranges, I then looked for patterns. Thanks to the continuous glucose monitoring, I also had food logs to use.

Here are some of the initial findings:

1. **Good sleep (8–10) was most dependent on the ratio of REM-to-total-sleep, not total REM duration.** The higher the percentage of REM sleep, the more restful the sleep. The higher the REM percentage, the better the recall of skills or data acquired in the previous 24 hours. Higher-percentage REM sleep also correlated to lower average pulse and temperature upon waking.
2. **I could increase REM percentage by extending total sleep time past nine hours, or by waking for five minutes approximately four and a half hours after sleep onset.** One waking of 5–10 minutes, approximately four and a half hours after sleep onset, dramatically increased REM percentage. It seems that one waking is not necessarily a bad thing, at least when intentional.
3. **Taking 200 micrograms (mcg) of huperzine-A 30 minutes before bed can increase total REM by 20–30%.** Huperzine-A, an extract of *Huperzia serrata*, slows the breakdown of the neurotransmitter acetylcholine.[2] It is a popular nootropic (smart drug), and I have used it in the past to accelerate learning and increase the incidence of lucid dreaming. I now only use huperzine-A for the first few weeks of language acquisition, and no more than three days per week to avoid side effects. Ironically, one documented side effect of overuse is insomnia. The brain is a sensitive instrument, and while generally well tolerated, this drug is contraindicated with some classes of medications. Speak with your doctor before using.
4. **The higher the percentage of deep-wave sleep, the better your subsequent physical performance.**

2. It is therefore called an acetylcholinesterase inhibitor. The *-ase* of acetylcholinesterase indicates it breaks down the preceding molecule.

5. **More than two glasses of wine within four hours of sleep decreases deep-wave sleep 20–50%.** Even four glasses *six* hours beforehand did not appear to have this effect, so the timing is crucial. Conversely, taking 15+ drops of California poppy extract appeared to increase deep-wave sleep up to 20%.
6. **Eating two tablespoons of organic almond butter on celery sticks before bed eliminated at least 50% of the "feel like shit" (1–3) mornings.** Ever wonder how you can sleep 8–10 hours and feel tired? The likely culprit: low blood sugar. Make a pre-bed snack part of your nutritional programme. One to two tablespoons of flaxseed oil (120–240 calories) can be used in combination with the celery-and-almond-butter to further increase cell repair during sleep and thus decrease fatigue. Flaxseed oil tastes like a mixture of raccoon urine and asparagus, so—if you opt to include it—I recommend pinching your nose while consuming it, per Dr. Seth Roberts, whom we'll meet later.

Turning Off Monkey Mind

Next, I moved on to the biggest problem: getting to sleep in the first place. No matter how theoretically restful my sleep should be, based on Zeo results, more than 30 minutes of onset insomnia negated it all.

What follows are the changes and tools that had the largest effects on time-to-sleep. Some of them are more convenient than others. I excluded drugs[3] from testing, and if a given improvement couldn't be replicated at least three times on consecutive nights, it was omitted.

TEST 19–21°C (67–70°F) AS YOUR BEDROOM TEMPERATURE.

This was the variable I experimented with the most while in Nicaragua for my medical tourism adventures (coming up later), and it was also the variable that had the most consistent effects. Specifically, using a single bedsheet at a room temperature between 19°C (67°F) and 21°C (70°F) produced the fastest time to sleep. Warmer temperatures never worked, but as low as 18°C (65°F) would work equally well *if* I wore

3. Except melatonin in one case.

socks to keep my feet warm. If you can't control the ambient temperature, testing socks of different thicknesses is the easiest variable to change for tweaking heat loss.

Ideal temperature is highly individual, and each person will have a narrow range, so experiment to find your own.

EAT A LARGE FAT- AND PROTEIN-DOMINATED MEAL WITHIN THREE HOURS OF BEDTIME.

I discovered this unintentionally while tracking testosterone changes. Consumed within three hours of getting under the sheets, meals of at least 800 milligrams of cholesterol (four or more large whole eggs) and 40 grams of protein produced dramatically faster time-to-sleep scores than meals of lower volume or lower protein and fat. Eating two rib-eye steaks, each about 350g (12oz), had the strongest tranquillizer-like effect.

USE LIGHT CUES – THE PHILIPS goLITE.

I bought this high-end blue-light emitter for a friend who suffers from seasonal affective disorder (SAD)—aka mild to severe depression during winter months.

He already owned the same device, so I began to use it as a replacement for coffee first thing in the morning. I set it to the side of my laptop, pointing at me for 15 minutes at about a 30-degree off-centre angle (if noon is my laptop, pointing at me from 10 A.M. or 2 P.M.). That evening, my time to sleep was less than 10 minutes for the first time in weeks. I was able to replicate the effect four nights out of five.

Though most often used for jet lag or winter depression, I've found the goLITE to be singularly most useful as a corrective sleep tool, even if I wake up late and need to go to bed at a normal hour. Battery life is long and, at the size of a small square book, the goLITE is portable enough to fit in a carry-on travel bag.

TAX THE NERVOUS SYSTEM WITH ISO-LATERAL MOVEMENTS.

Exercise is commonly recommended to improve sleep.

The problem for me was that results were unpredictable. I might exercise for 20 minutes and fall asleep in 10 minutes, or I might exercise for two hours and fall asleep in two hours. There was no repeatable cause and effect. It seemed like a coin toss.

This changed when I began to incorporate iso-lateral (one-arm or one-leg) resistance training. I logged faster to-sleep times after 8 out of 10 training sessions. The more complex the stabilization required, the shorter the to-sleep time. To experience this effect for yourself, do a single session of pre-hab testing from the "Pre-hab" chapter.

TAKE A COLD BATH ONE HOUR PRIOR TO BED.

The Japanese have longer average lifespans than most other nationalities, including Americans, whom they beat by more than four years. One explanation researchers have proposed is that the regular *ofuro*, or hot bath at bedtime, increases melatonin release and is related to mechanisms for life extension. Paradoxically, according to one of the Stanford professors who taught the sleep biology class I took circa 2002, cold is a more effective signaler (aka *zeitgeber*, or "time giver") for sleep onset.

Perhaps the ofuro effect was related to the subsequent rapid cooling? Not eager to kill my swimmies with hot baths, I opted for direct cold.

I tested the effect of combining shorter-than-usual 10-minute ice baths with low-dose melatonin (1.5–3 milligrams) one hour prior to sleep. The ice bath is simple: put two to three bags of ice from a supermarket ($3–6/£1.85–3.75) into a half-full bath until the ice is about 80% melted. Beginners should start by immersing the lower body only and progress to spending the second five minutes with the upper torso submerged as well, keeping the hands out of the water. (See "Ice Age" for other approaches and benefits.)

It was like getting hit with an elephant tranquillizer. Best of all, this was true even when melatonin is omitted.

USE AN ULTRASONIC HUMIDIFIER.

The Air-O-Swiss Travel Ultrasonic Cool Mist Humidifier is incredible. It is small enough to fit in a jacket pocket (590g/1.3lb), and its water source comes from any supermarket: a plastic water bottle turned upside down. The ultrasonic technology uses high-frequency vibrations to generate a micro-fine cool mist, which is blown into the room, where it evaporates into the air. This device is my go-to combination with the goLITE, especially after seeing how well it eliminates sinus problems while travelling. It also dramatically reduces facial wrinkles, which was an unexpected but pleasant side effect.

The Air-O-Swiss humidifier comes with a transcontinental travel AC adapter and exchangeable plugs that can be used in both the United States and Europe. My only complaint: it emits a stylish (but distracting) blue glow, so you'll need an eye-mask if you're light-sensitive like I am.

USE A NIGHTWAVE PULSE LIGHT.

The NightWave was introduced to me by a good friend named Michael, who also has severe onset insomnia.

During my testing, he started ranting and raving about this tiny device, a slow-pulsing light the size of a cigarette pack that helped him get to sleep in less than seven minutes. Dr. James B. Maas, Weiss Presidential Fellow and professor of psychology at Cornell University, is one of several researchers who have endorsed it.

From the NightWave website:

> *NightWave projects a soft blue light into your darkened bedroom. The "luminance" of the light slowly rises and falls. Lie with eyes open and synchronize your breathing with the blue wave as its movement becomes slower and slower. After a short time [the cycle Michael used was seven minutes long], NightWave shuts off and you roll over and fall asleep . . . unlike sound machines, the soft light does not disturb others.*

It does work, but I found it less consistent than Michael did (his hit rate was near 100%). I now travel with the NightWave but use it as a supplement to the goLITE when needed.

RESORT TO THE HALF MILITARY CRAWL POSITION.

Lie on your chest with your head on a pillow and turned to the right. Both arms should be straight by your sides, palms up. Now bring your right arm up until the top of your right elbow is bent at 90 degrees and your hand is close to your head. Alternative hand placement: the right hand is under your pillow and under your head. Next, bring your right knee out to that side until it is bent at approximately 90 degrees.

This is a last resort that works for one simple reason: you can't move.

It's like a self-imposed papoose, which the Inuits and other cultures have used to calm infants by immobilizing them. To toss and turn from the half military crawl position, you have to first lift your entire body off the bed. Less fidgeting means faster sleep.

TOOLS AND TRICKS

F.lux (http://stereopsis.com/flux/) It's possible that your computer screen is what's keeping you awake. F.lux is a free computer application that dims your computer screen when the sun sets. In the morning, it makes the screen return to its default sunlight-like settings.

California Poppy Extract (www.fourhourbody.com/poppy) This extract from the California poppy acts as a mild sedative, and I found it to increase my percentage of deep-wave sleep.

The Zeo Personal Sleep Coach (www.fourhourbody.com/zeo) Brad Feld's favourite sleep device. The Zeo uses a headband that measures electrical patterns generated in the brain and can wake you at a point of elevated brain activity. It was the only recording device that offered usable data and that consistently reduced grogginess.

Philips goLITE (www.fourhourbody.com/golite) This light is most responsible for my sub-10 minute sleep times after decades of futile effort. I'll usually set it to the side of my laptop for 15 minutes a day. Battery life is long, it's portable enough to take in a carry-on bag, and it can also replace your morning coffee if you give yourself 2–3 days to adapt.

NightWave (www.fourhourbody.com/nightwave) My friend Michael found that the NightWave (a slow-pulsing light the size of a cigarette pack) was a permanent fix to his sleeping problems. I travel with the NightWave and use it is a supplement to the goLITE.

Air-O-Swiss Travel Ultrasonic Cool Mist Humidifier (www.fourhourbody.com/humidifier) This device is my favourite pairing with the goLITE. It improves both time to sleep and depth of sleep, not to mention skin and sinus health.

Sleep Cycle iPhone Application (www.lexwarelabs.com/sleepcycle) The Sleep Cycle alarm clock analyses your sleep patterns and uses the iPhone's in-built accelerometer to wake you when you are in the lightest sleep phase. This has been the #1 paid app ($0.99/59p) in many countries, including Germany, Japan and Russia.

"Lucid Dreaming: A Beginner's Guide" (www.fourhourbody.com/lucid) Lucid dreaming, as clinically demonstrated by Stephen LaBerge of Stanford Univeristy, refers to becoming conscious during REM and affecting dream content. To facilitate lucid dreaming, I have used huperzine-A to increase REM percentage.

Lucid dreaming can help you accelerate skill acquisition, improve sports performance and reactivate "forgotten" languages. This article is a concise step-by-step how-to guide for beginners.

BECOMING UBERMAN

Sleeping Less with Polyphasic Sleep

Death, so called, is a thing which makes men weep, And yet a third of life is passed in sleep.

—Lord Byron

They say he only sleeps one hour a night. You know about this guy? Tyler Durden?

—Fight Club

Scientists know embarrassingly little about why we spend roughly one-third of our lives asleep.

It can't be as simple as tissue repair. Full-grown giraffes, as one example, weigh approximately 125.7st (798kg) but sleep an average of just 1.9 hours per 24-hour cycle.

Eight hours per night doesn't apply to most of the animal kingdom. Is there any reason why humans can't emulate giraffes?

Is it possible to cut your total sleep time in half, yet feel completely refreshed?

The short answer is yes.

In 1996, I once went almost five days without sleep to see (1) if I could make it a week (I couldn't), and (2) what the side effects would be. Hallucinations cut that little experiment short, but I've continued to play with different patterns of sleep cycles.

One of the most fascinating approaches is that of "polyphasic" sleep: breaking sleep up into multiple segments so you can perform well with as little as two hours of sleep per day. The potential advantages of this schedule for new parents—or anyone else forced to embrace insufficient sleep—

are tremendous. Beyond that, think of the books you could read, the things you could learn, the adventures you could have with an extra six hours per day. It would open up a new world of possibilities.

There are hundreds, if not thousands, who swear by the Thomas Edison approach to minimalist sleep, which bears little resemblance to "sleep" as you know it.

I have used both the "Everyman" and "Siesta", detailed in this chapter, with great success. I reserve anything resembling "Uberman" for emergency deadlines only. To explain the options and pitfalls of each, I'll let a more experienced polyphasic sleeper, Dustin Curtis, tell you his story.

Enter Dustin Curtis

My body is incompatible with Earth.

It has a daily sleep-wake cycle that lasts about 28 hours instead of 24, which means each day I stay awake about four hours longer than most people. In the middle of the week, I sometimes find myself waking up at 11:00 P.M. and going to bed in the early afternoon the next day. When I was younger, people thought I was insane. The only thing I remember of elementary school is being tired.

Eventually, I discovered that if I stuck to a 28-hour schedule, my body was happy. I woke up rested, went to sleep tired and everything worked great. Except that, well, my life was incompatible with the rest of the world. Living with a normal schedule was going to be tough, so I had to find a solution.

After some research, I discovered that what I probably have is called non-24-hour sleep-wake syndrome. The solution is polyphasic sleep, which anyone can use to shave six hours off their normal sleeping time (with a catch, of course).

HELLO, POLYPHASIC SLEEP...

The basic premise of polyphasic sleep is that the most beneficial phase of sleep is the REM phase. Normal sleepers experience REM for a mere 1–2 hours per night. To reap the benefits of polyphasic sleep, we'll need to engineer things so that REM is a much higher percentage of total sleep.

One of the ways to force your brain into REM sleep and skip the other phases is to make it feel exhausted. If you've gone 24 hours without sleep, you might notice that you drift away into dreams straight from being awake. This is because your body goes instantly into REM sleep as a protection mechanism. The way to hack yourself into entering REM sleep without being exhausted is to trick your body into thinking you're going to get a tiny amount of sleep. You can train it to enter REM for short periods of time throughout the day in 20-minute naps rather than in one lump at night. This is how polyphasic sleep works.

There are actually six good methods to choose from. The first one, monophasic sleep, is the way you've probably slept your whole life. The five others are quite a bit more interesting.

With monophasic sleep, you sleep for **eight hours** and you get about **two hours of good REM sleep**. This is the normal schedule most people use, and it means about five hours of the night are lost to (as far as we know) unnecessary unconsciousness.

There are five methods for polyphasic sleep that all focus on many 20-minute naps throughout the day and, in some cases, a couple hours of core sleep at night. The simplest is the **"Siesta" method,** which includes just one nap in the day and then a huge chunk of sleep at night. Remarkably, adding just one nap during the day **shaves an hour and 40 minutes off** your total sleep requirement.

The "Everyman" method is just a stepped ladder that offers different combinations of naps and core sleep. The amount of total sleep per day is drastically reduced for each extra nap you add.

The **"Uberman" method,** coined by PureDoxyk, has six naps and no core sleep. Amazingly, you can function with just **two total hours of sleep** using the Uberman method.

THE CATCH

How awesome would it be to sleep a total of two hours a day and feel rested? Very awesome, of course, but there is a catch. The more naps you have (and thus the less sleep you have total), the more rigorous you have to be regarding your nap times. You can't miss a nap by more than a couple of hours in the Everyman 2 and Everyman 3 methods, and you must have your naps within 30 minutes of their scheduled times for the Uberman method. If you miss a nap, the whole schedule is thrown off, and you'll feel tired for days.

The rigour of keeping the schedule makes most of these methods un-

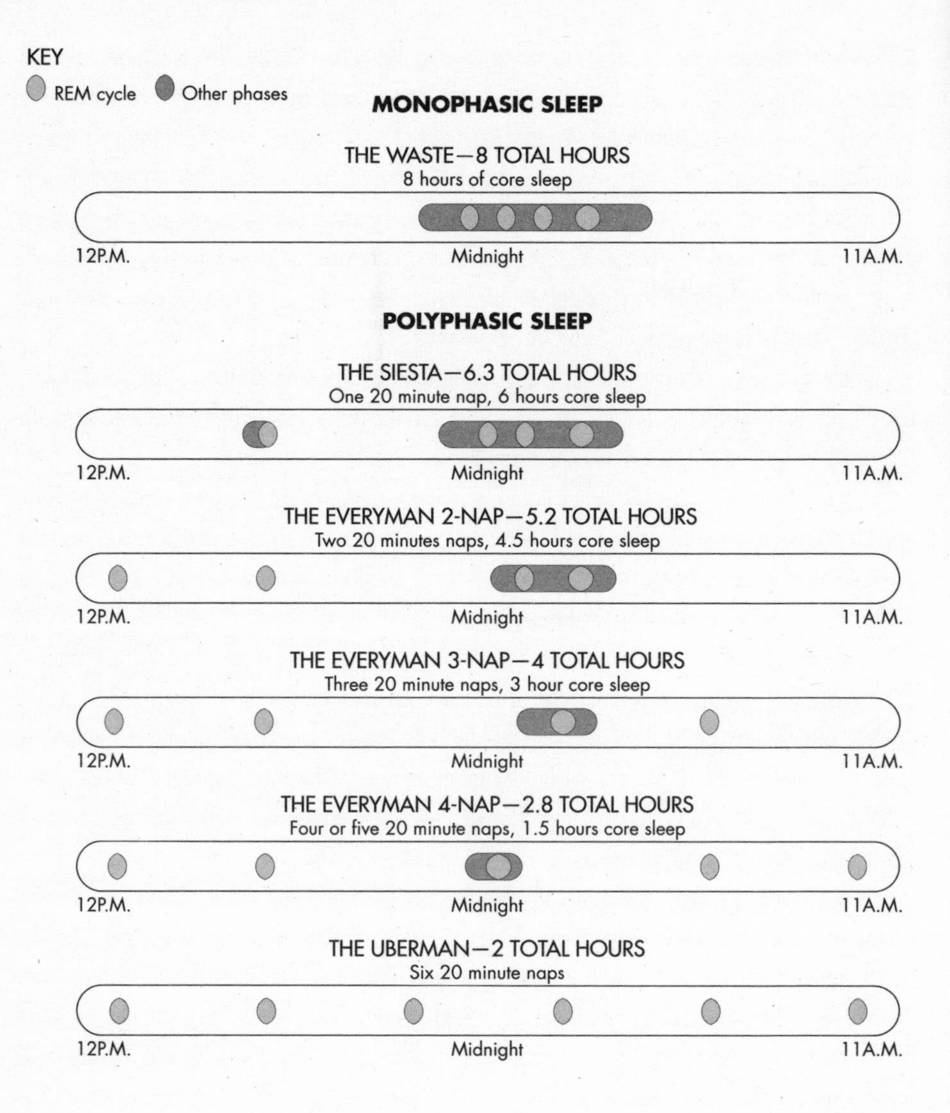

realistic for 9-to-5 employees. But if you have a flexible schedule and can manage to pick a method and stick with it for several months, you'll find that you feel amazing and have a seemingly unlimited amount of time during the day to get things done.

This, to me, is the ultimate brain hack.

UBERMAN 101

Step #1: Determine your sleep schedule. You will be taking 20-minute naps, every four hours, around the clock. That's six naps, evenly spaced over the course of 24 hours (e.g., 2:00 A.G., 6:00 A.G., 10:00 A.G., 2:00 P.G., 6:00 P.G.,ÄandÄ10:00 P.G.). This cycle will remain the same throughout your polyphasic sleeping period.

Step #2: Do NOT oversleep. By oversleeping just once, you'll upset the cycle and feel exhausted (for up to 24 hours) as a result. Under no circumstances should you sleep more than 20 minutes, as it can ultimately cause you to abandon the polyphasic schedule out of fatigue. Get a reliable alarm clock. If you're tempted to hit the snooze button, put the clock far away from where you sleep.

Step #3: Do NOT skip naps. Respect your schedule and follow it to the minute. Skipping them will have a compounding effect. Missing one nap results in a loss of energy that requires two more naps to return you to normal mental sharpness.

Step #4: Beat the initiation phase. The first week and a half is the toughest. If you follow your outlined schedule, don't oversleep, and don't skip naps, you should be well adjusted to your new sleeping regimen in just under two weeks, though some can take up to three weeks.

TOOLS AND TRICKS

Dustin Curtis (http://blog.dustincurtis.com/) The blog of the author of this chapter, interface designer, start-up design advisor and amateur neuroscientist Dustin Curtis.

Steve Pavlina's Sleep Logs (www.fourhourbody.com/pavlina) Steve Pavlina's trial of polyphasic sleep is what introduced me to Uberman. These are the most detailed polyphasic sleep logs you'll find anywhere on the web.

Uberman Schedule Success Stories (www.poly-phasers.com, www.fourhourbody.com/kuro5hin) Kuro5hin is what introduced Matt Mullenweg, lead developer of the popular blogging software WordPress, to the Uberman schedule, which he used for one year. He recounts the experience:

"It was probably the most productive year of my life. The first three to four weeks you're a zombie, but once you settle into the schedule, you don't even need an alarm to wake up after the naps. I probably wrote the majority of my code contributions for Wordpress.org during that time. Then, I got a girlfriend. That was the end of Uberman, and the beginning of a significantly less productive—but more romantic—phase. It's nice to be able to spend a normal night with someone instead of just sleeping 20 minutes."

Try Polyphasic (http://forums.trypolyphasic.com/) This forum covers common questions, and practical suggestions, from people around the world who are attempting polyphasic sleep.

"How the Everyman Sleep Schedule Was Born" (www.fourhourbody.com/everyman) Read about how the Uberman has been modified to make it more flexible with people's schedules.

"Polyphasic Sleep: Facts and Myths" (www.supermemo.com/articles/polyphasic.htm) This article compares polyphasic sleep to regular monophasic sleep, biphasic sleep, and the concept of "free-running" sleep.

HOW TO KEEP ON SCHEDULE

Kuku Klok (www.kukuklok.com) Once loaded, this online alarm clock will work even if your Internet connection goes down.

Clocky Moving Alarm Clock (www.fourhourbody.com/clocky) This patented alarm clock jumps 90cm (3ft) from your nightstand and runs away while beeping to get you up. You can only snooze once.

Wakerupper (www.wakerupper.com) Wakerupper is an online phone reminder tool. Schedule reminder calls to ring to your mobile phone at specific times.

REVERSING INJURIES

Hacking is much bigger than clever bits of code in a computer—it's how we create the future.

—Paul Buchheit, creator of Gmail

I recently went to a new doctor and noticed he was located in something called the Professional Building. I felt better right away.

—George Carlin

REVERSING "PERMANENT" INJURIES

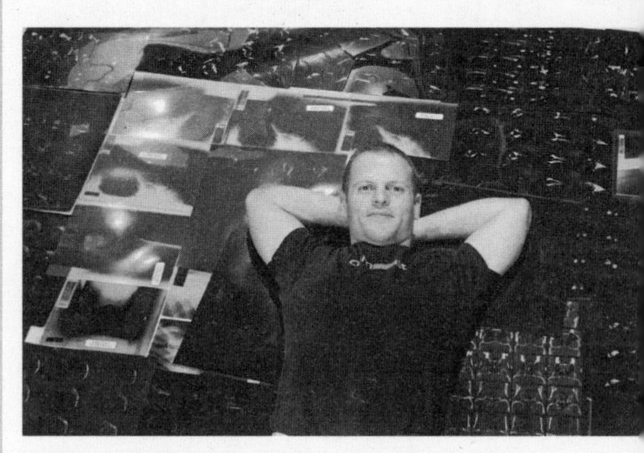

Less than half of my MRIs and X-rays from 2004 to 2009.

The French explorer and marine biologist Jacques Cousteau was once asked how he defined a "scientist". His answer:

> *It is a curious man looking through a keyhole, the keyhole of nature, trying to know what's going on.*

I had become a very curious man in June 2009 out of pain and desperation. The question I had in mind was extreme: what would happen if I tried to reverse a lifetime of injuries and physical abuse in 14 days?

If there were no financial constraints, if I had access to the doctors and drugs of Olympic and professional athletes, could I do it?

Or, perhaps more likely, would I just go bankrupt or kill myself?

In the end, I did come close to killing myself (easy to avoid, thankfully), but I reversed almost all of my "permanent" injuries. It took closer to six months, but the end result was well worth the hiccups along the way.

Let us begin with a cautionary tale, and then we'll move on to how to reap the benefits without the screw-ups.

The $10,000 (£6,250) Lesson

I was sitting on a doctor's table in Tempe, Arizona, battling the ice-cold air conditioning as I stared, not through Jacques' keyhole, but at a bulging transverse colon.

It was gorgeous.

The bulbous organ was right in the middle of an anatomical poster on the wall, and for some reason the artist had rendered it in such glistening realism that it dominated the entire chart. For lack of other decorations, I ended up fixating on the colon like a candle flame while I had 7.5cm (3in) needles stuck into my neck, shoulders and ankles.

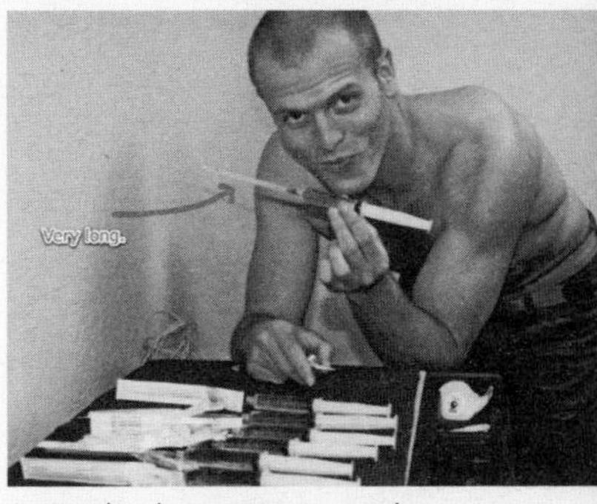

Setting the clinic injection record.

The first needle grazed my cervical spine, and I began to sweat. That was just the warm-up. Within two hours, I set the clinic record for single-visit injections.

There were two additional sessions over the next eight days, and I travelled the full spectrum of emotions, including abject terror. The needle taps on my spine, done to elicit additional growth factor release, sounded like small scratches on a blackboard. Less than an hour later, I watched on in perverse amusement (the cumulative anaesthetic of 10+ shots helped) as a syringe inserted in one side of my left ankle began to dance underneath the skin on the opposite side like a chest-popping foetus from *Aliens*. It then poked through the skin, and I was less amused. Not a party trick you want to show your patients.

We used everything but the kitchen sink.

The most potent of the chemical cocktails was a hybrid. It combined the ingredients used on the knees of an Olympic skier with the ingredients used on one sprinter who'd torn his Achilles tendon eight weeks prior to the world championships. The latter ended up winning a gold medal.

The final Frankenstein elixir was serious business. It included:

Platelet-rich plasma (PRP) PRP is an emerging treatment mainly used with elite athletes. It gained national attention in 2009 when used successfully to treat two Pittsburgh Steelers just weeks prior to their Super Bowl victory. PRP contains the plasma portion of your blood with concentrated platelets. Platelets are packed with growth and healing factors and are part of the body's normal tissue repair system. The PRP is prepared using a special centrifuge after whole blood is drawn from your arm, similar to getting blood drawn for lab work.

PRP formed the base to which the following were added:

Stem cell factor (SCF), flown in from Israel, which assists in blood cell production.

Bone morphogenic protein 7 (BMP-7), which helps adult stem cells (mesenchymal) develop into bone and cartilage. In retrospect, I believe this to be the most dangerous substance in all of the cocktails I tried.

Insulin-like growth factor 1 (IGF-1) IGF-1 has anabolic (tissue-building) effects in adults and is produced in the liver after stimulation by growth hormone. It is one of the most potent natural activators of cell growth and multiplication. It is also an expensive drug used at the higher levels of professional bodybuilding.

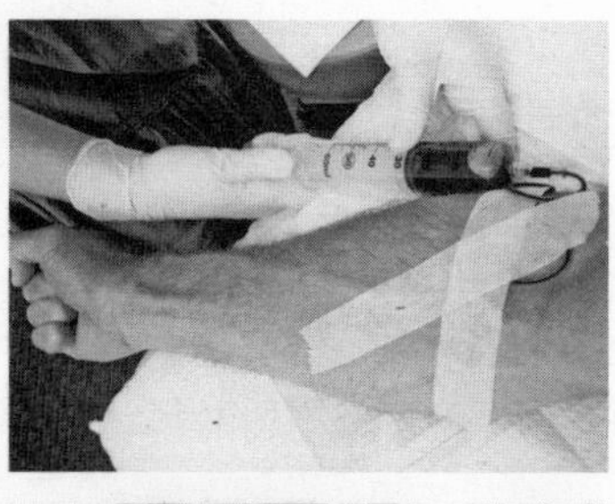

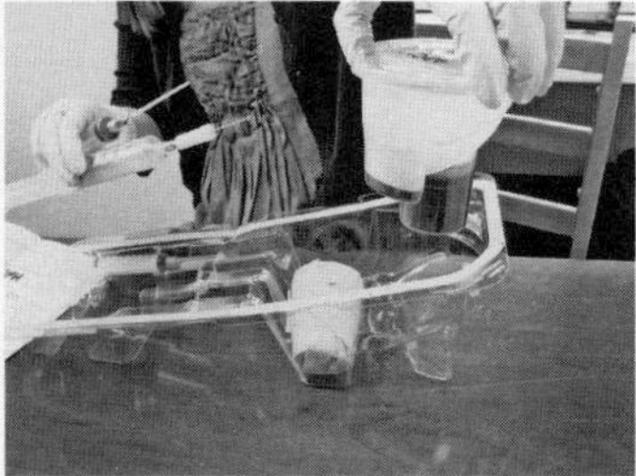

Making platelet-rich plasma.

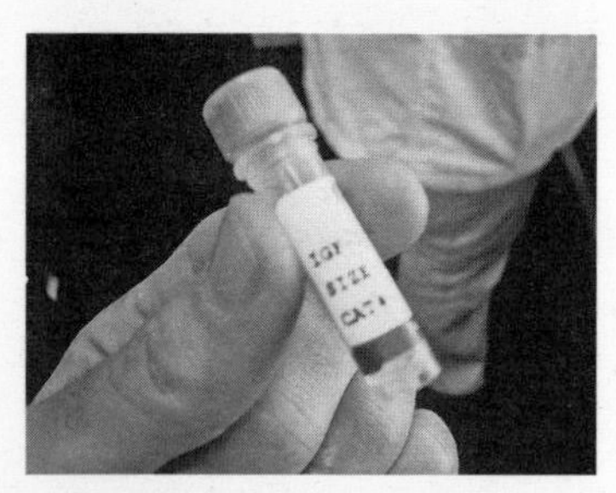

Insulin-like Growth Factor 1 (IGF-1)

So what happened?

The end result four months later, according to the world-class Harvard-trained spine specialist who looked at the before-and-after MRIs, was:

"I could not appreciate any before-and-after differences."

Now, there might have been microscopic changes (cytokines, etc.), but the MRIs reflected my pain: no change.

The three sessions had cost more than $7,000 (£4,350), and not only was the experience expensive, it ended up being a disaster.

One of the injections in my right elbow resulted in a staph infection and emergency surgery at the University of California–San Francisco Medical Center, almost two months of limited arm use, and more than $10,000 (£6,250) in hospital expenses.

When I contacted the sports scientist responsible for the injections to ask for $1,500 (£950) to help defray the costs, the e-mail response was as unorthodox as the treatment:

> Why would you even waste your time asking me for this when you can just go out and make far more money?

Wow.

In scientific parlance, the whole thing was a total cluster-fuck.

Not because PRP, for example, doesn't work (I believe it will completely revolutionize regenerative medicine), but because I didn't find the right person to administer it.

There are a lot of pitfalls when you seek out the cutting-edge: snake oil, and con artists who capitalize on the desperate, among other things. How then can you, the reader, with no desire to waste $7,000–20,000 (£4,350–12,500), weed out the junk science and charlatans?

The least painful option is to let a human guinea pig test them all for you.

That's my job.

The Reasons

First things first: why the hell would I do this to myself?

It's quite simple. There is a price to be paid for all of the envelope-pushing I've done over 15+ years. Namely, more than 20 fractures and 20 dislocations, two joint surgeries (shoulder and, now, elbow), and enough tears and sprains to last a lifetime. Decades of full-contact abuse and over-confidence in all sports ending in "-boarding" has made me, as one orthopaedic surgeon put it, "a 30-year-old in a 60-year-old body".

Though it was a depressing and fatalist diagnosis, it didn't appear uncommon. My closest male friends, also former competitive athletes, had all started creaking and groaning after age 30. The aches were turning into surgeries, small training injuries had become chronic pain, and we all recognized the pink elephant in the room: it was going to get worse. Much worse.

For me, the straw that broke the camel's back was a series of high-dose prednisone prescriptions and epidural injections in 2009. It started with an innocuous shoulder impingement. MRIs showed no shoulder issues but uncovered cervical spine degeneration in five discs.

"This is something you'll just need to live with" was the concluding remark, delivered with an inappropriate smile, from a spine surgeon who works with NHL and NFL teams. None of his recommended drugs or injections would fix the problem. They were nothing more than Band-Aids designed to mask symptoms, to dull the senses. I had graduated to terminal pain management.

My second day on prednisone, a strong immunosuppressant drug, I spent the entire afternoon stumbling around the Mission district in San Francisco in a daze, looking for a car I'd parked just an hour earlier. I gave up after three hours and took a cab to a dinner meeting.

The next morning, I woke up looking like a pug and couldn't remember who I'd had dinner with. Enough was enough. If conventional medicine couldn't fix the problem, it was time for more drastic measures.

If I was going to fix one thing, I wanted to fix them all.

The Menu

Looking at the ultimate results (what worked and what didn't) I could have saved myself a lot of expense by following a four-stage approach. Only when options in the first stage fail do you proceed to stage two, and so forth, up to the final stage and last resort: surgical repair.

Stage #1—Movement: Correcting posture and biomechanics through specific movements

Stage #2—Manipulation: Correcting soft-tissue damage or adhesion using tools or pressure with the hands

Stage #3—Medication: Ingesting, injecting or applying medication

Stage #4—Mechanical reconstruction: Surgical repair

Below is just a small sample of the approaches I tested for this book during a five-month period in 2009, as well as following shoulder reconstruction in 2004 (which accounts for most of the intramuscular injections). Injections were performed with blood test reviews every two to four weeks.

Part of the drive to experiment was fuelled by positive experience: I knew what was possible. Post-surgery in 2004, I used a careful combination of therapies that produced incredible results: my surgically repaired shoulder ended up superior to my uninjured "healthy" shoulder.

Sometimes it's possible to not just restore but exceed previous capabilities, making you "better than new". It can be life-changing.

I have put asterisks next to what had the most immediate and lasting effects, with the areas fixed in parentheses. The most effective of all will be explained in detail afterwards.

MOVEMENT

Feldenkrais
Pilates
Assisted stretching
Tai Chi Chuan
Yoga (Ashtanga, Bikram)
*Barefoot/Vibram walking (lower back)
*Egoscue (cervical/neck and mid-back)

MANIPULATION

Massage (from Swedish to Rolfing)
Acupuncture and acupressure
*Active-release technique (ART) (shoulders)
*Advanced muscle integration therapy (AMIT) (pectorals, glutes and calves)
Graston technique

MEDICATION

Topical
- Androgel® (crystallized testosterone)
- DMSO (a solvent popular among sprinters and racehorses) combined with MSM
- Arnica

Oral
- Cytomel® (liothyronine sodium = synthetic T3 thyroid hormone)
- High-dose L-glutamine (50–80 grams per day)
- High-dose bovine and chicken collagen (types 1, 2 and 3)

Intra-articular (in the joint) injections
- PRP
- Cortisone
- *Prolotherapy (left knee, right wrist)

Intramuscular injection
- *Deca-Durabolin® (nandrolone decanoate) (left shoulder)
- Delatestryl® (testosterone enanthate)
- Depo®-Testosterone (testosterone cypionate)
- Sustanon® 250 (testosterone blend)
- HCG (human chorionic gonadotropin)
- *Biopuncture protocol using microdoses of Traumeel and lymphomyosot (Achilles tendon, infraspinatus)

Subcutaneous (under the skin) injection
- HGH (human growth hormone)
- *Biopuncture protocol (same as above)

It's quite the laundry list.

The Chosen Few

All of them helped to some extent, but only a few of them produced relief that lasted more than 48 hours, and some of the exercises were impossible to perform alone.

There were just five treatments that reversed "permanent" injuries, either as 1–3 sessions or as viable solo exercises. Here they are:

1. SHOE HEEL REMOVAL AND VIBRAM TRAINING. AREA FIXED: LOWER BACK.

Ugly, and ultimately painful, postural compensation is unavoidable when wearing shoes that elevate the heels. This simple observation somehow escaped me for 30 years, until CrossFit Chicago instructor Rudy Tapalla introduced me to Vibram Five Finger shoes, which look like gloves for your feet.

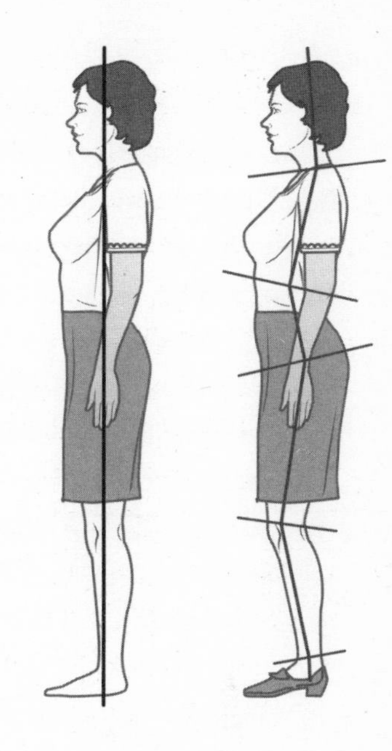

Chronic use of high-heeled shoes usually results in some degree of kyphosis-lordosis and related pains in the lower back and mid-upper back. Kyphosis-lordosis, seen in the second illustration to the right, is posture characterized by "convex curvature of the thoracic spine and an inwardly curved lower back resulting from the pelvis being tilted forward". This is an academic way of saying hunchbacked and sway-backed at the same time.

This is how both men and women with less than 10% body fat can end up looking potbellied. It's the overarching of the low back, not excessive body fat, that causes this unfortunate optical illusion.

The fix is simple: most of the time, wear flats or shoes with little difference in sole thickness from toe to heel. Shifting to wearing Vibram Five Fingers® and Terra Plana Barefoot Vivo shoes completely erased low-back pain I'd suffered from for more than 10 years. To the degree it was possible, the Vibrams also helped restore my feet. Restore to what? Their natural condition, illustrated below in the first set of photos, published in the *American Journal of Orthopedic Surgery* in 1905.

Don't get me wrong. Used on occasion, a nice set of heels can really accentuate the female form and give fellas some style and height.

Just use the elevation in moderation.

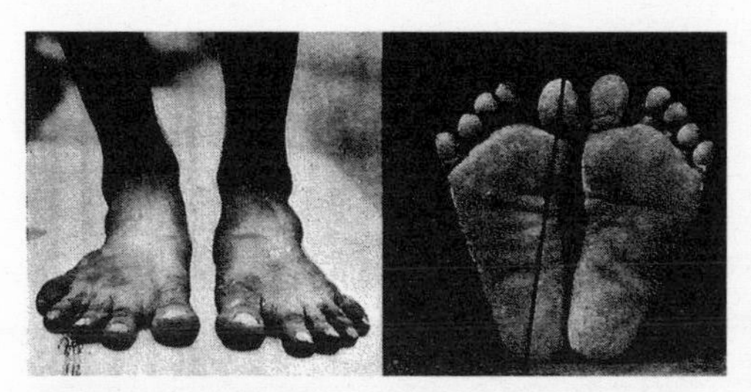

In barefoot walkers, the toes fan out, providing a stable base for walking. Notice the natural outward line from the centre of the heel to the big toe, which prevents excessive pronation (rolling of the feet inward) and related problems in the knees and lower back.

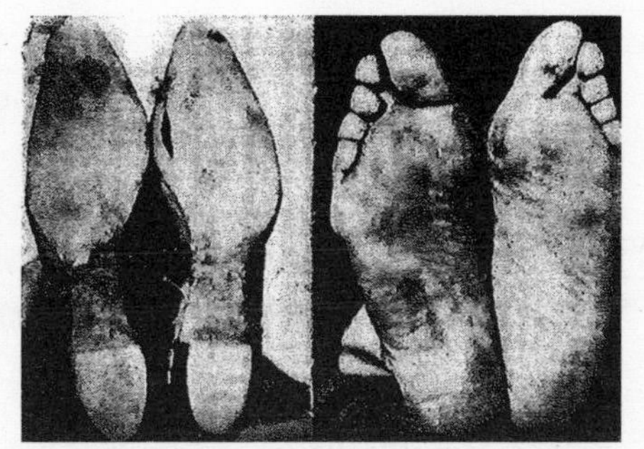

Much like in Chinese foot binding, the feet of this modern man have conformed to his shoes. The outward line from heel to big toe is non-existent.

2. THE EGOSCUE METHOD.
AREAS FIXED: CERVICAL/NECK AND MID-BACK.

Peter Egoscue (pronounced "Eg-*os*-cue", not "*E*go-scue") is the founder of the Egoscue Method, a postural therapy programme with 24 clinics worldwide. Peter is a former marine and self-taught therapist who became famous through experimentation on himself and athletes. One of his early experiences is lore among his trainers:

Peter found himself in the locker room of a professional wrestler after the athlete had sprained his ankle. Peter, only at the event because the producer was his friend, had the wrestler lie on the floor and place his extended and injured leg on top of a locker door. Unsure of what to do, he chose elevation. Peter then got a phone call and walked out, only to return 15 minutes later. The wrestler stated in no uncertain terms that the elevation had been a complete waste of time. His ankle still felt the same.

But, for whatever reason, his chronic back pain felt better.

Peter asked himself a simple question: "Why?" He then repeated and refined this unusual locker-room stretch until its success rate for back pain was impressive enough to warrant a formal name. It became the rather obscene-sounding "supine groin progressive", which I later fell in love with. Decades later, he still emphasizes the fundamental importance of basic questioning at Egoscue University: "Students, in my world, because I know nothing, everything is possible."

For me, the Egoscue Method was not love at first sight.

I had been exposed to Egoscue on half a dozen occasions via athletes before testing it myself in 2009. I held off for as long as I did because the early exposure left me with an aftertaste of cult.

Testimonials claimed everything from disappearing allergies to self-healing digestive problems, and I was shown videos of trainees going into full-body involuntary spasms like grand mal seizures during certain "e-cises" (exercises).

I decided I was just fine without a Pentecostal brand of Pilates. If I wanted to squeeze my pelvic floor while swinging a dead cat over my head, I could do that on my own. So I ignored the Egoscue Method, despite endorsements from golf legend Jack Nicklaus and Super Bowl ring-sporting NFL players like John Lynch.

Then, in June 2009, I found myself in Tempe, Arizona, eating lunch with a friend who was scheduled for an Egoscue session that very afternoon with John Cattermole, a well-respected and seasoned practitioner with 25 years of physical therapy experience. I agreed to accompany him and undergo an evaluation, fully prepared for a nice dose of voodoo.

Instead, I walked out 90 minutes later with no pain in my mid-back for the first time in six months. I couldn't believe it.

It would be one of many times that I slapped myself for prematurely throwing out the baby with the bathwater. This experience also reconfirmed two truisms: (1) some practitioners of any method will get the message wrong and broadcast it, creating confusion as representatives, and (2) it's critical, as Bruce Lee emphasized, to "absorb what is useful, discard what is useless, and add what is uniquely your own".

Based on several months of testing myself and other laptop hunchers, I can recommend six 80/20 exercises for desk-dwellers' postural imbalances. For the minimalists who work at home (or who have understanding coworkers), I suggest performing #1, #2 and #3 after every two or three hours at a desk or in a sitting position and performing all five movements at least once per week.

The supine groin progressive, the most inconvenient, unusual and time-consuming of the five, is the singular most effective tool I've found for eliminating psoas and other hip flexor tightness to unlock the pelvis and relieve hamstring tightness.

1. Static Back

Sets 1 | **Reps** 1 | **Duration** 0:05:00

Description

1. Lie on your back with your legs up over a block or chair.
2. Place your arms out to the sides at approximately 45 degrees from your body with palms up. Touch your thumbs to the floor.
3. Relax your upper back and ensure your lower back flattens to the floor evenly from left to right.
4. Hold this position for five minutes.

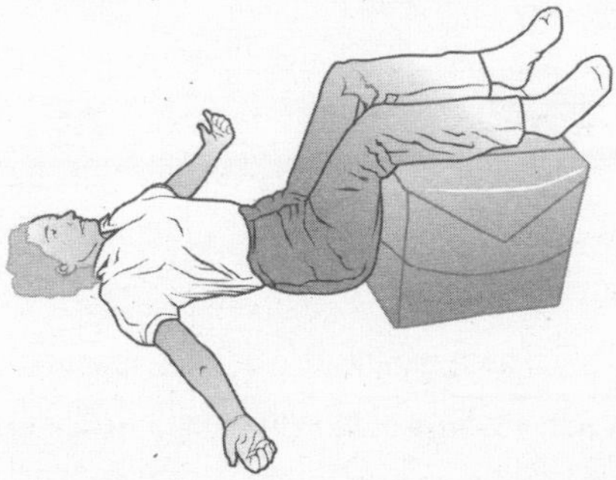

2. Static Extension Position on Elbows

Sets 1 | **Reps** 1 | **Duration** 0:01:00

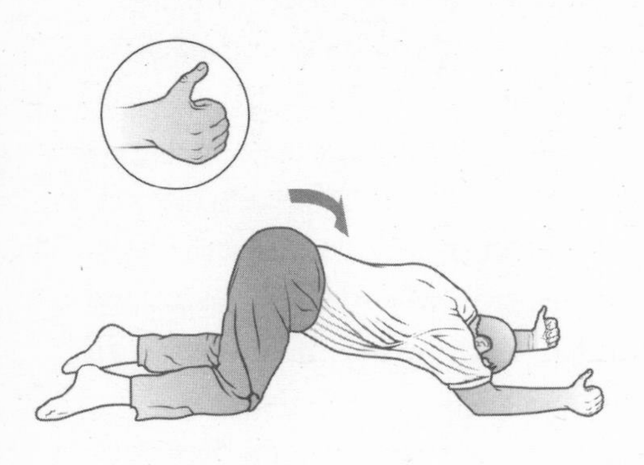

Description

1. Start on the floor on your hands and knees, ensuring your higher joints are aligned (i.e., shoulders, elbows and wrists in a straight line; hips directly above the knees).
2. Walk your hands forward about 15cm (6in), and then, noting placement of the hands, replace them with your elbows.
3. Make a light fist of each hand and pull them away from each other, pivoting on your elbows and turning the thumbs out.
4. Push your hips backward towards your heels to place an arch in your lower back.
5. Let your head drop down.
6. Hold for 60 seconds.

3. Shoulder Bridge with Pillow

Sets 1 | **Reps** 1 | **Duration** 0:01:00

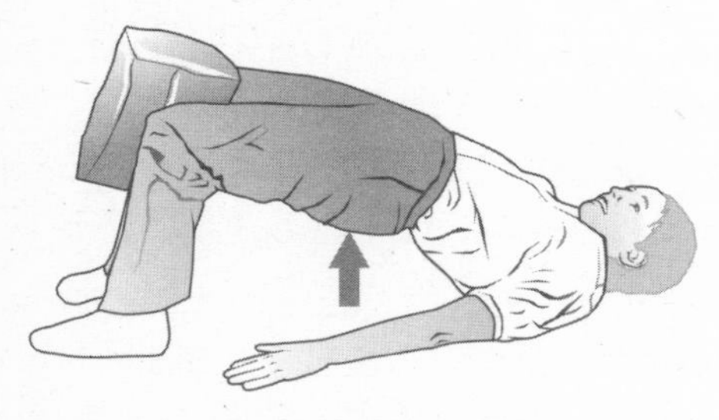

Description

1. Lie on your back with your knees bent and your feet pointed straight ahead.
2. Place a pillow between your knees and apply a constant pressure inward while executing the exercise.
3. Relax your upper body and lift your hips and back up off the floor.
4. Hold in top position for one minute.

4. Active Bridges with Pillow

Sets 3 | **Reps** 15 |

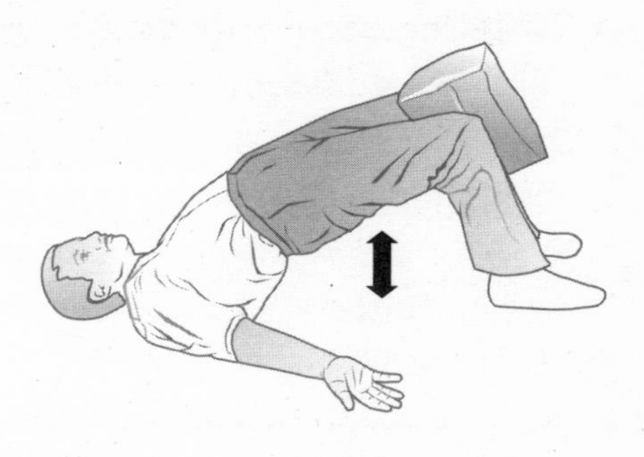

Description

1. Follow the instructions for the last exercise, but, instead of holding at the top of the movement, lift your hips as high as you can and slowly lower them back down. Keep the motion as smooth and continuous as possible.
2. Repeat 15 times for three total sets.

5A. Supine Groin Progressive in Tower

Duration 25 minutes each side

Description

1. Lie on the floor with one leg up over a block or chair, bent to 90 degrees (in the illustration, the right leg). Your arms should be out to your sides at 45 degrees, with palms facing up.
2. Place the other foot in the boot used with the tower.
3. Place your booted foot on the tower, starting at the lowest level and moving it up until an arch begins to form in your lower back. This is the level where you will complete your first 5 minutes.

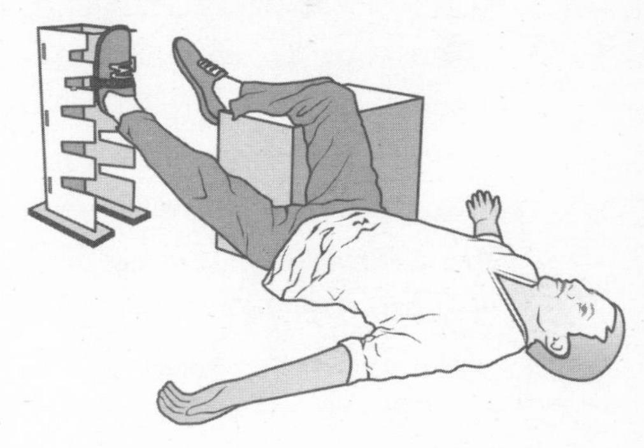

4. Hold until your back is flat on the floor. Pay more attention to the flattening of your back than the specified time.
5. After 5 minutes, lower your foot one level on the tower and again hold.
6. Continue this until your leg is extended straight out on the lowest level.
7. Switch legs and repeat the entire sequence.

5B. Alternative: Supine Groin on Chair

This is a far inferior version of the supine groin progressive, as it's not progressive, but it's more convenient.

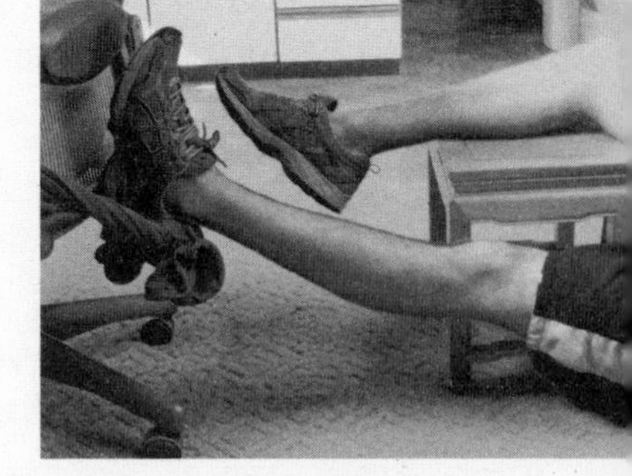

1. Tie a sweatshirt or pair of jogging bottoms around a chair or door knob.
2. Set a small chair or table, approximately knee height, next to the set-up from step 1.
3. Suspend the heel of one leg in the sweatshirt or jogging bottoms and rest the other leg on the chair or table. Hold for 10 minutes.
4. Repeat on the opposite side.

6. Air Bench

Sets 1 | **Reps** 1 | **Duration** 0:02:00

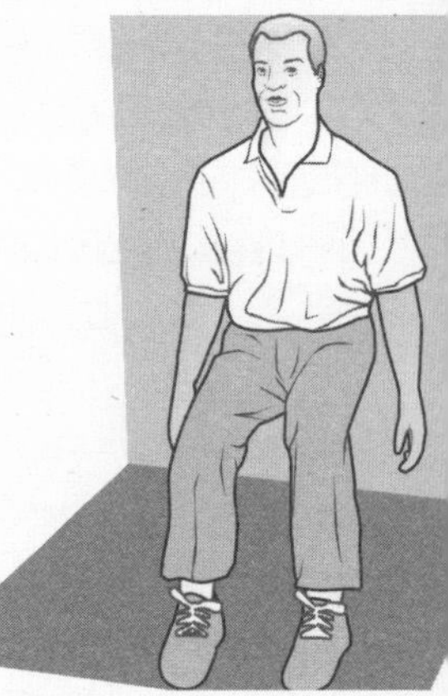

Description

1. Stand with your back against a wall with feet and knees hip width apart. Feet point straight ahead.
2. Walk your feet away from the wall while sliding your body down at the same time until your knees are bent at 90 degrees. Ensure your ankles are slightly ahead of your knees. Your lower back should be completely flat against the wall. Your arms can hang down to your sides, or you can rest your hands gently on your lap. Keep the weight in your heels and do not press forward on your toes.
3. Hold for two minutes.

3. ADVANCED MUSCLE-INTEGRATION THERAPY (AMIT). AREAS FIXED: PECTORALS, GLUTES, CALVES.

I split guinea pig duties for injury reversal with a semi-professional athlete we'll call "Seabiscuit". He had torn his hamstring in sprint training. I took the bullet for biochemical experiments and injections, and he tested the unusual therapies and painful mechanical corrections. From Mexico to Miami, we'd seen a lot and spent more than $100,000 (£62,500) already. Few things paid off.

"Dr. Two Fingers" was Seabiscuit's single best find, and I received a text message to that effect, which ended with:

"Mate, you need to break something just so Dr. Two Fingers can fix you. Trust me."

I'd already taken care of the breaking things, so I booked a flight to Salt Lake City and drove almost an hour to the small Mormon-dominated town of Kaysville, where the ChiroMAT office of Craig Buhler—"Dr. Two Fingers"—is located.

The walls of his waiting room are covered with thank-you letters and signed jerseys from the best of the best in their respective sports: four-time Super Bowl star linebacker Bill Romanowski, NBA players John Stockton and Karl Malone, and alpine ski star Picabo Street, among others.

Buhler approached injuries differently than most.

Unlike the majority of therapists, who treat the tight or painful muscles and joints themselves (i.e., sore lower back? → work on the lower back; painful Achilles? → rehab the Achilles), Buhler's sought to unpeel the onion of *proprioception*, how the nervous system, in this case, turns muscles on or off.

Seabiscuit had nicknamed Buhler "Dr. Two Fingers" because of his unusual approach to isolating and reactivating individual muscles that had been injured or deactivated. For his highest-level athletes, this could be done for up to 700 muscles. With one finger pressed deep into the end of a given muscle (a tendon insertion point) and another finger of the opposite hand pressed into the opposite end, he would progress through a series of tests to return a dormant muscle to its previous function.

From a brochure at his clinic:

> *We have found that when a body part is overloaded or stressed past its capacity to handle the load, there is a predictable result. Either the muscle or connective tissue is injured, or the proprioceptive system deactivates parts of the tissue, much like a circuit breaker in an electrical circuit.*
>
> *The body adapts, recruiting other muscles to take over the load. With repetition, the adaption advances. Recruited tissues get stronger, impaired areas atrophy.*

It didn't take long to demonstrate this "reactivation" in practice. Dr. Two Fingers first tested the strength of my supraspinatus (the most commonly injured rotator cuff muscle) using an FET force sensor, showed that

I had the strength of Dakota Fanning, and then proceeded to reactivate it, more than quadrupling my strength.

I went from lifting 2.7kg (6lb) to lifting 12.7kg (28lb) in less than five minutes.

"Do you have pain at the bottom of your right Achilles tendon?" Buhler asked. He hadn't even looked at this location, and he had pinpointed one of my most serious problem areas. He could see I was confused, so he explained:

"Your gastrocnemius [calf] isn't firing properly—it's turned off—so it makes sense that you have Achilles and knee pain, and most likely referral pain in your hamstring."

And so he continued, proving again and again that what I thought was the problem wasn't the problem. It was a muscle that had taken over for another muscle, which had taken over for yet another muscle. The original muscular deactivation could be on the opposite side of the body, nowhere near the site of pain.

His spotting ability was incredible. One world-class powerlifter who'd visited Buhler shared an anecdote from his first visit: "He hadn't even touched me and he announced that I had weak quads. I responded back with 'Weak quads?! I deadlift 408kg (900lb)!' to which Craig just shrugged and went to work." The lifter later reviewed slow-motion footage of his pulling technique in competition and realized that, undeniably, his technique clearly indicated he was straightening his legs quickly to compensate for weak quadriceps.

Time spent with Dr. Two Fingers added up. Fifty dollars (£31) per muscle reactivated means that function doesn't come cheap. I had a total of four sessions and covered more than 50 muscles.

I couldn't accept all of his supplemental programmes, but I knew that exploring the fringes required casting a wide net. To find the few things that worked, it was sometimes necessary to bite your tongue and withstand things you knew didn't work, even within the same offices.

In the end, I tested his treatments with the only jury that really mattered: objective weights.

The changes were not subtle.

Take the pectorals, for instance. Since fracturing both collarbones in my teens, I have had disproportionate trouble recruiting the chest, making the bench press and similar movements my weakest exercises.

Twenty-four hours before my second session with Buhler, I performed decline flies with 18kg (40lb) dumbbells for a maximal five repetitions.

Twenty-four hours after the session, I performed slow decline flies with 23kg (50lb) dumbbells (20% increase) for 14 repetitions (180% increase).

Incredible.

Before you aim to improve a muscle's output (weight or repetitions lifted) by increasing size, it's important to ensure that the input (neural system) is functioning properly. Do you really need "stronger muscles", or is the wiring just not conducting the signal properly?

If you can't make a trip to Dr. Two Fingers, see the MAT resources at the end of this chapter for a local option.

4. ACTIVE-RELEASE TECHNIQUE (ART).
AREA FIXED: SHOULDER INTERNAL ROTATORS.

Dr. P. Michael Leahy's engineering education began with aeronautics in the air force. His fascination with structural mechanics only fully expressed itself much later, in 1985. This was the year ART was formalized and patented, the year he applied his engineering to human soft-tissue injuries. Leahy, a veteran of 25 Ironman triathlons, has since been doctor to, among others, Olympic gold-medal sprinter Donovan Bailey, Gary Roberts of the NHL Toronto Maple Leafs and Mr. Universe Milos Sarcev.

The basic premise of the method is simple: shorten the tissue, apply manual tension, and then lengthen the tissue or make it slide relative to its adjacent tissue. Simple does not mean easy; as Leahy explains, "It's as simple as playing a piano and just as difficult."

What does this look like in practice? If muscles are adhered to one another or to bone, it looks a lot like tearing muscles apart. See the visual preview to the right.

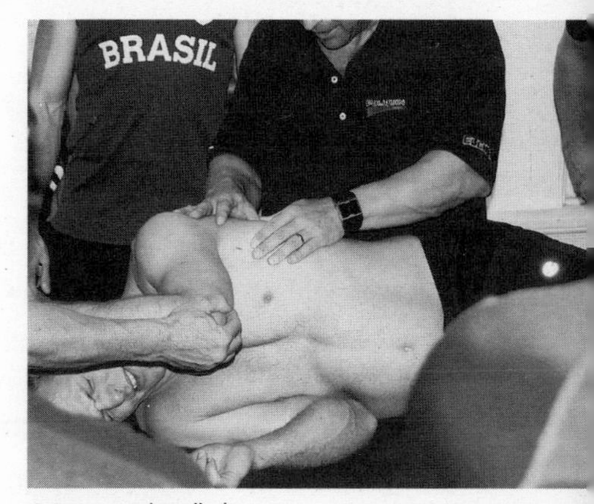

Getting manhandled.

I first encountered ART in 2001 through Frank Shamrock, five-time middleweight Ultimate Fighting (UFC) champion.

Frank had his first ART treatment in July 2001 following an acute lower back injury during training. He was unable to walk and didn't expect much:

I had seen more than 30 chiropractors throughout the world over a 16-year period for lower back pain and numbness in my leg. With the training injury that prompted my visit, I couldn't raise my head above waist-level, and I was sleeping on the living room floor in the fetal position. I had always been told one of two things by orthopedists and various MDs: I would need to have my vertebrae fused, or simply tolerate the pain of an injury that was irreversible. Based on past experience, I was certain that I would need to cancel the K-1 kickboxing fight I had scheduled for one month later.

In four sessions of approximately 10 minutes each, the doctors at the Janzen & Janzen Sports Health Clinic in San Jose, California, eliminated the cumulative scar tissue and adhesions that had created the pain in Frank's lower back. He was carried out of the gym on his trainer's shoulders on Thursday and was training at 100% the following Tuesday.

Three weeks later, Frank won his K-1 fight by first-round KO. Frank then recommended ART to B. J. Penn, Brazilian Jiu-Jitsu World Champion, who used ART to restore full range of motion to his left shoulder (preventing surgery), right shoulder and hamstring, among other areas. Two weeks prior to the 2 November 2001 UFC championship, B. J. Penn's lower back pain was treated successfully in two 15-minute sessions. B.J. proceeded to knock out a heavily favoured Caol Uno in just 11 seconds of the first round.

Experimenting with ART

Flash-forward to an overcast and dreary afternoon in New York City, December 2009.

Freezing rain was falling in sheets outside of the Peak Performance gym where 20 or so strength trainers, coaches and I had been taking an all-day seminar on PIMST (Poliquin Instant Muscle Strengthening Technique), developed by professional and Olympic trainer Charles Poliquin. For each diagnostic and training exercise, we paired off with partners and tested range of motion. For the first exercise, we'd looked at both external and internal shoulder rotation (for the latter, imagine the motion of arm wrestling or pitching a baseball). My external rotation was excellent, but my internal rotation was so close to immobile that my partner thought I was joking: "Wow. You're kidding, right?"

Unfortunately, I wasn't kidding. I couldn't remember the last time I'd been able to touch most of my back. Reminded of this handicap and a bit demoralized, I approached Charles during a break to ask him for recommendations. He paused for a second and looked at me:

"Would you like me to fix it?"

I wasn't sure how to answer.

"That would be incredible" was all I could get out. Charles led me to a massage table on one side of the gym and asked me to lie down. He gathered all of the students for a demonstration of removing adhesions and restrictions.

Quite the demonstration it was.

Though I was the weakest male in the entire group, the big boys and Westside-style powerlifters had more respect for me 20 minutes later. It was clearly the most painful thing they had seen in a long time. Poliquin, who'd used ART on his athletes under Mike Leahy for four years, had to use two hands: "You know it's bad when I have to use two hands. I *never* have to use two hands."

He had two 14.3-plus-stone (90.7-plus-kilogram) assistants guiding my arms through movements as he applied enough pressure to put his fingers a good centimetre in between muscles that had either fused to bone or fused to adjacent antagonistic muscles. I felt like a Christmas turkey.

The before-and-after photos on the following page tell a more complete story.

Charles estimated he'd need three or four more sessions to fix the restriction in both shoulders completely. It wouldn't be the first time he'd helped resurrect shoulders:

"A few years ago, my good friend and IFBB professional bodybuilder Milos Sarcev called me out of the blue. He mentioned that he was scheduled to have arthroscopic surgery the following week for both of his shoulders. He was understandably upset. For one thing, the surgery would cost him about $18,000 (£11,250). Additionally, he'd have to undergo an extensive rehab programme, and this would keep him from competing and earning an income for a long time. I told him to get his ass over to my office right away and see [Dr. Mike Leahy] before letting a surgeon anywhere near his shoulders.

"When Milos came to the office, he hadn't trained in over four months because of the excruciating pain. Even lowering an unloaded Olympic bar (20kg/45lb) caused him to recoil in pain. However, after working on him [on adhesions around his subscapularis muscle] for just 45 minutes, Dr. Leahy told Milos to go to the gym and give his shoulders a trial run. Somewhat reluctantly, Milos allowed me to take him to the local World Gym. In total disbelief, he bench-pressed 143kg (315lb) for two reps. Five days later, he did 6 reps with 143kg (315lb) without feeling any pain!"

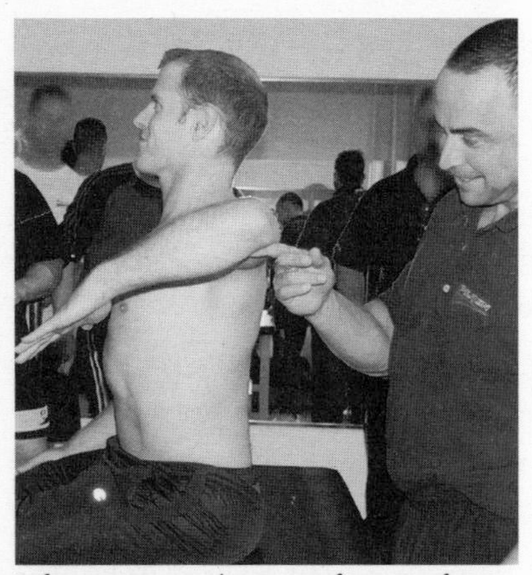

Before treatment—the range of motion of a piñata. Notice Charles laughing.

ART sessions are typically 5–15 minutes in length and cost $45–100 (£28–62) each. Most client injuries are treated in one to six sessions. Soft-tissue injuries eligible for ART treatment include rotator cuff impingement, tendinitis, low-back strain, ankle and wrist sprain, shin splints, hip flexor impingement and carpal tunnel syndrome.

But ART isn't perfect.

As Charles noted: "ART is 100% effective in 70% of patients."

Fixing chronic pain often requires a combination of therapies. Sometimes that involves needles, which brings us to the next stage: medication.

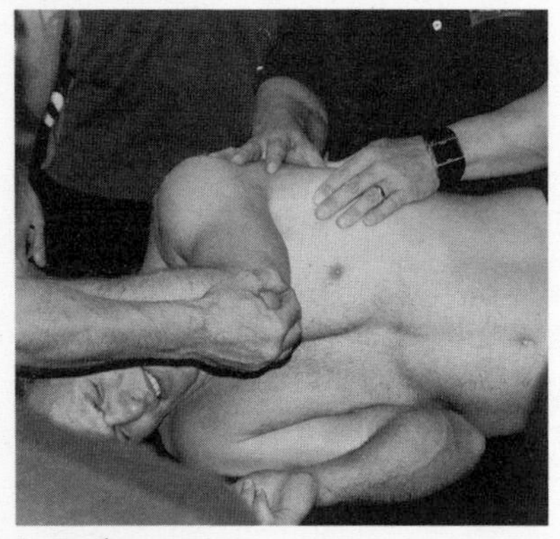

During the treatment.

5. PROLOTHERAPY.
AREAS FIXED: LEFT KNEE, RIGHT WRIST.

In prolotherapy (so named for the "proliferation" of collagen fibres it's supposed to produce), a mixture of irritants are injected into tendons, ligaments and inside joints themselves. The objective is to create a mild inflammatory response that stimulates tissue repair.

The simplest of prolotherapy cocktails, and the one with the longest track record, was developed by the founder of the technique, George Hackett MD. His mixture is, in effect, "sugar water": dextrose mixed with a local anaesthetic (lidocaine) and saline (saltwater).

Dr. C. Everett Koop, the 13th surgeon

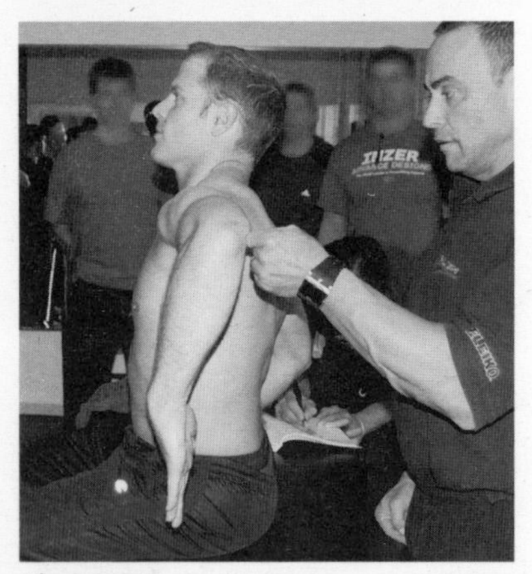

After treatment.

general of the United States, opened the doors for wider research on prolotherapy when he publicly endorsed it:

> *Prolotherapy, unless you have tried it and proven its worth, seems to be too easy a solution to a series of complicated problems that afflict the human body and have been notoriously difficult to treat by any other method....*
>
> *When I was 40 years old, I was diagnosed in two separate neurological clinics as having intractable (incurable) pain. My comment was that I was too young to have intractable pain. It was by chance that I learned that Gustav A. Hemwall, MD, a practitioner in the suburbs of Chicago, was an expert in prolotherapy.... To make a long story short, my intractable pain was not intractable and I was remarkably improved to the point where my pain ceased to be a problem.*
>
> *The nice thing about prolotherapy, if properly done, is that it cannot do any harm. How could placing a little sugar-water at the junction of a ligament with a bone be harmful to a patient?*

In 2005, doctors at the Mayo Clinic began testing prolotherapy and identified the most responsive injury sites as the knees, elbows, ankles and the sacroiliac joint in the low back. They concluded in their newsletter that "unlike corticosteroid injections—which may provide temporary relief—prolotherapy involves improving the injected tissue by stimulating tissue growth".

The prolo cocktail I used at the clinic mentioned at the opening of this chapter had a few additional ingredients:

Dextrose
Marcaine (anaesthetic)
B-12
Proline
Lysine
Glucosamine sulphate

My first session entailed 12 prolo injections. It wasn't all fun and games. For 45 minutes after the first session I had vertigo and a cold, numb right hand.

On the positive side, decade-old pain in my right wrist (from impact in gymnastics) and my left knee (wrestling) both disappeared approximately 21 days after the last session.

The dangers of the ingredients are minimal, particularly when a simple dextrose-based version is used, but there is always the risk, albeit small, of infection. If a needle passes through the skin, it can carry bacteria from the skin into the target site. This is most serious when the infection occurs inside a joint and turns it septic, a process that can cause the joint cartilage to deteriorate in as little as 72 hours.

A survey in France reported an overall risk of sepsis of 13 per 1 million injections, with a much lower incidence if pre-packaged syringes are used.

That said, after one staph infection, I was eager to explore less invasive injections, which led to the next therapy: biopuncture.

6. BIOPUNCTURE.
AREAS FIXED: INFRASPINATUS, ACHILLES TENDON.

"Can you hear that?"

I could, and it was disgusting. Dr. Lee Wolfer was in the process of giving me between 40 and 60 injections[1] with small needles commonly used for tuberculosis tests. Each injection was no more than 1cm (½in) under the skin, but the noise emanating from my infraspinatus, one of the rotator cuff muscles in the shoulders, sounded like someone walking on hard snow: audible crunching.

"That's calcium deposited where it shouldn't be."

Lee, one of the foremost spine and back specialists in the United States, then got back to work. The injections weren't close to done. I'd given her a laundry list—neck, upper back, shoulders, ankles—and we had a lot of ground to cover.

Lee is now a die-hard fascist. "Fascist", that is, in the sense of someone who treats the long-neglected fascia as more than just anatomical glue. The results have, so far, been impressive:

"I'm finally happy as a doctor. I'm helping my patients' bodies to heal themselves."

The "fascia" comprise a three-dimensional web of fibrous connective tissue that maintains the structure of the body. Think of fascia as the ropes that hold the tent in its shape. Ropes that help to bind muscles together and keep internal organs suspended, among other things. Ever heard runners complain of plantar fasciitis? It's a fascial problem, and a painful one. The plantar fascia of the foot is a thick band of connective tissue that extends

1. Similar to the pioneering Hackett-Hemwall protocol of prolotherapy, often referred to as the "sewing machine" approach.

from the heel to the five toes. It supports the arch of the foot, and when it becomes inflamed and compromises that arch, chronic pain is the result.

It's not just a foot issue. The fascia exist throughout the body and also have biochemical roles.

Lee's journey started with a research paper on lower-back pain, where she noticed the researchers had observed something odd: the patients' fascia looked like those of diabetics. There were unusual calcium deposits throughout the tissue, which she later saw in her own patients.

The area of greatest concern was the Grand Central Station of the entire back: the thoraco-dorsal fascia. This fascial sheath connects prime movers like the lats and the glutes in the lumbar area, and problems in Grand Central can cause pain almost anywhere. Fascia are masterful at misdirection. Fascial slings can connect areas like the right shoulder to the left lower back, and pinpointing the actual problem requires a Sherlock Holmes-like ability to connect seemingly unconnected dots, often outside of the body.

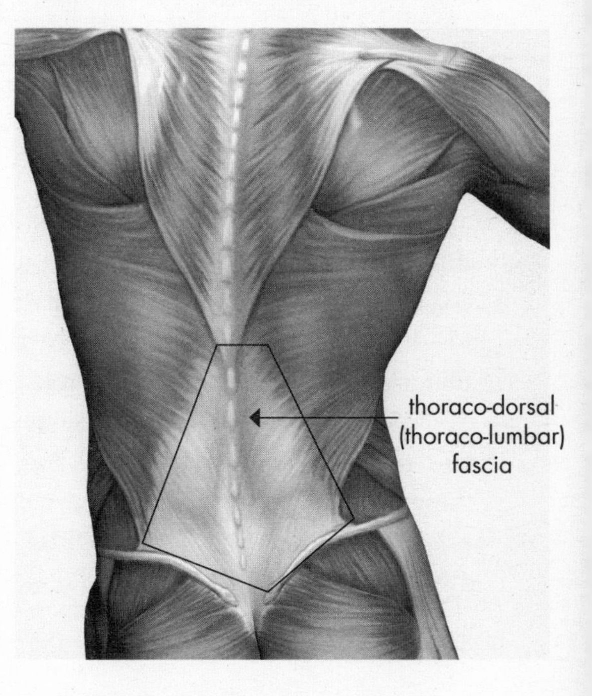

Just one example from diet: Lee had come to realize the importance of eating nutrient-dense animal foods with adequate fat-soluble vitamins (A, D, E and K) to restore function in chronically inflamed tissues with abnormal calcium deposits.

Now, Lee was using me to test her latest and greatest: biopuncture.

Coined in 1991 by Jan Kersschot MD, a Belgian physician, "biopuncture" involves shallow injections of different substances, including Traumeel, zdeel and lymphomyosot. Traumeel is typically used for acute inflammation from sports injuries, and lymphomyosot is utilized for lymphatic drainage in chronically swollen or congested tissue. Traumeel has been shown in some peer-reviewed journals to shorten recovery time from acute sports injuries and inhibit the secretion of immune mediators

(IL-1B and TNF-alpha) that are associated with tissue damage and increased inflammation.

Though biopuncture solutions aren't diluted to the extent that they contain no active product (like most homeopathic medicine), they are diluted and referred to as "microdoses". Lee used both Traumeel and lymphomyosot in my treatments.

In addition to the drug treatments, we also tested a saline solution with 20% dextrose. It was just like prolotherapy but with shallower injections.

The results of dozens of "baby jabs" with a small 30-gauge 1cm (½in) needle were amazing.

Twelve hours after the first treatment of both infraspinatus muscles, I had zero pain at the rear of either shoulder. I had suffered through persistent pain and soreness at the back of both shoulders for more than six years, and one 15-minute session fixed both of them. To date, no pain has returned.

The biopuncture was repeated for the right Achilles tendon, with similar results.

I think the mechanisms of action, while unclear, could be different for different locations. In the case of the infraspinatus, it seemed to be mechanical: the breakdown of calcium deposits with a needle, much like hacking at ice on your windshield. For the Achilles tendon, Lee hypothesized that it was some form of cutano-muscular or cutano-neural response.

Given their homeopathic origins, I remain sceptical of lymphomyosot and, to a lesser extent, Traumeel. But, given the minimal downside of biopuncture and the results I've experienced, I would recommend testing biopuncture before prolotherapy or PRP. For most musculoskeletal problems, a series of four to eight injection sessions are recommended.

TOOLS AND TRICKS

This chapter will encourage a slew of con artists to become self-proclaimed experts. Though you might miss some good practitioners, I suggest focusing on those who were treating patients before this book was first published in December 2010.

Vibram Five Finger and Terra Plana Shoes
(www.fourhourbody.com/vibram, www.fourhourbody.com/terra) These are the two brands of shoes I used to eliminate low-back pain. The Vibram Five Fingers are ideal but look like gecko feet. The Terra Plana Vivo Barefoot shoes, on the other hand, can double as dress shoes without anyone noticing that the soles are practically non-existent.

Healthytoes Toe Stretchers (www.fourhourbody.com/toe-stretch)
These toe stretchers are like soft brass knuckles for your toes. They help restore natural toe spread and relieve pain from overlapping toes and toe drift. Start with five minutes each evening.

Active Release Technique (ART) Practitioner Database (www.activerelease.com) Use this site to find local ART specialists.

Finding a Prolotherapy Practitioner Here are the three organizations recommended by those I trust in the field:

Hackett-Hemwall Foundation (HHF) (www.hacketthemwall.org)
American Academy of Orthopedic Medicine (AAOM) (www.aaomed.org)
American College of Osteopathic Sclerotherapeutic Pain Management (the old term for "prolotherapy") (www.acopms.com)

ChiroMAT (www.chiromat.com) Founder of the AMIT technique, Craig Buhler (aka "Dr. Two Fingers") has helped elite-level athletes from the NBA, NFL and PGA to maximize their performance.

Muscle Activation Technique (MAT) Specialists (www.fourhourbody.com/mat) If you can't get to Utah to see Dr. Craig Buhler, use this site to find a MAT practitioner in your area. Though there is some contention between groups about the best technique, this organization provides the widest certification and is thus most accessible.

Southern California Orthopedic Institute (www.scoi.com) Dr. Stephen Snyder at SCOI has developed many new techniques and technologies for arthroscopic shoulder surgery. Referred to me by friend and fellow patient Scot Mendelson, who bench-presses more than 454kg (1,000lb).

Video of My Reconstructive Shoulder Surgery with Dr. Snyder (www.fourhourbody.com/surgery) The pre-surgery shoulder dislocation while I'm sedated is disgusting. Fun watching if you enjoy YouTube videos of folks face-planting off Swiss balls, etc.

Biopuncture: Common Questions and Answers (www.chiromedicalgroup.com/biopuncture)

Overview of Biotensegrity (www.fourhourbody.com/biotensegrity) This explains the fascinating functions of fascia. Steven Levin, an orthopedic surgeon, explains how the principles of tensegrity seen in R. Buckminster Fuller's geodesic domes apply in the human body, with bones acting as the compressive elements and the soft tissues as the tension elements. If you are at all geek-inclined, read "The Importance of Soft Tissues for Structural Support of the Body". It's outstanding.

Egoscue (www.egoscue.com) Egoscue is a postural therapy programme with 24 clinic locations worldwide. The programme is designed to treat musculoskeletal pain without drugs, surgery or manipulation. It was instrumental in reducing and eliminating my back pain.

***Atlas of Human Anatomy* by Frank H. Netter (www.fourhourbody.com/netter)** This is THE most beautiful and (mostly) comprehensive anatomy book I've ever encountered. It was suggested to me by multiple doctors, including Dr. Lee Wolfer, who described this book thusly: "Netter is single-handedly responsible for the anatomical knowledge of the majority of doctors out there. He just missed the fascia and complexity of ligaments." I also own the flashcards based on the book, which are designed for medical students.

HOW TO PAY FOR A BEACH HOLIDAY WITH ONE HOSPITAL VISIT

I wish we were all naked all the time. I have always believed it's what's underneath that counts.

—Celine Dion

Edwin loved Celine Dion and seemed happy to tell someone about it.

During his radiology training in Iowa, he'd seen Stone Cold Steve Austin at the WWE, one dream fulfilled, but Celine Dion was still on his to-see list.

"We have a lot to do! Please don't move. Here we go . . ." Edwin was also my MRI technician and companion for the next four hours. It was a long time to be horizontal, but the surroundings were beautiful. Hospital Metropolitano Vivian Pellas, a pristine private hospital in the centre of Managua, Nicaragua, couldn't have been nicer.

I'd come to Nicaragua almost three weeks earlier to focus on writing and world-famous surfing. The Kiwi, of Perfect Posterior fame, and I had rented a hillside villa with a pool overlooking the ocean. To skip the crowds at the beaches, we chartered a boat with a captain to the best secluded surf spots up the coast. En route home, the captain also helped us catch and clean fish our private chef could prepare for dinner.

Now, it was 12 hours before my return flight to San Francisco, and I was going to pay for the whole thing with one trip to the hospital.

An Introduction to Medical Tourism

Let's look at the maths to see how this is possible. First, the per-person expenses in Nicaragua:

EXPENSES

Round-trip Orbitz air fare to Nicaragua from San Francisco (one stop in Houston)—$385 (£240) + taxes

Chartered boat (per trip per person)—$20 (£12.50)

First week housing ($2,000 per week for nine people in a 14-bed villa owned by a former NBA player)—$222 (£139) per week

Second week housing onward (gorgeous two-bed villa closer to downtown [www.palermohotelandresort.com])—$129 (£80) per night

Land Rover rental (per person)—$140 (£84) per week

Total for two and a half weeks, excluding food—$1,812 (£1,130)

I've excluded food above to show costs above what I would have spent in the U.S. anyway, as I eat out at least two times a day in San Francisco. Here is the grand total:

Total for two and a half weeks, including food and wine (+$600): $2,412 (£1,500)

So how do we get back to break-even and make the trip, in effect, free?

MEDICAL SAVINGS

I had seven MRIs taken at a negotiated price of $400 (£250) each. For comparison purposes, similar MRIs in San Francisco would have cost approximately $750 (£468) each, so 7 × $350 (£218) savings = $2,450 (£1,530) total cost savings.

I also saved roughly $640 (£400) on comprehensive blood and urine testing by having it done in Nicaragua rather than the United States. Thus, my total savings on medical expenses came to **$3,090 (£1,930).**

I enjoyed a surfing trip in luxury, got a ton of writing done, and then took care of testing and imaging that I wanted to do anyhow. The total cost savings of $3,090 (£1,930) put me ahead (in essence, gave me a profit on the trip) of $687 (£430).

"But," you might rightly point out, "what if I'm not a freak who wants seven MRIs?"

First, despite urban myths to the contrary, there is no radiation risk with MRIs, and I would therefore suggest one or two of them for nagging pains or injuries. Not to mention the preventative value: ask any cancer survivor if they wish they'd had MRIs earlier.

But MRIs aside, the beauty of this geographic arbitrage is the menu of options.

I never seriously considered medical tourism before 2009, as I didn't have pending surgeries I couldn't afford, nor did I want cosmetic procedures (buttock implants, anyone?), which medical tourism agencies have made popular.

Testing and prevention, though, opened up a world of combining world-class travel with world-class medicine.

Due for a dental cleaning and check-up? Perhaps you want to run comprehensive blood work, which I recommend no less than every six months? Consider making a kick-ass trip out of it. That same exotic dream trip, something you might otherwise postpone forever because of expense, could end up as good as free.

Perhaps the lure of travel is exactly the incentive you need to take a closer look at your health?

To get a full appreciation of how easy it was, and how much my experience contrasted with most U.S. hospitals, let me recount the process.

As Easy as 1, 2, 3

I showed up at the private hospital emergency room at 10:30 P.M. on a Sunday night with no advance notice. The Kiwi had swimmer's ear and needed to get it drained prior to his flight, and I wanted to cover the costs of the trip at the same time. The easiest option: take MRIs of all joints with residual pain from sports injuries.

I asked The Kiwi's doctor if I could have MRIs taken, and she informed me that I needed to speak with a supervisor, whom she called in. The list price was $600 (£375) per MRI. I asked for her best volume discount for five MRIs: she responded with $2,400 (£1,500). I told her I would pay in cash (credit card) instead of insurance if she could do $2,800 (£1,750) for seven MRIs, or $400 (£250) per MRI. She agreed. The entire transaction was cordial and pleasant.

The supervisor authorized the MRIs in five minutes and had a car service sent to pick up technician Edwin, who was at home, and bring him to the hospital. I would not be charged for the pick-up. The doctors, realizing we had some time to wait, invited me to sit down with them and share their favourite indigenous fruit, called *jocote* (Red Mombin), which I'd never tasted.

I then asked them what else I could do to fill the remaining 60 minutes of time. Urinalysis? Blood tests? Two doctors pulled out a list of tests I could order and we went through them together, ticking off 25 boxes I wanted, as well as a few the doctors suggested as often-neglected but important. They priced each item for me, I had blood drawn 10 minutes later, and they promised results from the lab within three hours. Three hours?! This amazed me, as I usually wait seven to ten days for blood test results in the United States.

Then I remembered: I was in the A&E department. It was a far cry from the UCSF Parnassus equivalent, where I'd once been chastised by a doctor because I looked at my own chart after waiting for more than three hours in an empty room: "That's property of UCSF. Patients aren't allowed to look at charts. Give it to me."

This spotless and friendly environment in Nicaragua felt so much like a private club that I'd forgotten I was in an A&E department. I was the only person there.

Edwin came in, we completed the MRIs, and, at his insistence, we then took several X-rays for reference images, which I was not charged for. He handed me all of the images and showed me back to the front desk, where I had my blood test, urinalysis reports and a glass of water waiting for me. The supervisor explained that there were few cabs at this late hour—around 3:00 A.M.—so she ordered a car service, at the hospital's expense, to take me back to my hotel.

She gave me a hug and wished me safe travels.

Back in the U.S., when I began to reverse more injuries with the help of MDs (the last chapter), the MRIs from Nicaragua were invaluable. Each saved me expensive imaging orders, as well as guesswork that would have led to weeks of inappropriate therapies. Sadly, the 11-minute visit average per patient in the United States produces a lot of mistakes, but most

MDs will not order just-in-case images to prevent them. Why? Because, as a clinic or doctor, ordering a lot of images increases the likelihood of being audited by insurance companies. In my case, if a hasty diagnosis was made in 11 minutes, I was now able to pull MRIs out of my bag and say, "Let's make sure, shall we?"

This, I believe, is a very prudent thing to do.

Putting off those white sand beaches you've fantasized about? Consider treating yourself to some relaxation and defraying the costs with a visit to a clinic or two.

You might even get some tasty *jocote.*

TOOLS AND TRICKS

***Patients Beyond Borders* by Josef Woodman (www.fourhourbody.com/woodman)** The most comprehensive print guide to medical tourism. This 400+-page book contains 40 of the top medical travel destinations, lists hundreds of hospitals around the world and has an index that matches your medical condition to the best clinics.

***International Medical Travel Journal* Medical Tourism Guide (www.imtjonline.com/resources/patient-guide)** The *IMTJ*'s 10-step guide to medical tourism is a useful starting framework for those considering a fun but productive trip abroad. The plethora of options can be daunting, and this checklist will minimize the paradox of choice.

Bumrungrad Hospital (www.bumrungrad.com) This world-class hospital in Thailand has been featured in the "Top 10 World's Medical Travel Destinations" (*Newsweek*) and is one of the "Top 4 Medical Tourism Pioneers" (*Wall Street Journal*). The pictures on their website will probably make your own US hospital look like a third-world hovel.

Med Retreat (www.medretreat.com) Med Retreat can walk you through the decision-making process and help you find the best international clinic for your needs. Popular destinations include Argentina, Costa Rica and Turkey.

MedTrava (www.medtrava.com) Similar to Med Retreat and based in Austin, Texas, MedTrava can introduce you to hand-picked facilities around the world and save you up to 70% on common procedures.

PRE-HAB

Injury-proofing the Body

I never struggled with injury problems, because of my preparation. In particular, my stretching.

—Edwin Moses, two-time Olympic gold medalist in the 400-metre hurdles; winner of 122 consecutive races

Preface: *This is the longest and most difficult chapter in the book, and for a high percentage of readers, it will be the most important.*

Pursuing rapid increases in performance without doing "pre-hab" for injury prevention is like getting in an F-1 racing car without checking the tyres. The small up-front investment of time (even two to four weeks) will allow much faster progress while avoiding serious setbacks.

Skim it now or return to it later, but don't forget to read this chapter if you're incorporating strength or speed training.

1:30 P.M., CAPE TOWN, SOUTH AFRICA

The security guard at Virgin Active Health Club was not impressed. In a country with 25% official unemployment, violence was less common than you'd expect, but it still paid to be vigilant.

I explained my idea again, which involved taking a thick 90cm (3ft) metal pipe into the gym. The plan was to saw off the base of an umbrella stand and drill a 1cm (½in) hole in one end.

"No, really. It's for my workout. Not for hitting receptionists."

The last part didn't seem to help my argument.

"But, but, Gray Cook told me to do it!" I wanted to pout. "Don't you know Gray Cook?!"

He wouldn't know him.

The real shame is, most people don't, even if he could make their bodies indestructible.

Gray's Anatomy: From the NFL to Special Ops

Michelle Wie was, for several months, arguably the most famous injured athlete on the planet.

During a brief time in 2008, her injuries prevented her from doing a single push-up or holding steady on one foot for 10 seconds. Not exactly what you would expect from the youngest woman ever to qualify for an LPGA golf tour event. Sponsored by Nike and heralded as "one of 100 people who shape our world" by *Time* magazine, it seemed that she had been forced past her prime. She wasn't even 20 years old.

"Before [training], Michelle could drive 293m (320 yards) with the wind at her back. Now, one year later, she can still drive the same 293m (320 yards). The difference is that she can now do it 300 times a day."

Gray Cook, the mastermind behind Michelle's rapid recovery, was schooling me from his quiet base in Danville, Virginia.

He saw what the general public missed. Even injured, Michelle could crush the ball. Most assumed that, if power was there, all was well. But she was inconsistent. Power was just one piece of the puzzle.

Fixing professional athletes in his human durability factory, Gray has become perhaps the world's most sought-after injury-prevention specialist. In 2007, both the Chicago Bears and the Indiana Colts used him as their secret weapon to keep athletes on the field, and both teams ended up at Super Bowl XLI.

Gray wasn't limited to the ranks of the NFL, MLB, NHL or NBA. The special forces also placed their bet on this soft-spoken southerner. Gray explains:

"The Pentagon puts as many millions into someone on the Special Ops as an NFL team puts into a player, but an NFL career might last three years, whereas a Delta Force career should be more than ten."

Millions. That's a lot of money.

How on earth do *you* injury-proof yourself if you don't have access to someone like Gray?

Revisit beating my favourite dead horse, of course: the 80/20 principle.

80/20 Functional Screening

According to Gray the most likely cause of injury is neither weakness nor tightness, but imbalance. Think doing crunches or isolated ab work is enough to work your core muscles? Think again. "The core, as just one example, often works fine as long as one's hips aren't moving. It's when the hips are moving—a more realistic scenario—that the core starts to compensate for left–right differences." That's when you get injured.

Gray's fundamental tool for identifying imbalances is his brainchild: the Functional Movement Screen (FMS). The FMS is a series of seven movement tests administered by a certified professional. Each test is scored on a three-point scale.

For self-assessment, his professional FMS can be abbreviated to five movements with simple pass-fail evaluation:

1. Deep squat
2. Hurdle step
3. In-line lunge
4. Active straight leg raise
5. Seated rotation

This self-FMS is designed to identify two things: left–right imbalances (asymmetry) and motor control issues (wobbling and shifting).

Even if you can bench-press 272kg (600lb), it doesn't mean you won't dislocate a shoulder five minutes into a game. More weight with more reps does not equal stability.

"Most people can press more weight overhead for a set than they can walk with overhead for the same period of time. Strength [the former] should *never* exceed stability [the latter]," Gray Cook explains. "It's a recipe for disaster. The biggest misconception is that you can strengthen stabilizers [like the rotator cuff for the shoulder] alone to prevent injury. Even 10% stronger is like pissing in the ocean."

Working muscles in isolation will change muscles, but it's not likely to make movement safer. In contrast, working on basic movement patterns will make muscles stronger and it will also make movement (whether running a 37-metre/40-yard dash or carrying luggage) safer. To use an analogy of Paul Chek's, the basic movement patterns are like the 0–9 keys on a calculator. All other numbers, complex movements in this case, are still combinations of the basics.

Does the FMS work?

The Atlanta Falcons professional football team suffered seven season-ending injuries in 2007. In the 2008 season, there was just one minor surgery late in the season. The difference: their new director of athletic performance, Jeff Fish, made the FMS mandatory. Once players are "diagnosed" with the FMS, they receive personalized programmes to correct imbalances and improve range of motion.

Then there's the Colts. The Indianapolis Colts have been the smallest NFL team in the nation for the last nine years. They've also had the fewest injuries of any NFL team and the highest total of games won in the last nine years. This is an unusual combination. Jon Torine, their head strength coach, has used the FMS for that entire period of time.

The Critical Four

Initially, this chapter was going to be dedicated to the FMS. That was, until I realized that isolating the problems with the FMS was just the first step. Step two was prescribing the corrective actions for each major mistake in each of the five movements, and that would easily take 50 pages of dense material.

So I e-mailed Gray to reduce the seemingly irreducible:

> Assuming people do the screen, what are the 2–4 corrective exercises that you'd suggest to best fix the most common imbalances/weaknesses? If you had a gun to your head and had to pick 2–4 exercises for correction across the board, what would you choose?

Gray's picks were, without hesitation, the following critical four:

Chop and lift (C&L)
Turkish get-up (TGU)

Two-arm single-leg deadlift (2SDL)
Cross-body one-arm single-leg deadlift (1SDL)

I've put the exercises in the order that you should learn them, as greater coordination is required as you move down the list. There is no shame in sticking with just the C&L for two to four weeks if the other three prove awkward to incorporate at the beginning.

I'll first summarize the exact schedule I used to find and fix my imbalances in "The Critical Four Schedule" below. This provides the big picture before we dive into details, and it should serve as an easy-to-find reference later. Then I'll describe the exercises, using primarily Gray's words.

The exercises are not complicated, but using text instead of video can make it seem so. Use the videos listed in "Tools and Tricks" to become familiar with the Critical Four, and return to the below summary if overwhelmed.

The Critical Four Schedule: Finding and Fixing

Here is a potential schedule for putting it all together.

WEEK 1: TUESDAY, 30–45 MINUTES

COORDINATION

This is not a workout. This session is about practising the movements, just like a dance or karate form. For this purpose, light weights are used, even for movements that use heavier loading in training (like the deadlift).

Developing a base level of coordination with these patterns will ensure that you do not base an entire training programme on massive imbalances that could have been fixed with a few minutes of practice and neural adaptation.

Practise both the TGU and variations of the SDL with no weight until you can perform the movement on both sides, then add light weight. In all exercises, use the minimal weight needed to help stabilize the body.

WEEK 1: THURSDAY AND SATURDAY, 45–60 MINUTES PER SESSION

TESTING

Now we will test to find your weakest quadrant and weakest sides in each movement. Perform the TGU and SDL only if you can execute them flawlessly without weight:

C&L (like my example on page 338)

Chop down to left knee × 6–12 reps
Chop down to right knee × 6–12 reps
Lift up to left knee × 6–12 reps
Lift up to right knee × 6–12 reps

TGU

5 TGU each side (16kg/35.2lb kettlebell)
5 TGU each side (24kg/53lb kettlebell)

These TGU weights are what I used. Read the TGU description that follows for suggested male and female starting weights. Dumbbells can be used in place of kettlebells.

2SDL

5 reps each leg

1SDL

5 reps each leg

FULL-RANGE SQUAT

10 reps

I've added the full-range squat because it's important to at least maintain (or have) the ability to perform this movement, even if our focus is on the deadlift.

Repeat this testing both Thursday and Saturday to ensure that you haven't misdiagnosed imbalances. Use the same weights on Saturday, but don't look at the number of reps completed on Thursday. Saturday is, once again, to confirm that imbalances aren't just mistakes of some sort.

WEEKS 2–6: MONDAY AND FRIDAY, 30–45 MINUTES PER SESSION

FIXING

Once you've identified your imbalances, the exercises for weeks 2–6 are designed to fix them.

If you can perform 10 bottom-to-heels squats with no weight, do the following in each workout (sets and reps are explained next):

1. Half-kneeling C&L
2. TGU
3. 1SDL

If you cannot perform 10 full-range squats, perform this instead:

1. Half-kneeling C&L
2. Full-kneeling C&L (this is a symmetrical addition, both knees down, that will help you develop proper squatting form)
3. TGU
4. 1SDL

SETS AND REPS: For all exercises for weeks 2–6, use a 2:5 ratio of sets for strong:weak sides and a repetition range of 3–5. This means that you perform a total of seven sets, two for the stronger side and five for the weaker side, as follows:

Strong side × 3–5 reps (I aim for 5 on all)
Weak side × 3–5 reps
Strong side × 3–5 reps
Weak side × 3–5 reps
Weak side × 3–5 reps
Weak side × 3–5 reps
Weak side × 3–5 reps

Take one minute between sets. If you can't complete five repetitions in the later sets, decrease the repetitions rather than decreasing the weight. Record everything.

I suggest a one-second or two-second concentric (lifting) speed and a four-second eccentric (lowering) speed. No matter what speed you use, make it consistent.

OPTIONAL WEEKS 7+: MONDAY AND FRIDAY, 30–45 MINUTES PER SESSION—SUSTAINED PRE-HAB AND STRENGTHENING

For weeks 7 and beyond, you can incorporate the full-kneeling C&L and 2SDL for symmetrical corrections and pure strength. Perform this sequence twice a week if you'd like to further reduce injury risk. I simply retest every 4–6 weeks and fix accordingly.

But to continue with the programme, once 10% or greater strength differences are corrected, use two sets of 3–5 reps (I prefer 5) per side for each exercise.

TGU
Full-kneeling C&L
2SDL
Half-kneeling C&L
1SDL

The 2SDL is performed exactly like the 1SDL but instead of lifting with one arm you either hold a barbell with both hands, or, my preference, hold a dumbbell/kettlebell in each hand.

Taking 30–45 minutes twice per week to do these exercises takes less time, and sacrifices less progress, than 6–24 months of recovery after a major injury.

Four exercises can keep you stable and strong. Too busy? Do whatever you can, as every bit helps.

Focus on pre-hab so you never have to do rehab.

Exercise Details

EXERCISE #1—CHOP AND LIFT (C&L)

Chopping is a downward diagonal movement across the body from a high position to a low position, and lifting is the upward diagonal movement from a low position to a high position. They are essentially mirror images of one another.

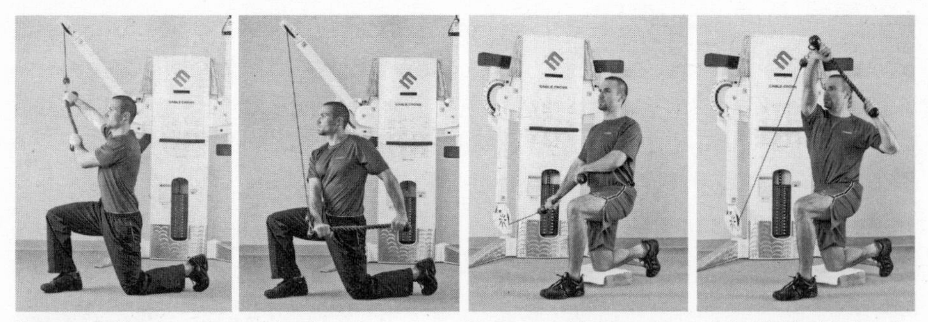

The start and finish positions of the chop.

The start and finish positions of the lift. The block under the knee, which I did not use, is optional and used here to achieve a more acute upward angle.

There are two stances commonly used when performing the C&L, seen above.

We will focus on the "half-kneeling" C&L for two reasons.

First, it is important to address asymmetrical (left–right) problems before any issues present on both sides, and the half-kneeling position addresses both upper and lower asymmetries. Second, of the six people I tested with a single-leg flexibility assessment (see sidebar), all had major left–right differences.

Half-Kneeling Description

One knee is down and one knee is up, with thighs and calves at 90-degree right angles to each other.

You will always chop to the down knee and lift toward the upward knee. Each move is a pull-to-a-push movement, and keep the hands close to the chest on the transition. In the chop, for example, you pull the bar to your sternum and press it to the floor. The cable should travel in a straight line.

Both the front foot and down knee should ideally be placed in a straight line, and tape on the ground (or any line) can be used to ensure this is the case.

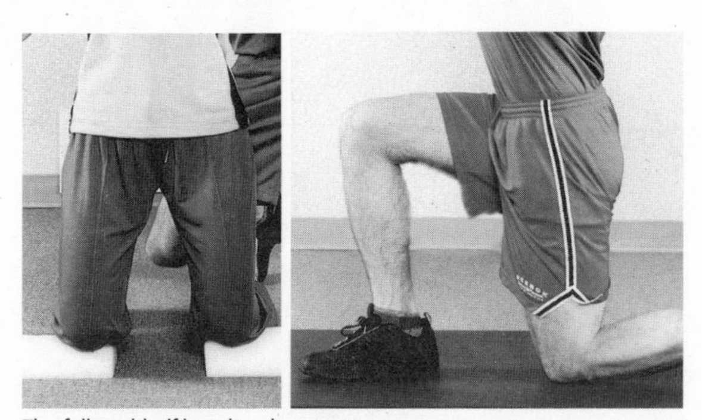

The full and half-kneeling leg positions.

If this narrow stance proves too difficult, use a wider base. Put your front foot 10cm (4in) off the knee line and bring it in closer over several workouts. Just ensure that the width is the same for the left and right sides in each individual workout, which is critical for keeping your comparisons accurate.

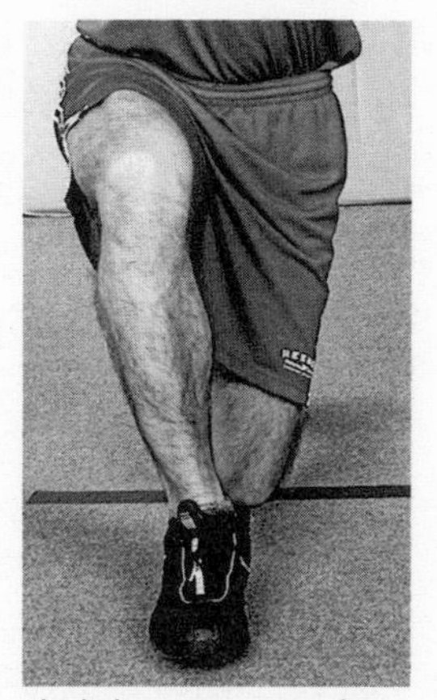

Ideal placement on one line.

The 80/20 Chopping and Lifting Programme

Guidelines

1. **Stick with a "bar" for the first month or two.** Both the half-kneeling chop and the half-kneeling lift will be performed on cables using either an attachable bar or, as in our photographs, the more common "tricep extension" attachment with the rope fully slid to one side to imitate a bar. This is what I used.

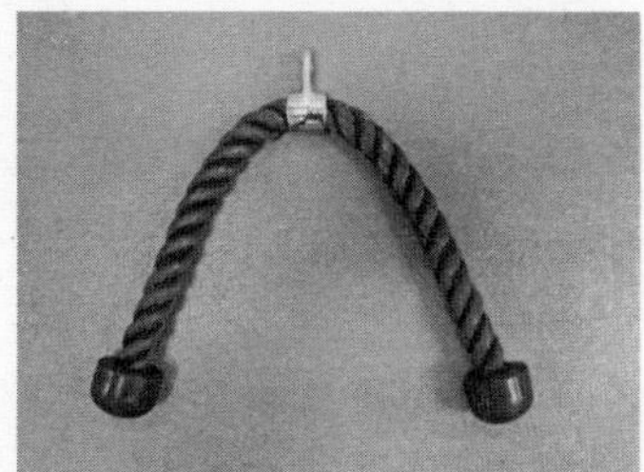

Tricep rope attachment (normal).

This bar or fake-bar approach forces you to use your core to counteract the mechanical disadvantage, rather than cheat through the movement with arm strength.

If you want to perform the C&L at home or while travelling, you can use resistance bands.[2] If using bands, the movement becomes more of a press to the front of the body as opposed to across the body.

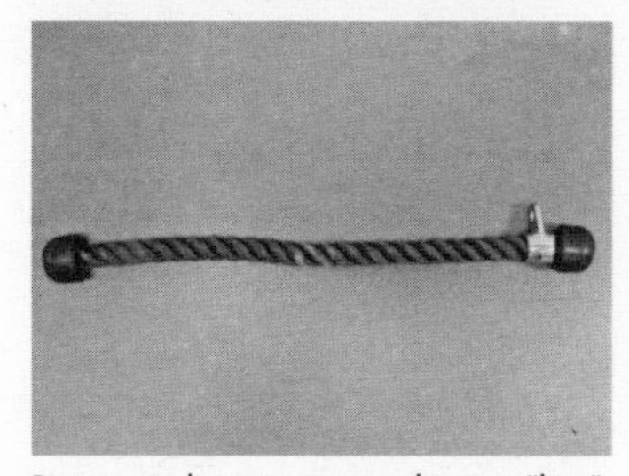

Rope attachment converted into a "bar".

2. **Unload between repetitions if possible (rest the weight stack).** This is something I missed in my first several workouts, as I was overseas and incommunicado. I still doubled my strength and corrected my imbalance within four workouts without unloading, but I made faster progress later with it. If you find it overwhelming to coordinate, you can start without it.

2. See "Tools and Tricks" at the end of the chapter.

SINGLE-LEG FLEXIBILITY ASSESSMENT

Try it yourself:

1. Keeping your feet together and knees locked, attempt to touch your toes with both feet on the ground. If that's too easy, attempt to touch the heel of your palms to your toes.

2. Now test the same stretch again on each side independently. Place one foot on a step or block, and remember to keep your knees fully locked to prevent cheating. Perform on both sides.

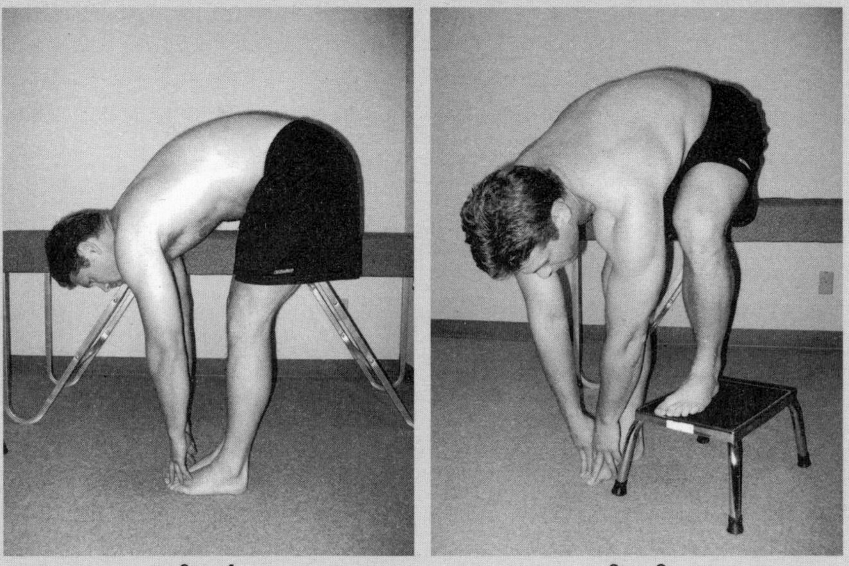

Step 1 Step 2

How did you fare? My reach was a full 7.5cm (3in) shorter on my right side.

Gray explains the concept: "Imbalance is not just a strength problem. It is a motor control problem. Going from unloaded to loaded and vice versa is the whole point. Re-engaging is where the money is, and where you stimulate more neurons."

But how do you get in the proper position, which requires having the rope in hand at a distance from the machine, without automatically lifting the weight stack? In other words, how do you rest the weight without falling over? You need to extend the cable. The best option involves carabiners, the metal clips used in rock climbing.

First option: use a link of chain from a hardware shop and two carabiners to extend the cable. One end of the chain will connect to the cable, and the other end will connect to the tricep attachment. This works. **The second option,** and the one I prefer, is to use a nylon sling (or "pocket daisy chain") designed for rock climbing in place of the chain. The nylon sling is a flat strip of material with loops on it. This webbing is light enough to fold up and put in your pocket, but it's plenty strong enough to hold the weights in the chop-and-lift movements. I travel with this.

If you don't want to bother with extending the length of the cable, you can train with a partner who takes the weight from you for a second after each repetition, or simply train without unloading, as I did for four workouts, which was enough to correct my largest imbalance.

3. **Don't hold your breath.** Once I progressed to heavier weights, I ended up holding my breath on the lifting portion and then exhaling slowly on the lowering. This is referred to as the Valsalva Technique, and though it can be valuable for maximal lifts, it is cheating in the C&L. Do your best to breathe as follows and keep your face relaxed:

a. Inhale a large amount of air at the start of the movement and pressurize your abdomen by tightening all the muscles in your hips and torso. Stiffen and brace your body but stay as tall as possible.
b. Begin the pulling portion of either movement and force air out between your clenched teeth to produce a hissing sound. Continue this slow continuous hiss as you transition into the pushing and reach full extension. Upon full extension, you should still have more than 50% of the air in your lungs. Continue the hiss on the return, using the remaining air, until the weight stack comes to rest.

c. Take two normal breaths, the weight stack resting, and start the next repetition.

4. Make your positioning 100% consistent workout to workout.

Foot placement: To standardize position from one workout to the next, Gray suggests using a stretching or yoga mat, narrow end against the machine, and then setting your down knee approximately one-third of the way from the far end of the mat.

If you own the mat (yoga mats can be rolled up and are a smart investment), use something like a marker pen to mark knee placement for both movements. If you don't own the mat, use tape.

Here's a diagram showing Gray's ideal placement and what I ended up doing:

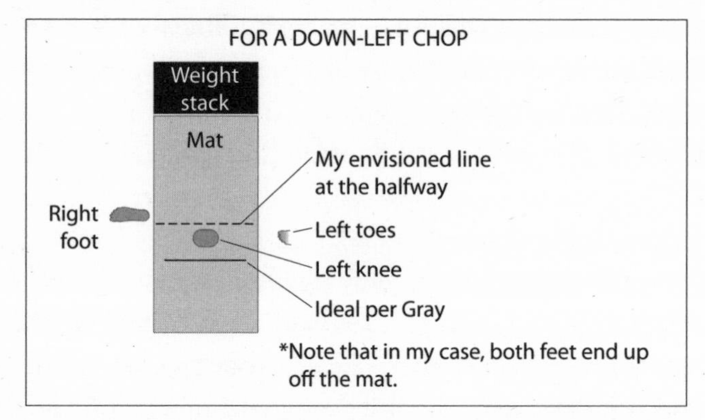

I started using a standard stretching mat to prevent mat burn on my knees, not for placement. Then I realized, no big surprise, that using a mat made replicating the exact positions much easier. I placed my down knee at the midpoint halfway from the weight stack, as I didn't have tape and halfway was easier to visually determine. I then ensured that my hips were approximately in front of the centre of the weight stack. While not precisely what Gray recommended, it made the positioning for both sides and movements easy to remember.

For foot and down knee alignment, as seen in the diagram, I put my knee down on one side of the imaginary halfway line, and my foot on the other.

The hips don't need to face exactly at a 90-degree angle from the weight stack, but I found this easiest to remember and replicate.

Hand positioning: For hand positioning in both the chop and the lift, I placed the hand farthest from the machine exactly three hand-widths up from the dangling end of the rope "bar". My hand nearest the machine grabbed the rope as close as possible to the cable.

Head and shoulder rotation: The head should not rotate independently of the shoulders. If we imagine the hips and shoulders square with each other in the starting position, you shouldn't rotate the shoulders more than 15–20 degrees off the hips. More rotation will not get more activation out of the abs, and it could force you to lose the proper lower back and "tall spine" position.

Let the Testing Begin

Finding imbalances in the C&L is done by testing the four quadrants: lower left, lower right, then upper left, upper right. The goal is to identify your single weakest quadrant. The chop is always done before the lift, as you will use heavier weights for the former.

TESTING

Chop down to left knee × 6–12 reps
Chop down to right knee × 6–12 reps
Lift up to left knee × 6–12 reps (be sure to move slowly for the lowering portion of the lift, or the weight will pull you over)
Lift up to right knee × 6–12 reps

The test is best done at the beginning of a workout. For the lift portions, subtract half or even two-thirds of the weight used for the chop. Choose a weight for both movements that you believe you can perform for no more than 6–12 repetitions, and then look for discrepancies in quality and your ability to hit maximum repetitions on either side.

It should be a mild struggle. You want to do a complete "rep-out" within 6–12 repetitions, so that **you test to the point of loss of appropriate posture and/or smooth movement, or to the point where a struggle is demonstrated that compromises technique.**

Thus, you're lifting to "failure" of posture or technique, not muscular failure.

Keep the back straight, the hips neutral and your head as tall as possible. "Loss of posture" occurs when you cannot maintain this tall position and your head drops or moves to the side. Stop your repetition count when you can no longer correct this. Though not required, it is helpful to have someone watch you or record the test on video.[3] For both sides, count the maximum number of repetitions until the movement is no longer smooth and fluid.

If you happen to miscalculate the weight and exceed 12 repetitions, keep going and record the repetition when posture fails. Just use the same weight on both sides.

Once the test is complete, you should have an assessment of four quadrants—the right and left chop and the right and left lift. Imbalances are defined as a greater than 10% difference in weight (if the same number of reps) or number of repetitions (if the same weight) between left and right sides.

Find the weakest quadrant and work there until symmetry is restored.

Here are the results from my first day of testing:

Chop down to left knee:	9kg (20lb) × 7.5 reps
Chop down to right knee:	9kg (20 lb) × 15 reps(!), and I could have done 3–4 more
Lift up to left knee:	4.5kg (10lb) × 13 reps
Lift up to right knee:	4.5kg (10lb) × 14 reps

I tested again two days later, as I wanted to confirm my imbalance before planing an entire programme. I did confirm it, but you can already see an incredible motor control improvement, which is reflected in the strength gains:

Chop down to left knee:	9kg (20lb) × 16 reps
Chop down to right knee:	9kg (20lb) × 20 reps, and I could have done 7–8 more (I stopped, as the first test had been confirmed)
Lift up to left knee:	6.8kg (15lb) × 6–7 reps (the heavier weight made the weakness on this side clearer than in the first test)
Lift up to right knee:	6.8kg (15 lb) × 11 reps

3. I used a Flip Cam mounted on a nearby machine with a bendable Joby Gorillapod tripod.

Two workouts later, I was using 20kg (45lb) for both sides in the chop. The worst imbalance had been corrected, and the back soreness I experienced from extended writing had all but disappeared along with it.

You will be amazed at how many other core issues clean themselves up by simply finding the weakest quadrant and addressing it.

EXERCISE #2—TURKISH GET-UP (TGU)

If Gray could pick just one movement from our Critical Four, he would pick the Turkish get-up.

The TGU can be a complex move, and it should be viewed as a long-term investment. If it gets frustrating, view it as a low-weight warm-up that you practise for a few minutes before each workout, and just focus on increasing resistance with the other movements until you're 100% comfortable.

This is the movement that Gray used most with Michelle Wie, along with the basic swing.[4] The TGU is an elegant solution that includes nine discrete movements which, in combination, address all of the major muscle groups and planes of movement. Gray underscores why the mainstream usually doesn't see it:

"The Turkish get-up and swing just aren't sexy enough for the glossy magazines. Am I actually saying that you can be a world-class athlete and only do TGU and swings for injury prevention? Yes, pretty much."[5]

Once Michelle was able to do a full TGU with a 16kg (35.2lb) kettlebell, supervised by TGU phenom Dr. Mark Cheng, the gains she'd made with rehab, chopping and lifting, and the single-leg deadlifts were integrated and locked in place. The TGU can be thought of as your "Save Document" function. In other words, the C&L moves the upper body while freezing the lower body; the SDL (coming next) moves the lower body while freezing the upper body; and once both halves have been strengthened, the TGU is what pieces them together. If you don't "Save Document" at the end of a workout with the TGU, the lower-body and upper-body gains aren't incorporated for full-body movement.

The TGU is also stunningly effective as a stand-alone exercise.

4. The swing is not one of the Critical Four but a personal favourite. It is fully described in "Building the Perfect Posterior".

5. Do you need sports-specific skills training? Of course. But if you don't own these basic motor patterns, you shouldn't be doing other exercises until you fix them. These are the foundation.

Jon Torine, head strength coach of the Indianapolis Colts, states in no uncertain terms: "My job is exercise, injury prevention and performance enhancement. I start with the TGU. I finish with the TGU. I check progress with the TGU."

The amount of weight you should use depends on your TGU experience, not your strength in other exercises. For dumbbells or kettlebells:

FEMALE

Beginner: 4–6 kg (8.8–13.2 lb)
Intermediate: 6–8 kg (13.2–17.6 lb)
Advanced: 8–12 kg (17.6–26.4 lb) or larger

MALE

Beginner: 8–12 kg (17.6–26.4 lb)
Intermediate: 12–16 kg (26.4–35.2 lb)
Advanced: 16–24 kg (35.2–52.8 lb) or larger

Though there are many versions of the TGU, on page 341 is one designed as a systemic corrective exercise. It provides the most detailed feedback. Some other forms—those that omit certain pauses, for example—allow for more compensation and make it easier to miss weak links.

Demonstrated by Brett Jones from the left side on the following page, steps 1–9 are illustrated in the photo sequence, which would then be reversed in exact order to return the kettlebell to the ground.

The photos can be used for reference and for spot-checking, but please view a video of proper execution before attempting (www.fourhourbody.com/tgu).

If the complete TGU is too difficult, you can stop at the arm post (step 5) and identify the left-right discrepancies up to this point. This "half-TGU" is outstanding for shoulder rehabilitation, and is now prescribed in some high-end physical therapy clinics specifically for this purpose.

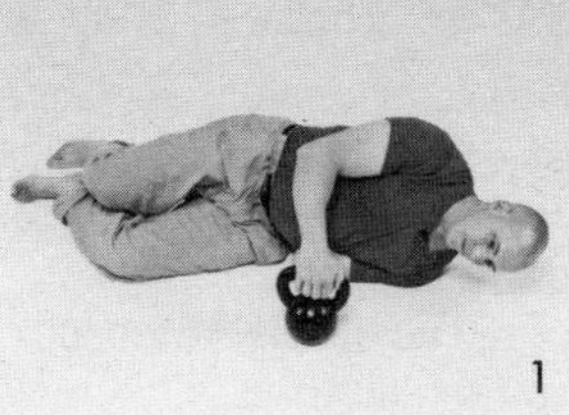
1

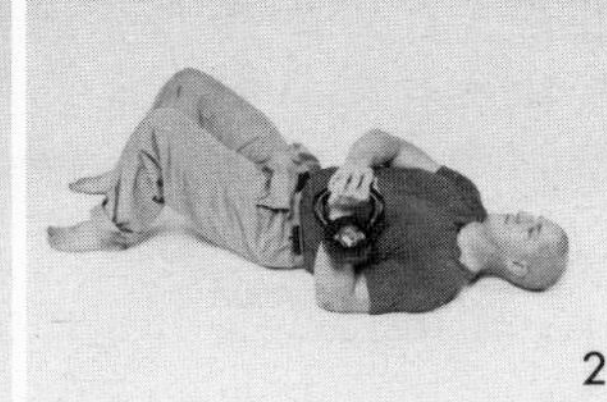
2

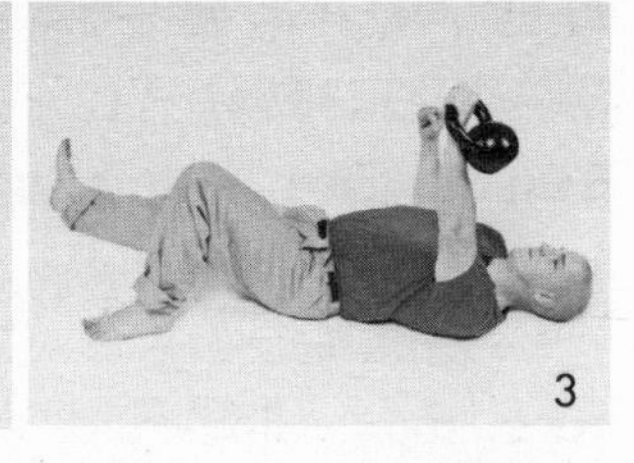
3

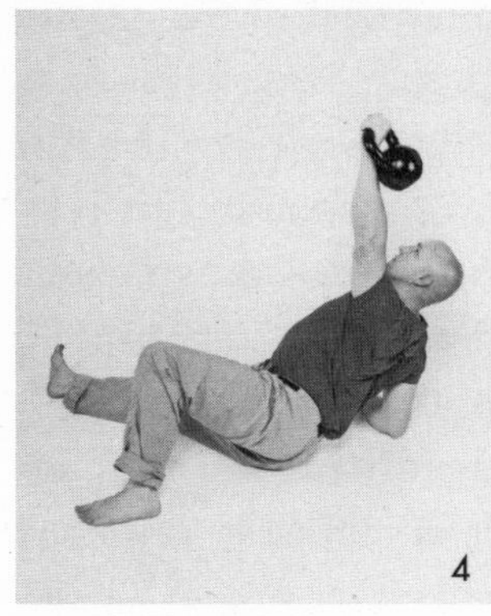
4

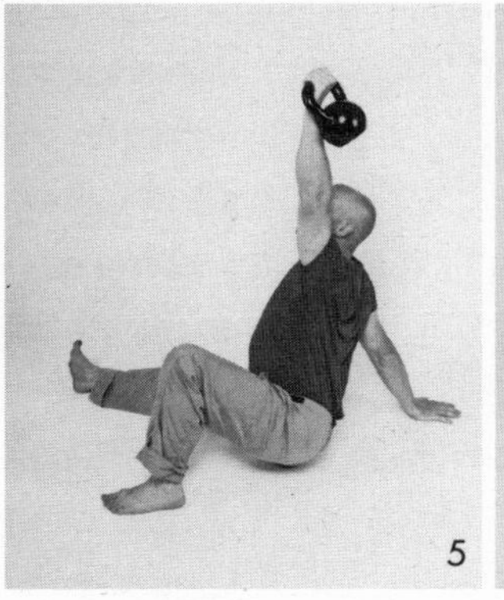
5

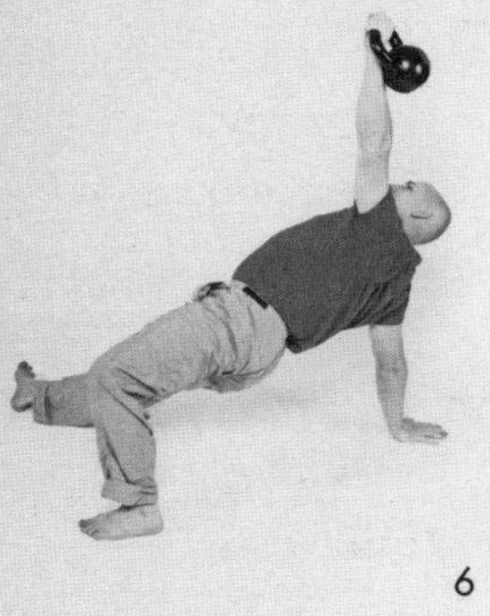
6

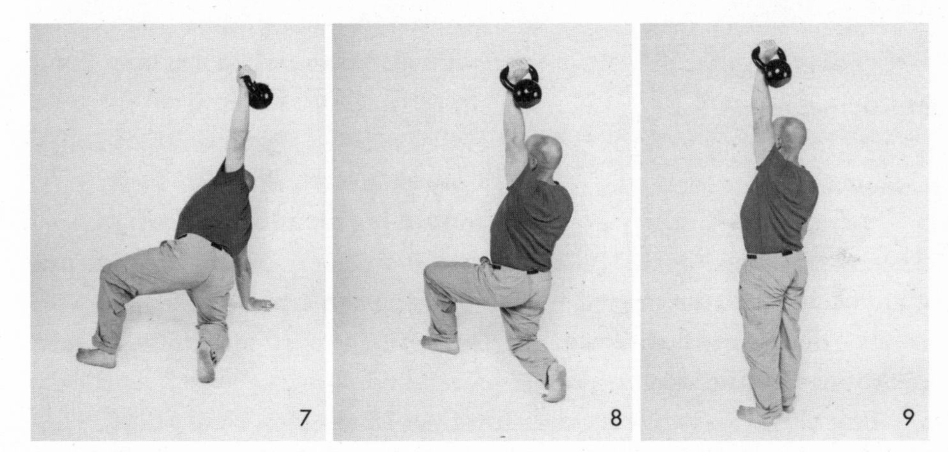
7
8
9

EXERCISES #3, #4—THE CROSS-BODY ONE-ARM SINGLE-LEG DEADLIFT (1SDL)

The standard deadlift is simple: grab a barbell just outside of the knees with both hands and stand to a fully erect position.

The single-leg deadlift, as the name implies, is this movement performed on a single leg.

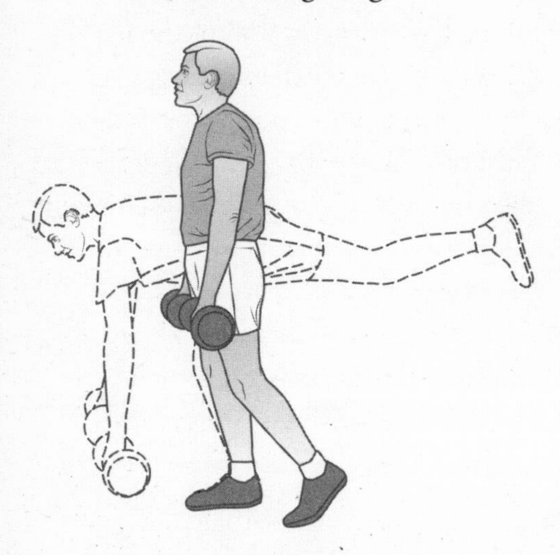

Start and finish of the 2SDL. Note that the toes of the rear foot must be pointing at the ground, not outwards.

The deep muscles of the hip are designed to be stabilizers as much as movers, and the single-leg deadlift allows them to function in this role, making left–right imbalances obvious at the same time. The variation we'll focus on—the **cross-body one-arm single-leg deadlift (1SDL)**—involves a single dumbbell or kettlebell instead of a barbell.

Before using just one arm, though, you need to become comfortable on one leg.

Learning with the Two-arm Single-leg Deadlift (2SDL)

Though we'll use the 1SDL in training, it's a good idea to first become comfortable with the single-leg deadlift using two arms. Two loaded arms create balance, and this allows you to focus on the most important element of the deadlift: the hip.

Learning with two arms takes less than 15 minutes. Here's how:

Using a set of light dumbbells (4.5–13.6kg/10–30lb each), do 3–5 sets of 3–5 reps of the 2SDL to become comfortable with core stabilization and balance on one foot. The guidelines are identical to those for the 1SDL below but involve two hands and two dumbbells.

It will feel unusual. Prepare for your arches to be sore afterwards. This brief time with the 2SDL will help prevent undue frustration when you move to the 1SDL, which involves many more forces, such as counter-rotation and counter-sidebending.

Use the below guidelines for practising the 2SDL first, with two hands and two weights.

Performing the One-arm Single-leg Deadlift

- Stand on one foot, with about a 20-degree knee bend, and with the dumbbell or kettlebell placed to the inside of the supporting foot (elevated if needed to accomodate flexibility). The other leg is in full extension behind the body and is not allowed to be externally or internally rotated. In other words, the toe of the rear leg should point towards the ground at all times. External rotation of the leg will allow the hip to open up and throw off the mechanics.
- Hinging at the hip, mimic a sitting movement and push your buttocks backwards. Reach down and grab the weight with the arm opposite the standing leg. Use the free arm to balance. Imagine lifting the weight in a see-saw-like motion.[6] A significant amount of rotational torque is generated when you stand on one leg and pull a weight with the opposite arm. Preventing this rotation requires core stability, which is exactly what we're trying to develop.
- Set the weight down between each repetition. Gray works with high-profile athletes, and his deadlifting injury rate is zero. This rule (sets of one) is why.

If you are aiming for a set of five repetitions, for example, what you're really performing is nine repetitions, five loaded and four unloaded interspersed between them. Here's what it looks like: Reach down, deadlift the weight up to standing, set it back down under control, stand back up without the weight, regain your composure and posture, clear a breath, then go back down and repeat. Learn to hinge the hip and push into the floor with your foot before regrabbing—setting up the rep is as important as the rep itself. Just as with the chop and lift, going from unloaded to loaded is the whole point.

Deadlift Guidelines from Gray

1. The deadlift is a **forward bending motion in appearance only. It is actually a sitting-back motion that puts the rear end far behind the heels.** If deadlifting with one or two legs, the tibia (shin bones) should remain as close to vertical as possible.

6. Like a perpetual motion bird. If you haven't seen one, look at: www.fourhourbody.com/bird.

2. **Keep the grip strong, as that will keep your shoulders safe.** Retraction (pulling back) of the shoulder is not necessary. Using a heavier weight, and therefore a firm grip, will allow proper reflex contraction of the rotator cuff musculature.

3. **Fully extend and straighten the back leg. It should look like an extension of the spine.** If your chest goes down 5cm (2in), you lift your back heel 5cm (2in). If your chest goes up 5cm (2in), you lower that back heel 5cm (2in). They should be perfectly connected.

4. **Lift a respectable amount of weight, even if you must reduce the range of motion to do so.**

Gray is constantly amazed how some personal trainers use 2.3kg (5lb) chrome dumbbells on individuals who routinely carry children or suitcases that weigh 16–20kg (35–45lb). In bending and lifting motions like the deadlift, a light weight will encourage elbow flexion (bending) and shoulder shrugging, all of which is bad news.

The point of the deadlift is to keep repetitions low, elicit neuromuscular reactions, and create core stability in a hip drive. The repetitions should be kept between one and five, evoking strength. This is not done for hypertrophy (muscular growth); it is done to create a stable base from which to pull.

It's possible to restrict the range of motion of the deadlift as you work up to full range of motion. You can, for example, deadlift a kettlebell off a crate or lift a dumbbell off a step or platform. If it's a significant weight and you are demonstrating the proper hip hinge, you're going to benefit, even if the weight travels a short distance. Rather than skip the exercise, just elevate the weight until you have control. As you progress, lower it gradually and eventually lift it off the ground.

How do you put it all together? Just revisit the synopsis on page 328.

TOOLS AND TRICKS

Find a Functional Movement Screen (FMS) Expert (www.fourhourbody.com/fms) The FMS is Gray Cook's primary tool for identifying imbalances. Use this site to find local FMS experts who can run you through the complete assessment. Scores of 14 or fewer total points—the "danger zone"—correspond to 35% higher injury rates. My first FMS score was 17 and computed by Eric D'Agati at the One Human Performance Center in New Jersey, which is the FMS home of the Giants NFL team.

FMS Self-Screen (www.fourhourbody.com/fms-self) Eager to test yourself without a pro? Use this stripped-down version as a starting point.

Chop and Lift Video (www.fourhourbody.com/cl)

Turkish Get-Up (www.fourhourbody.com/tgu) Zach Even-Esh demonstrates the Turkish get-up. Take note of his timing in this sequence. It's not one continuous motion, but rather a specific set of movements with brief pauses. The slower you can do this, the better your technique is. Do not rush.

Cross-Body One-Arm Single-Leg Deadlift (www.fourhourbody.com/1SDL) This video demonstrates the proper execution of the 1SDL.

Squat (www.fourhourbody.com/squat) This is an outstanding tutorial on how to correct the lower back rounding common at the bottom of the squat.

Kayaking Dry Bags (www.fourhourbody.com/kayak) A kayaking dry bag is designed to keep water out. It can also be used to hold water in, and it's a great way to travel and still do your TGU. I use the SealLine Baja Dry Bag 30, which holds up to 30 litres. One litre = 1 kilogram (2.2 pounds). Thirty litres gives you up to 66 pounds.

Bands for Mobile C&L: Gray Cook Bands (www.fourhourbody.com/cl-band) For those who want to do the C&L on the road or in their home, these resistance tubes are an effective and affordable substitute for exercise machines.

Metolius Nylon Daisy Chain for the C&L (www.fourhourbody.com/chain)

Black Diamond HotWire Carabiner for the C&L (www.fourhourbody.com/carabiner) Extremely lightweight carabiner rated "Best in Gear" by *Rock and Ice* magazine.

RUNNING FASTER AND FARTHER

HACKING THE NFL COMBINE I

Preliminaries—Jumping Higher

The more technique you have, the less you have to worry about it.

—Pablo Picasso

GARDEN STATE INDUSTRIAL PARK, WYCKOFF, NEW JERSEY

"What is that?" I asked.

Tom, whose arms were bigger than my legs, was rubbing something on his elbows in between sets of pull-downs.

"It's horse liniment."

Ha ha. Sure.

The fumes were so strong that they cleared my sinuses from 3m (10ft) away. I weaved around trainees to get to the shelf where the bottle stood on end.

"McTarnahan's Absorbent Blue Lotion"
Methyl salicylate 3%
Menthol 1.7%
Camphor 1.7%

There was a huge horse head on the front of the label, mane flowing in the wind. It was, after all, racing horse liniment.

In Joe DeFranco's gym, slotted invisibly in the back of an industrial park next to a Chevy dealership, the tools are chosen without regard to popularity. If it works and it's legal, it's fair game.

The Science and Business of Running Faster

The NFL Scouting Combine is the ultimate job interview.

Once a year in February, the 330 best college football players are invited to Indiana's Lucas Oil Stadium, and the top NFL coaches and talent scouts spend a week determining their worth. At the top of the list in importance are the "measurables"—physical tests that allow each of the 330 players to be measured against every other. These tests include a vertical jump, the 37-metre (40-yard) dash, a three-cone agility drill, and the bench press for repetitions with 102kg (225lb).

The NFL draft, later held in Radio City Music Hall, is the first time the teams can make offers and negotiate contracts with potential players. Players are picked over seven rounds, and with rare exceptions, the earlier you are picked, the more you are paid.

How much can Combine results affect ultimate pay? A lot. One inch or one-fifth of a second can make the difference between millions of dollars and nothing at all.

Almost all of the players come into the Combine signed with sports agents, whose job it is to make sure their clients are worth as much as possible. The sales pitches of many top agents, intended to snag the cream of the crop, include a name: "If you sign with me, I can get you trained with DeFranco."

Joe DeFranco, the Yoda of the Combine, is best known for creating monsters who jump higher and run faster than they should. The NFL has had to change the rules to keep up with him. To wit: the three-cone drill.

The rules of the three-cone drill are straightforward. First, the athlete must get in a three-point stance (both feet and one hand down) behind the line, just like the start of a 37-metre (40-yard) dash. Second, the athlete must run 4.5 metres (5 yards), touch the far-side line with his right hand (*not* left), then immediately run back and touch the starting line with his right hand, after which he sprints across the opposite line.

One of Joe's athletes, Mike Richardson of Notre Dame, ran the fastest three-cone drill ever recorded at an official NFL Combine or Pro Day:[1] 6.2 seconds. Joe explains how he did it:

> *Since the rules of the test dictate that you must touch both lines with your RIGHT hand, I discovered that it would be much more efficient to get in a less-common "left-handed" stance when performing this test.... Simply put, the left-handed stance enables the athlete to cover the 1st 9 metres (10 yards) in two fewer steps; when you're talking about TENTHS of a second, two steps makes a huge difference! Taking 2 less steps can shave up to 4 tenths of a second off of this test. And when we're talking about the NFL Combine tests, 4 tenths of a second is an eternity that can mean millions of pounds for an athlete.*

Some of the NFL scouts now disallow left-handed starts at the Combine. This is amusing since some athletes are, well, left-handed. Unhindered, DeFranco continues to produce record-breakers, always one step ahead. Pros on all 32 teams have been through his machine.

But was DeFranco really that good? Or was he using the favourite trick of PR-savvy trainers: babysitting genetic freaks for a year and then basking in their performances?

Amid 272kg (600lb) tyres and chains, I had come to his storage facility to find out.

Forty-eight hours later, I had:

- increased my vertical jump 7.5cm/3in (matching the gym's single-session improvement record)
- improved my 37-metre (40-yard) dash by 0.33 seconds (beating the previous single-session record of two-tenths of a second).

This chapter and the next will explain how you can replicate what I did, starting with my personal nemesis (there's a reason I chose wrestling over basketball):

The vertical jump.

1. Pro Days, organized by top football universities, allow NFL scouts to watch players participate in the Combine's various tests on university grounds prior to the Combine. Coaches rightly assume that players will often have better performances on home turf.

The Vertical Jump

DeFranco started me off with an abbreviated warm-up, videos of which can be seen at www.fourhourbody.com/defranco:

Normal jumping jacks × 10
Seal jacks × 10 (open and close the arms in front of the chest)
Reverse lunge × 5 (each side)
Side lunge × 5 (each side)
Leg swings forward and backward × 10 (each side)
Pogo jumps × 20 secs (jump on the balls of your feet with legs straight as fast as possible)

We then approached the altar of air: the Vertec.

It is, Vertec's marketing department forgive me, a pole with sticks that rotate when struck. The highest stick you hit determines your vertical leap.[2]

"Show me your best."

So I did. 53cm (21in). My second and third attempts yielded an equally unimpressive 56cm (22in).

STARTING POINT: 56CM (22IN)

As I prepared to receive my first set of instructions, the asshole walked in. Correction: The Asshole.

"Hey, Asshole!" DeFranco shouted over his shoulder.

"What's up!" The Asshole offered back.

DeFranco looked back at me and explained, "It's not derogatory at all. That's just what he is. It's his name." Outside the gym, The Asshole is known as Mike Guadango. His story was typical of DeFranco's acolytes. He had been cut from the University of Delaware baseball team his freshman year. He responded by transferring to William Paterson University and sacrificing his body to DeFranco. Twelve months later, he was first-team All-American. The Asshole could now do 50 consecutive military chins and, at 175cm (5ft 9in), had become a YouTube celebrity for a jump from

2. The starting height—0cm (0in)—is the height of your fingertips extended overhead when your feet are flat on the ground. This allows scouts to compare a 178cm (5ft 10in) player to a 193cm (6ft 4in(player.

standstill onto a face-height 140cm (55in) box.[3] Not bad for someone known in DeFranco's clan for his lack of natural gifts.

The Asshole took a comfortable seat to enjoy the spectacle.

DeFranco's first round of training began with corrections.

Flaw #1: Too Little Shoulder Drive

"Shoulders are prime movers in the jump and contribute up to 20% of your height. Try running a 37-metre (40-yard) dash with your arms by your sides and you'll get the idea. For the vertical jump, the speed of your descent into a half-squat will correlate to the max height. Really use your upper-body strength and throw your arms down as fast as you can, recoiling with the same speed."

DeFranco encouraged me to start with my arms overhead like an Olympic diver, using the additional distance for increased velocity downwards. This would maximize elastic recoil. My dominant right arm would then be the only arm extended overhead to hit the sticks.

Flaw #2: Pulling the Extended Arm Back at the Apex of the Jump

My arm was retracted at the highest point, as if I were spiking a volleyball, and I was hitting the sticks on the way down. It needed to be retracted on the way up.

Flaw #3: Too Wide a Squat Stance

My squat stance, just outside of hip width, was too wide and decreased my standing height by 2.5–5cm (1–2in). I needed to place my feet just inside the hips and keep my back flat as I squatted.

I had to keep my eyes on the sticks at all times, except for at the very bottom on the squat.

Shaking out my arms and legs, I ran through the checklist and took a few deep breaths.

Then I jumped again.

3RD ATTEMPT: 61CM (24IN)

I had just gained 5cm (2in) on my vertical.

"Who taught you to jump with your feet together?" The Asshole shouted from behind me.

3. www.fourhourbody.com/asshole

It seemed that, in an effort to start with my arms overhead like an Olympic diver, I'd also stood like an Olympic diver, with my feet firmly together. I didn't even notice. How had I managed to squat like that?

Four or five things might not seem like much, but it's a hell of a lot to keep in your head for a maximal-speed movement.

DeFranco pulled out a stretching mat. It was time for more corrections.

Flaw #4: Tight Hip Flexors

"Normally, we don't use static stretching. The hip flexors are the one exception. The objective is to put them to sleep, as they can restrict maximal leg extension."

Static stretching is what most people think of as stretching—go into a stretch and hold it for 10 seconds or more. It turns out that this de facto approach can temporarily decrease the strength of the muscles and connective tissue being stretched, increasing the likelihood of injury. In this unusual exception, we wanted to temporarily elongate and weaken one area and one area only: the hip flexors.

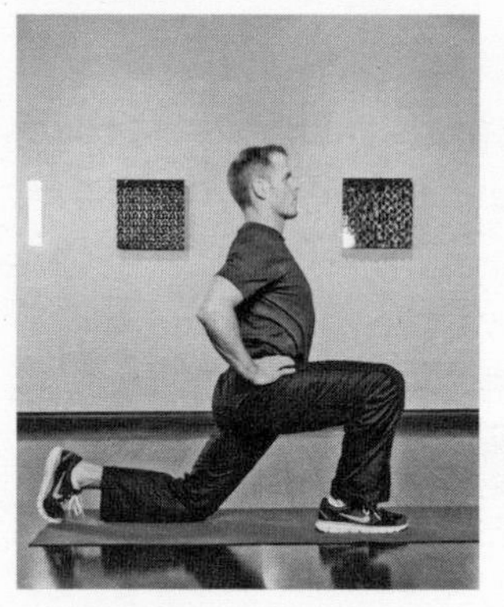

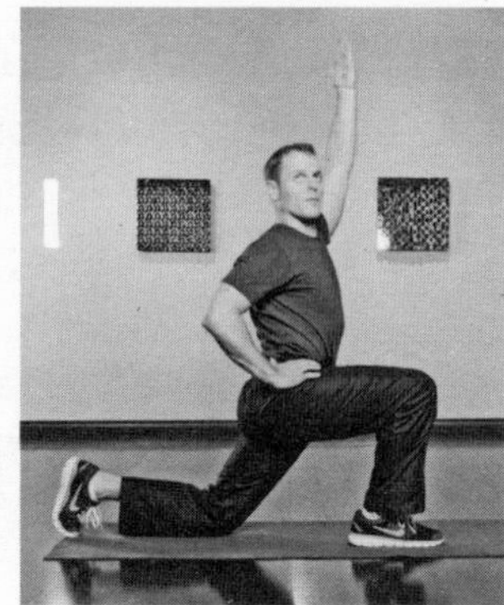

Hold this position.

The hip flexor stretches are performed 30 seconds to two minutes before a jump, and the non-dominant side is stretched first. In my case, that was my left side. Each side is held for 30 seconds.

4TH ATTEMPT: 64CM (25IN)

I was pleased with our progress, and so was DeFranco: "That'd be a million pounds if you could play football and were in the NFL.

"Mid to low 20s is the average for high school players in this gym. Going from 74cm (29in) to 76cm (30in) in the Combine puts you in a new bracket altogether. A new tax bracket too."

One of his protégés, Miles Austin, had a 107cm (42in) vertical at 15.4st (98kg). Brian Cushing, who was then leading the AFC in tackles, weighed 17.8st (113kg) and had a 89cm (35in) vertical. "Cush" had started with DeFranco at age 17 and was a first-round draft pick. Cush could now bench-press 102kg (225lb) for 35 reps. He could also put on a 9kg (20lb) weight vest, sit in a chair and jump directly from the seated position onto a 127cm (50in) box. Yep, a freaking mutant.

My performance didn't compare well, but I had gained 7.5cm (3in) on my vertical in 20 minutes and tied the gym record for single-session improvement.

The next morning, however, a much bigger challenge awaited: Sprinting.

TOOLS AND TRICKS

Probotics Just Jump Mat (www.fourhourbody.com/jump-mat) This portable mat measures vertical jump based on air time. It's used by Rich Tuten, the Denver Broncos' strength and conditioning coach, during their annual tryouts and can fit under a bed.

***Mastering the Combine Tests*, DVD (www.fourhourbody.com/combine-dvd)** DeFranco dissects every aspect of the NFL Combine tests in this DVD, including the 18-m (20-yard) shuttle, the three-cone drill, the bench-press test and the broad jump.

McTarnahan's Absorbent Blue Lotion (http://store.allvet.org/abblloga.html) Pain and stiffness relief for horses... and elite athletes. Makes Ben-Gay seem like water.

Videos of Mutants:

Adrian Wilson Jumping 66 Inches (www.fourhourbody.com/wilson): Watch the Arizona Cardinals' safety jump over the 167.64cm (5ft 6in) mark.
Keith Eloi Jumps into a Flatbed Truck (www.fourhourbody.com/flatbed): No run-up, no expression of effort, and he's in goddamn slippers.
Keith Eloi Jumping Out of a Swimming Pool Backward (www.fourhourbody.com/pool-eloi)

Every morning in Africa, a gazelle wakes up. It knows it must move faster than the lion or it won't survive. Every morning, a lion wakes up, and it knows it must move faster than the slowest gazelle or it will starve. It doesn't matter if you're the lion or the gazelle. When the sun comes up, you'd better be moving.

—Maurice Greene, five-time world champion 100-metre sprinter

HACKING THE NFL COMBINE II

Running Faster

KING GEORGE DINER, 721 HAMBURG TURNPIKE

It was 8:00 A.M. EST (5:00 A.M. PST on my physical clock), and Joe and I were waking up to a classic New Jersey diner breakfast: omelettes and never-ending cups of strong, bitter coffee. I pulled out a pad and started the questions.

"Who's the best strength coach no one knows?" I asked.

Answer: Buddy Morris from the University of Pittsburgh.

"Favourite coach for functional strength?"

Answer: Louie Simmons of Westside Barbell.[4]

"Favourite stretching expert?"

Answer: Anne Frederick, whose clinic, Stretch to Win, I had visited in Tempe, Arizona, just six months earlier. I'd left a session with her husband with more hip mobility than I'd experienced in a decade.

"Favourite sprint or speed coach?"

Answer: Charlie Francis.

Ah, Charlie. Charlie Francis is also my favou-

4. A common answer among those interviewed for this book.

rite speed coach. Unfortunately, he's most famous for training 100-metre gold medalist Ben Johnson, who tested positive for steroid use (stanozolol) in the 1988 Olympics. Few realize the sophistication of Charlie's training techniques.[5] He was a legitimate genius.

Francis was first and foremost a biomechanics and training expert, not a chemist. One of his innovations involved using extremely short distances and training at 95% or more of max effort—never between 75% and 95%. Less than 95% was too slow to be speed work, and the higher volume accompanying slower speeds was too hard to recover from within 24 hours.

Joe DeFranco adapted these concepts, among others, and prospered. Case in point:

Rather than running 400 metres or more to build a base for sprinting and then working down, as is common, DeFranco had one of his Division III football players, the aforementioned Miles Austin, spend more than 80% of this sprint training on 9m (10-yard) dashes. Miles focused on perfecting the starting stance, the exact number of steps for optimal speed, and the precise posture for sustained acceleration. Despite the fact that Miles ran just *three* 37m (40-yard) dashes among more than 100 9m (10-yard) dashes, he ran 4.67 seconds in the 37m (40-yard) dash at the Combine and was later clocked at an official 4.47 seconds.

If Joe was a Combine specialist, he appeared to be a 37m (40-yard) dash savant:

"For improvement, the vert is 9 out of 10 people. The 40 is 1,000 out of 1,000."

Them's strong words.

I had visions of breaking Ben Johnson's record on little more than a Greek omelette and several litres of shitty coffee. It was going to be a good day.

5. Fewer still realize that when Ben's gold medal was rescinded, it was passed to our great American hero Carl Lewis, who tested positive for three banned stimulants (pseudoephedrine, ephedrine and phenylpropanolamine) in the very same Olympics. Lewis was initially disqualified, but this decision was overturned with an appeal of "inadvertent use". In other words, he had consumed a herbal supplement but was unaware that it contained the stimulants. Not to imply a world-class athlete knew what he was ingesting, but ephedrine plus testosterone was a favourite combination of sprinters throughout the 1980s, a decade often referred to as the "golden age" of steroid use in sports. In fact, four of the top five Olympic finishers of 100 metres in 1988 (right alongside Ben Johnson) had tested positive for banned drugs at some point in their careers.

The Warm-up

First things came first: warm-ups. I used basic football cleats without spikes, and Joe underscored the importance of mimicking the habits of good sprinting in the warm-ups themselves:[6] using arm action, etc.

GENERAL MOVEMENT PREP

18m (20yd) of skipping × 2
Reverse lunge × 6 reps one side, then 6 reps on the other side
Backward cycling[7] (for quadriceps and hip flexors) 18m (20yd) × 2
Side shuffle in half-squat[8] 18m (20yd) × 2

REVERSE LUNGE DEMONSTRATION

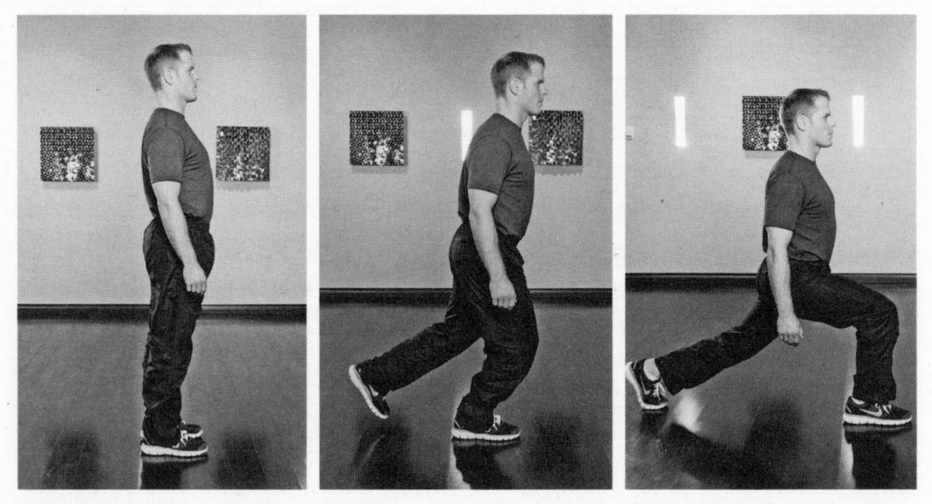

Notice that I bend the supporting knee first, bringing the knee over the toes before I extend the opposite leg backwards.

6. No amount of text can do the movements justice, but free video of each is available at www.fourhourbody.com/defranco.
7. Think of this as trying to heel-kick someone standing 90 or 121cm (3 or 4ft) behind you, aiming for hip height and alternating legs.
8. For the side shuffle, get into a half-squat and push off with the big toe of your trailing leg. Don't let your head bob up and down, and ensure 20m (67ft) is done to both the right and left sides.

GROUND-BASED DYNAMIC STRETCHING AND MUSCLE ACTIVATION[9]

10 × roll-overs into V-sits
10 × fire hydrants (to each side)
10 × mountain climbers[10]

FREQUENCY DRILLING TO PREP THE NERVOUS SYSTEM

Perform as many repetitions as possible of each exercise in the time allotted:

Pogo jumps × 20 secs.
Half-squat deep "wide-outs" × 2 sets of 5 secs (10-sec rest between)[11]

Joe kept the warm-up short and gave me time to recover. One of the oldest tricks in the training world, he explained, is to fatigue an athlete prior to their "before" testing with an extensive warm-up, then retest them later with a minimal warm-up. Voilà, instant measurable improvement.

Trixy coaches.

The Set-up

My times wouldn't depend on DeFranco's eyesight or judgement. We'd be using the Brower system, the same technology used at the "big show" of the Combine.

My finish time would be clocked automatically when I passed between two paired laser detectors at the 37m (40-yard) line, both of which were synced to his hand-held counter.

As a baseline, I ran two 9m (10-yard) dashes with no coaching:

Dash #1: 2.12 secs.
Dash #2: 2.07 secs.

9. See these in motion at www.fourhourbody.com/mobility.
10. For the mountain climber, don't put your heel down on your front foot. Stay on your toes and keep your knees in front of your feet at all times. Putting the heel down encourages a long stride when running, which leads to heel striking and hamstring tears.
11. See the demo at www.fourhourbody.com/wideouts.

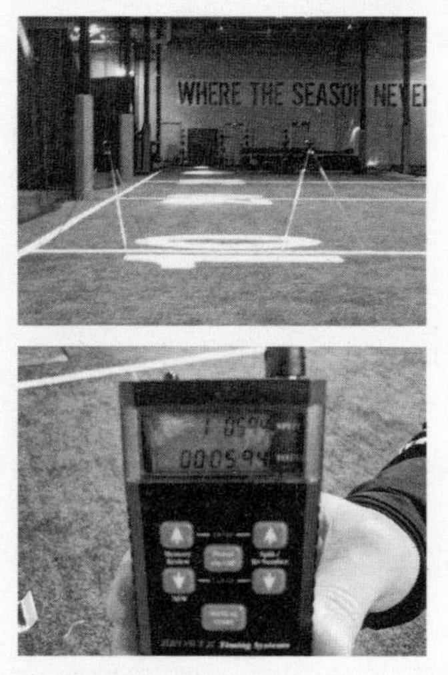

The Brower system.

Then I impressed Joe with a blistering starting 37m (40-yard) dash of . . .

5.94 seconds.

"The good news is that you broke six seconds," Joe announced as he pointed to the screen on the hand-held. "To paint that in a positive light, it's not bad if you're a below-average 22.8st (145kg) lineman."

Pacing back and forth with a bounce in his step, he looked up at me with an ear-to-ear smile:

"Where to start. . . . You are going to make me look good today! Big day for Joe!"

It was time to let Joe work his magic. The "where to start" was easy: the start position.

The Devil's in the Details

My first step had gone nowhere. Quite literally. My leg had gone from behind the line to the start line, the zero-metre mark. Losing a step might not impact a marathon, but it's an enormous handicap in the 37m (40-yard) dash.

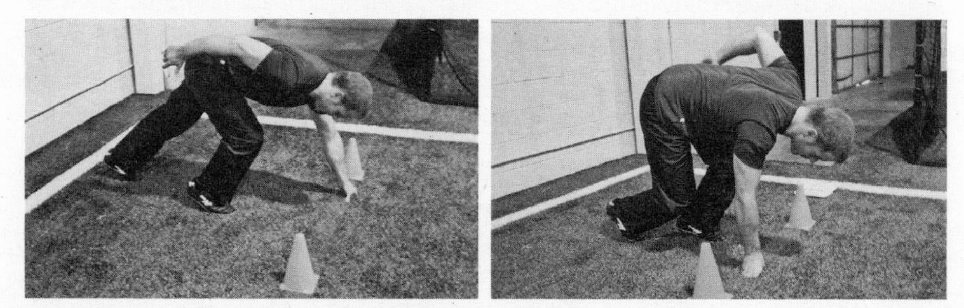
My untrained start position compared to the trained start position.

THE FIRST ROUND OF POSITIONAL CORRECTIONS

1. If right-handed, put your right hand down and left leg forward. Left-handers do the opposite. This will be optimal 90% of the time.
2. To set up as a right-hander: stand with the toes of the left foot roughly one foot behind the line, then touch the toes of the right

foot to the back of the left heel. Next, spread the right foot out so both feet are hip width and no wider. Support yourself on both hands, placed in front of the line (to place your weight forward), then bring the right hand to the line.

3. Put three fingers of the right hand on the line: index finger and middle finger together, plus the thumb. This caused too much pain in my thumb, so I used the index and middle knuckles with the thumb.
4. Just before you take off, the left arm, bent at a 90-degree angle, will come up so that your hand is next to your hip (see photo on previous page).
5. Drive and aim the first step with your rear leg to land 90cm (3ft) from your lead toe.

The result: my first trained 9m (10-yard) attempt clocked at 1.99 from a 2.07-second original, a 0.08 second improvement.

ADDING CORRECT ARM POSITION AND MOVEMENT

I had placed most of my weight on my legs, resulting in a *negative arm angle*. In other words, the line from my fingertips to my shoulder pointed up and behind me. This is bad. It meant I had to pause and lift my arm before taking the first step.

To correct this, I attempted to have my shoulder slightly ahead of my fingers and *replace* my arms. In Joe's words, I was to "leave the lead arm behind" and drive it backwards instead of lifting it. I would naturally fall forward as I removed the third leg of the tripod, and driving the right arm back would help me drive my right leg forward.

More weight forward, however, meant less sole contact with the ground, and my rear foot slipped both times I practised this. The solution Joe suggested was Nike Vapors, which, unlike common cleats, have small teeth at the toe of the shoe. Stuck with my standard football booties, I hoped the new forward pressure would compensate for less traction.

It did: the next 90m (10-yard) attempt clocked at 1.91 from a 2.07 original—a 0.16 overall improvement.

FOCUSING ON SUSTAINED RUNNING POSITION AND FEWER STEPS

Joe placed a string about 90cm (3ft) from my lead toe and prescribed the following:

1. From the start position, keep your head down but your eyes on the string, where you want your first step to land.
2. Ensure that your knee is ahead of your toes when you land that first step.
3. For the entire 9m (10 yards), keep your chin tucked and your upper body ahead of your lower body.
4. Take the fewest steps possible (seven steps or fewer for my limb length), which will paradoxically feel slower due to more ground contact.

I took a breath. The checklist was getting long and the setup was taking correspondingly longer. When I passed the 9m (10-yard) mark, it felt a lot slower.

It wasn't: this fifth attempt clocked at 1.85 from a 2.07 original—a 0.22 overall improvement.

Now it was time to retest the 37m (40-yard) dash.

"Just Run Your 9m (10 yards)"

"To transition to the 37m (40 yards), people forget all they learnt in the 9m (10 yards). Just run your 9m (10 yards). Run the best 9m (10 yards) you can. Don't worry about the rest but finish to the 37m (40-yard) line. But . . . run that 9m (10 yards) like it's for Olympic gold."

That was it? Five 9m (10-yard) dash practice runs and less than 15 minutes of coaching?

I took one warm-up run at about 60% of max effort to shake out the cobwebs.

"Ready?" I asked Joe.

"Ready."

Then I hovered in the starting stance for what seemed like an eternity, making tiny adjustments, trying to keep the dozen or so points straight.

And I was off.

For the first time in a long time, I felt fast. I kept my head down and body forward as I blew past the 9m (10-yard) mark. I could sense I was nearing the finish and looked up, at which point I felt a sharp pull. Before I could blink, I had passed the 37m (40 yards) and was decelerating into a jog.

My right hamstring felt odd.

"Nice!" Joe yelled out from the start line, and I headed over.

"5.61 seconds." He showed me the reading on the hand-held receiver and smiled. "You've broken the gym record for a one 1-session improvement. It was two-tenths of a second, and this is more than three-tenths of a second."

"My hamstring feels a little tight," I mentioned as I headed back to the starting line. Joe stopped and looked at me.

"In that case, we're done for today."

He continued:

"I've learnt from experience—I'm older and wiser than I once was—that you stop when the hamstrings feel tight. That's a sign of a pending tear."

"But it feels so tight. Shouldn't I stretch it a bit?"

"No, that's the biggest and most common mistake. It feels like it's contracting, so people stretch it, but it's already overstretched. You need ice and Hannah Montana."

Hannah Montana?

"Excuse me?"

"Ice and arnica montana."

I'd misheard him, of course. Arnica montana, not Hannah Montana, is also known as wolf's bane. It's a European flowering plant that contains a flavonoid called helenalin, which has made it popular among professional athletes for anti-inflammation.

DeFranco believed that, had I not pulled my hamstring, I would have reached between 5.51 and 5.53 that session and then dropped another one- to two-tenths after a week of additional training.

Lesson learnt: keep your chin tucked and don't look up. It pulls your torso upright and leads to striking with the heel, which can cause hamstring tears. The forces generated in the 37m (40-yard) dash are obscene. Keep in mind that DeFranco coaches athletes who can deadlift 272kg (600lb) for repetitions, and his advice to bodybuilders who want to develop their "hammies" is simple:

Sprint.

I'd be getting back to sprinting, but the first order of business was ice and Hannah Montana. I needed to heal.

The next leg of my journey was going to require a hell of a lot more than 37m (40 yards).

HIP THRUSTS AT THE COFFEE SHOP: PREVENTING HAMSTRING TEARS

Is there anything I could have done to prevent my hamstring pull?

If there is one injury Joe understands, it is the hamstring pull. His pre-hab prescription was effectively threefold:

1. **Train the natural glute-ham raise.** Nothing in the weight room can mimic the demands of sprinting. The next best thing, though, is the natural glute-ham raise, which builds an incredible foundation of eccentric strength in the hamstring. This helps prevent pulls and tears during the foot-strike portion of sprinting, when the load is greatest. The Asshole demonstrates proper form here: www.fourhourbody.com/asshole-demo.

According to Joe, athletes who can perform strict natural glute-ham raises rarely pull hamstrings. If you don't have the equipment, a partner can hold your ankles for this movement, which is much harder than it looks. Start slow and keep your hands in front of your face to avoid plastering it on the floor. See the Sorinex machine, which I have at home, in the "Tools and Tricks".

2. **Focus on hip extension strength.** Forget leg curls and knee flexion, with the one exception of the glute-ham raise. Otherwise, you should focus on strong hip extension. To prevent pulls and increase sprint speed, focus on these movements:

Reverse hyperextensions (reverse "hypers")
Regular hyperextensions
Kettlebell or dumbbell swings
Sled dragging (train both upright posture and a 45-degree "acceleration" lean)
Supine hip thrusts (see www.fourhourbody.com/hip)

If you can't do reverse hypers or a natural glute-ham raise, or if you lack the equipment, DeFranco and his acolytes recommend supine hip thrusts (see the video demo above), which can also be done with a barbell for added resistance (see my video with 188kg (415lb) here: www.fourhourbody.com/hipthrusts).

I love this exercise. It is also the money move for quickly relieving back pain from too much time at the laptop. Random digression: as I write this at 1:45 A.G. in a hotel café in South Africa, I have just finished a nice set of supine hip thrusts between a couch and a coffee table. I am the only night owl here.

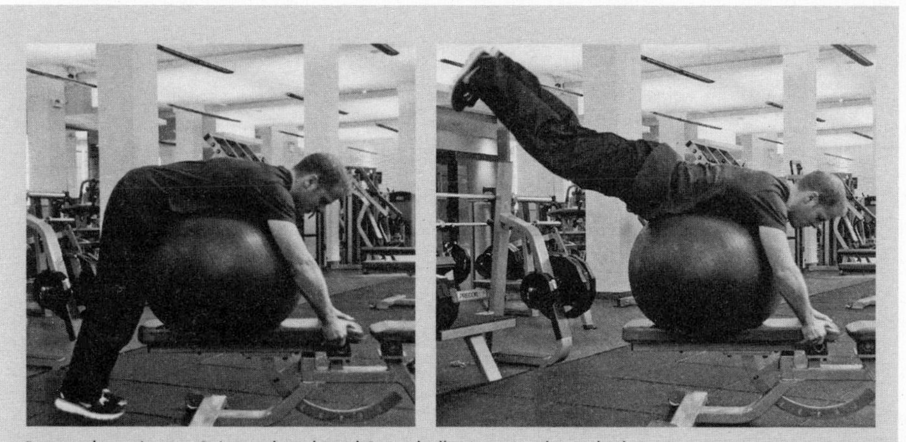

Reverse hyper(extension) on a bench and Swiss ball. It's easier than it looks.

A native Amaxhosa[12] cleaning woman just stopped to look at me as if I had lobsters crawling out of my ears, so I told her that the waitress had promised me free water, but only if I did the sexy booty dance.

She was not impressed.

3. **Keep your hip flexors flexible.** The most underrated way to improve stride length and prevent hamstring pulls is to (and this should sound familiar) keep your hip flexors flexible. See the hip flexor stretches in the last chapter.

When your hip flexors are tight, it creates constant tension and a constant pull on the hamstrings, which is a recipe for tears.

Tight hip flexors also prevent you from reaching full stride length. Upon extending your leg back into the turf, the stretch-reflex in your hip flexors causes them to contract prematurely and pull your leg back up. People with tight hip flexors take short, choppy steps when they run. Sometimes they look fast due to a high stride rate, but Joe calls it "going nowhere fast" because they are not covering any real ground.

Stretch those sons-a-bitches.

12. Speaker of Xhosa, the famous "click language".

HOMEOPATHY: THE PROBLEM AND PARADOX OF ARNICA MONTANA 30C

So what happened with Hannah Montana?

I had used topical arnica before, and it had worked well.

This time, I was taking Boiron Arnica Montana 30C pellets, an oral version that was the only option at the closest GNC. I started at five pellets, six times a day—twice the recommended dose. Risk of overdose? Not likely.

"30C", which I looked up that evening, tells you all you need to know.

This consumable version of arnica, unlike the creams I'd used in the past, was a *homeopathic* remedy. Samuel Hahnemann, a German physician, pioneered the field of homeopathy in 1796, if the term "pioneer" can be applied to alternative "medicine" founded on concepts like mass dilution and beatings with horse-hair implements:

> *Homeopaths use a process called "dynamisation" or "potentisation" whereby a substance is diluted with alcohol or distilled water and then vigorously shaken by ten hard strikes against an elastic body in a process called "succussion." . . . Hahnemann believed that the process of succussion activated the vital energy of the diluted substance.*

Riiiight.

Back to 30C. 30C indicates a 10^{-60} dilution, the dilution most recommended by Hahnemann. 30C would require giving 2 billion doses per second to 6 billion people for 4 billion years to deliver a single molecule of the original material to any one person. Put another way, if I diluted one-third of a drop of liquid into all the water on earth, it would produce a remedy with a concentration of about 13C, more than twice the "strength" of our 30C arnica.

Most homeopathic remedies in liquid are indistinguishable from water and don't contain a single molecule of active medicine.

I found this particularly bothersome. Bothersome because I appeared to heal faster using oral 30C arnica.

There are a few potential explanations:

HOMEOPATHIC REMEDIES WORK AS ADVERTISED

The water actually retains some "essential property" of the original substance because of the beatings and shakings. I give this a 0% probability. It violates the most basic laws of science and makes my head hurt.

THE PLACEBO EFFECT

I didn't realize it was a homeopathic remedy until after four or five doses, and I had been told it could reduce pain by up to 50% in 24 hours. Placebo is strong stuff. People can become intoxicated from alcohol placebos, and "placebo" knee surgeries for osteoarthritis, where incisions are made but nothing is repaired, can produce results that rival the real deal. This explanation gets my vote. Now, if I could just forget what I read on the label, I could repeat it next time.

REGRESSION TOWARDS THE MEAN

Imagine you catch a cold or get the flu. It's going to get worse and worse, then better and better until you are back to normal. The severity of symptoms, as is true with many injuries, will look something like a bell curve.

The bottom flat line, representing normalcy, is the *mean*. When are you most likely to try the quackiest shit you can get your hands on? That miracle duck extract Aunt Susie swears by when not talking about crystals? Naturally, when your symptoms are the worst and nothing seems to help. This is the very top of the bell curve, at the peak of the roller coaster before you head back down. Naturally heading back down is *regression towards the mean*.

If you are a fallible human, as we all are, you might misattribute getting better to the duck extract, but it was just coincidental timing. The body had healed itself, as could be predicted from the bell-curve-like timeline of symptoms. This is a very common mistake, even among smart people.

SOME UNEXPLAINED MECHANISM

'Tis possible that there is some as-yet-unexplained mechanism through which homeopathy works. Some mechanism that science will eventually explain. Until something even remotely plausible comes along, though, I'll do my best to scratch my *psora* (an itch "miasm" that Hahnemann felt caused epilepsy, cancer and deafness) with at least one molecule of active substance.

TOOLS AND TRICKS

DeFranco Training on Video (www.fourhourbody.com/defranco) These are the actual videos I took during our training day, in which DeFranco covers some of the more important dynamic warm-ups and stretches, in addition to sprint stance setup.

40-Yard Dash: Average Joe vs. Pro Athlete (www.fourhourbody.com/40yard) This is a clip of Rich Eisen, one of ESPN's newscasters and "every man" representative, running the 37m (40-yard) dash against professional athletes in the NFL Combine. It's hard to appreciate how fast NFL players are until you watch this.

Parisi Speed School (www.parisischool.com) Founded by Division I All-American javelin thrower Bill Parisi, this school has trained hundreds of professional athletes in increasing their speed. The Parisi NFL Combine programme has produced more than 120 successful NFL draftees.

Sorinex Poor Man's Glute-Ham Raise (www.fourhourbody.com/ghr) I first learnt of this (relatively) inexpensive GHR machine from Parkour athletes. It's a fraction of the cost of alternatives, small enough to be wheeled into a closet, and perfect for DeFranco's favourite exercise for hamstring development.

ULTRA-ENDURANCE I

Going from 5K (3 miles) to 50K (31 miles) in 12 Weeks—Phase I

"Beyond the very extreme of fatigue and distress, we may find amounts of ease and power we never dreamed ourselves to own; sources of strength never taxed at all because we never push through the obstruction."

—William James

(Quote from e-mail signature of Scott Jurek, seven-time consecutive 161 km (100-mile) Western States race champion)

IN THE SHADOWS OF A LARGE U.S. BRIDGE

"Drop your balls onto the bar."

Testicles and steel are like oil and vinegar: they don't usually mix well.

But I was being told, not asked, so balls were dropped.

Kelly Starrett, founder of San Francisco CrossFit, nodded in approval as I set myself up for the "sumo" deadlift. Kelly, nicknamed "KStarr", was echoing the advice of powerlifting icon Dave Tate: keep your hips as close as possible to the bar on the descent, as if you were aiming to set your twins between your hands. Romantic, n'est-ce pas? This birthing-hip position requires a near side split and is about as comfortable as it sounds.

The setting, the waterfront Presidio at San Francisco Bay, was more pleasant. Red and white homes, former officers' quarters, dotted the hills around us. Above the green expanses of Crissy Field, the sun was burning off the fog enveloping the Golden Gate Bridge. Kelly's next client was running late, and our conversation drifted from metabolic conditioning to how Kelly defines "athletic preparedness".

Before tackling the latter, he stopped to pose a question: "What'd you do for your RKC snatch test?"

The "snatch" is an Olympic weightlifting manoeuvre whereby you whip the weight from the floor to overhead in one clean motion, no pressing allowed. The snatch test was part of a Russian kettlebell certification (RKC) I had completed, and we had to complete X number of snatches (X being your weight in kilograms) with a 24kg (53lb) kettlebell. The time limit was five minutes, and we weren't permitted to put the weight on the ground.

"I weighed 77 kilograms and did 77 reps in 3 minutes and 30 seconds," I answered.

"Okay. Here, we do things like that as a finisher to a workout."

I wasn't sure exactly where the conversation was headed, but it sounded like he was calling me a big p***y.

He continued:

"I just turned 36, but I can still power clean 300, do a standing backflip, and also just ran the Quad Dipsea Ultramarathon, which is 48km (28.4 miles) with 5,639m (18,500ft) of elevation change. Rather than being laid out for weeks like most runners, I was fully able to lift heavy and train hard the next week."

Maybe he had a point with the girly-man comment. Then he dropped the bomb:

"And I never ran more than five kilometres in preparation for it."

My brain stopped there:

"Wait . . . Hold on. How the hell did you train then?"

"Lots of 400-metre repeats."

Suddenly he had my full attention.

Like many people, I'd fantasized about running a marathon before I died. Not running and walking, but running.

Not because I think it's good for you. It's not. Completing a gruelling 42km (26 miles)—a goddamn marathon!—was just one of the those things in the bucket list that wouldn't go away, along with skydiving (done), snorkelling the Great Barrier Reef (soon) and dating Natalie Portman (call me).

Sadly, jogging more than 1.6km (1 mile) made me look and feel like a drunk orangutan. I'd long ago assumed a marathon wouldn't happen.

But 400 metres? Even I could do that.

Kelly smiled, paused to enjoy my confused look, and handed me the holy grail:

"You need to talk to Brian MacKenzie."

Two and a Half Weeks Later

I could tell Louisville, Colorado, wasn't going to be kind to me.

My first glass of wine was only half empty, and the 1,600m (5,300ft) of elevation made it feel like my third.

The clock read 10:00 P.M., and the lobby of the Aloft Hotel was buzzing with Goth teens and ravers getting ready for the massive Caffeine Music Festival the following night. Platform shoes and coloured leather circled around the bar and lounge, filling the waiting hours with Facebook and text messaging, interspersed with shouts of "Dude!" and whispers of "Do you have any E?"

I was admiring the face piercings when a 187cm (6ft 2in), 13.8st (87.5kg) punk rocker sat down in the red plush chair in front of me. He looked like a cross between Henry Rollins, Keanu Reeves and a Navy SEAL.

Brian MacKenzie.

He shook my hand with a smile and I noticed the word "UNSCARED" tattooed across both hands, one letter on each of eight fingers. Within minutes, it became clear that we shared a similar brand of enthusiasm. The absurd kind that often overrides self-preservation.

In the early days of his endurance experiments, he had wanted to test the effects of 20-second sprints with 10-second rest intervals—the famous Tabata protocol.[13]

Brian somehow decided it was a good idea to start on the treadmill at an obscene 16km (10 miles) per hour at a 15-degree incline. He was forced to downshift to 14km (9 miles) per hour on a 10-degree grade after one and a half minutes. Then he flew off the back of the treadmill frozen in form, like a human gingerbread man. He landed on the floor with his legs locked, where he remained for more than five minutes at near-fibrillation. His two training partners, rather than help him up, stood over him laughing and pointing at his face, repeating over and over again:

"Dude, that was AWESOME! Buahahaha!"

My kinda guy.

I downed the last third of my Merlot and got down to business.

13. Named after Dr. Izumi Tabata, who demonstrated that these short sprints produced dramatic improvements in both short-duration *an*aerobic (without oxygen) performance and, surprisingly, longer-duration aerobic performance.

"So, what do you really think you could do with me in eight to twelve weeks?"

I explained my apparent handicaps, and he leant forward on his elbows:

"None of that matters. I could get you to a half marathon in eight weeks. That's assuming you have a baseline and can run a 5K in less than 24 minutes [3.1 miles at 8 minutes per mile or less]."

"What if I have never run 5Ks?"

"Fine. I'd have you do intervals first and build up to it. You have no shin splints or plantar fasciitis, right?"

"Right."

"And we have 12 weeks?"

"Yes."

"Well, then we can make miracles happen."

He'd taken one trainee, nicknamed "Rookie", to a mountainous 50K (31.2 mile) ultramarathon in 11 weeks. Prior to that, Rookie had never run more than 6km (4 miles) at a stretch.

Another trainee, a 43-year-old marathoner with an 8:30 mile pace, couldn't even complete three 400-metre sprints at the beginning of training. She had "no gears", as Brian put it: she couldn't maintain a 7:30 mile pace for even three minutes.

Two months prior to the New York City marathon, Brian had her do 16 minutes of total sprint training per week, in addition to four conditioning workouts per week using weights and calisthenics. Total workout volume was less than three hours per week. She called him daily the week prior to the marathon, often crying, pointing out the obvious:

"This will never work."

It worked.

She finished the marathon in 3 hours and 32 minutes—an 8-minute pace, 30 seconds per mile less than her previous time—and she would have finished much sooner had she not stopped to help another runner at the end.

Had she not stopped, Brian estimated her truer finish time at 3:30, a 7:28.8 per mile pace.

Brian had given her gears with 16 minutes per week.

The Journey from High Volume to Low Volume

Brian started in sports as a short-course swimmer. His coach couldn't get him to swim more than 100 metres without blowing apart at the seams.

In late 2000, he was conned into a short-course "sprint" triathlon by a 47-year-old friend who was a 13-time Ironman finisher. It was short but sweet: a 500-metre swim, a 21km (13-mile) bike and a 5km (3-mile) run.

He didn't blow apart this time, partially because he wasn't competing against swimming specialists. Much to his surprise, he loved it so much that he signed up for the Ironman the next day. He'd been bitten by the bug.

Brian climbed up the ranks of the triathlon world with an Olympic-distance race, a half-Ironman and then the Canadian Ironman. He trained 24 to 30 hours per week, just as his competitors did, including roughly 13km (8 miles) of swimming, 322+ km (200+ miles) of cycling and 80+ km (50+ miles) of running. It was par for the course in the endurance world, but it wasn't good for the body, his relationships, or much of anything else. He was severely overtrained, his wife was unhappy, and he had no life.

In 2001, he was introduced to the controversial Dr. Nicolas Romanov, a figure we'll revisit, which marked a turning point. Brian began to question the logic of high-volume, low-speed aerobic training and started to commit sacrilege in the world of long-form punishment. He decided to focus on less.

In June of 2006, he ran the Western States 161km (100-mile) endurance race, which has more than 5,180 vertical metres (17,000 vertical feet) of climbing and more than 6,700m (22,000ft) of downhill knee destruction. He finished in just over 26 hours. Compared to the mere 11-hour Ironman, he'd reduced his training from 30 hours per week to 10.5 hours per week.

But the 10.5 hours per week was still too much, and his body was still suffering, as was his marriage.

On 15 September 2007, after further refinement, Brian completed what is considered the fourth-toughest 161km (100-mile) run in the world, the Angeles Crest 100.[14] This time, he averaged just 6.5 *hours* of training per week, which included strength training (almost three hours), CrossFit, intervals and pace work. His body had learned to become aerobic at the

14. The Western States 100 doesn't even qualify in the top ten.

higher paces, even during speed training. Just before adopting this training mix, his one-rep max in the squat was 113kg (250lb).[15] Three weeks before the race, he could easily squat 108.8kg (240lb) for six consecutive reps, and he hadn't put on a single pound of body weight.

Now he was faster at every distance. It didn't matter if it was 100 metres or 161km (100 miles).

So You Want to be a Runner? Let's Try 400-metre Repeats

Back in Louisville, Colorado, 14 hours after my poor decision to drink wine, I was experiencing a unique clarity of thought.

It was the clarity of thought that only comes from repeatedly feeling as though your lungs and head are going to explode.

First, I ran 400 metres × 4, at 95% max effort, with 1:30 of rest in between.

Then I ran (or attempted to run) 100-metre repeats for ten minutes straight with ten seconds of rest in between runs.

I didn't stand a chance in either trial.

Halfway through my second 400-metre repeat, I was breathing entirely through my mouth like an asthmatic German Shepherd, and after the last I had to crouch down like Gollum and hold my knees to keep from vomiting.

For the 100-metre repeats, I had to stop after six and hold onto a picnic table to keep from falling over, and though I jumped back into the drill, I had to skip four repeats out of a total of about 20.

There were a few things I realized at that moment.

Namely, to run anything approaching an ultramarathon without doing myself permanent damage, I would need to ace a trifecta of preparation, biomechanics and training. The training would also need to redefine discomfort.

Thankfully, according to Brian, it would be brief.

15. Compare this to his maximum leading up to his very first Ironman, when the training made him weaker instead of stronger: 34kg (75lb) × 4 reps.

Preparation: The Undercarriage

4 WEEKS

It isn't your lungs or your slow-twitch muscle fibres that will fail first in long-distance running. It's your suspension.

To sustain the repeated impact of a mere 5K (3 miles), between 2,000 and 2,500 foot strikes for most runners, you need to ensure that your ligaments and tendons are both thick and elastic enough for the abuse; and you need to ensure that the proper muscle groups are firing in the right sequence.

I suffered a minor hamstring pull after the 400s (same leg as at DeFranco's) and experienced excruciating lower back pain for the next three hours, as did several other aspiring long-distance runners.

Why?

GA

My hip flexors and quads were too tight, common among desk workers, which made me bend forward at the hip during sprints. This then forced my hamstrings to attempt the job of the much larger and stronger glutes, which were inhibited. There you have it—overloading and a hamstring pull. The tight hip flexors pulled on the lower lumbar spine, which explained the sore back.

I also had pain on the inside of both knees after practising foot pulls (coming shortly), which appeared to be caused by two problems: tight quads and weak vastus medialis obliques (VMO), the teardrop-shaped muscle on the inside of the front of the legs.[16]

Last but not least, I had acute soreness throughout both feet and ankles. The ligaments, tendons and small muscles of the feet and ankles were underdeveloped.

In other words, I wasn't ready to run.

Before I could consider serious training, I needed good suspension. To do otherwise would be asking for injuries that could plague me for months or even years.

16. More precisely, the VMO is used to refer to a horizontally oriented group of fibres in the vastus medialis that should stabilize the patella (knee cap) and keep it tracking properly. Some physiologists believe that the importance of these horizontal fibres is overstated.

OF MARATHON MONKS AND ANTELOPES: THE ENZYMATIC EQUATION

The "marathon monks" of Mount Hiei in Japan run and walk the equivalent of an ultramarathon every day for six years, some averaging 84km (52 miles) per day for the last 100 days of training.

I wasn't looking promising as a monk.

"Am I ready for the Olympics, coach?" I jokingly asked Tertius Kohn PhD as he sat me down in his office at the Sports Science Institute of South Africa. Five days earlier, I'd had a biopsy tube the size of a pencil jammed into the side of my thigh[17] to skip the theory and look directly at the limits of my muscle. Much teeth grinding, three muscle samples, and a myography lab later, I finally had answers. Tertius looked at me with a serious expression.

"I'm a doctor, so I like to speak plainly. You might not like what I'm going to tell you, but I'm going to tell you anyway."

"Ummm . . . Okay."

"You'd have trouble finishing a 10K."

I nodded.

"In fact, I think you'd have trouble finishing a 5K."

This wasn't exactly what I wanted to hear, but three months of obsessing over ultra-endurance had taken me many places, and this was one of them: enzymes.

CS, 3HAD, LDH and PFK are all enzymes that limit energy production through different pathways.

South African Xhosa mid- and long-distance runners, for example, have high levels of lactate dehydrogenase (LDH), which allows them to recycle lactate at higher than normal rates. More LDH appears to mean less accumulation of plasma lactate (more commonly referred to as "lactic acid"), which means less debilitating muscle burn. In Kenyan runners, higher levels of another enzyme, 3-HAD, mean a greater ability to use fat instead of carbohydrate during sub-maximal exercise.

How did I measure up? I am the one under the line. Hear me roar:

17. Vastus lateralis. See the video of this at www.fourhourbody.com/biopsy.

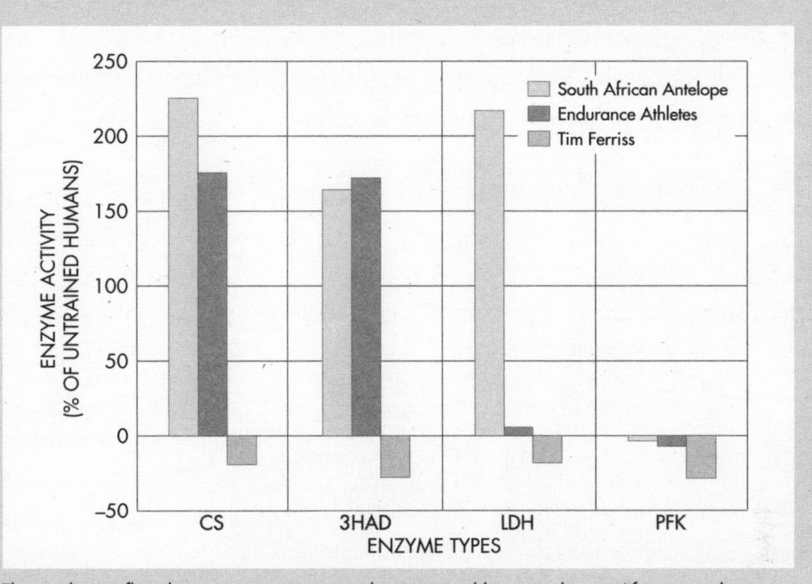

The numbers reflect the percentage compared to untrained human subjects. African antelopes and trained endurance athletes are in the mix for contrast. (Credit: Tertius A. Kohn PhD from the UCT/MRC Research Unit for Exercise Science and Sports Medicine. Special thanks also to Prof. Tim Noakes and the staff at ESSM.)

As Tertius showed me the numbers, I couldn't help but laugh out loud. How the hell did I have *negative* numbers? Despite all of my training and all my efforts, my enzyme levels were worse than a Homer Simpson couch potato.

So much for the "endurance preference" conclusion from the genetics testing.[18] Based on my raw materials, I seemed screwed for both endurance and power. In my mind, I flipped through the suitable sports: Competitive eating? Going down slides?

"You are . . . very, very average," Tertius would repeat several times over the next 30 minutes of discussion. "I hope you're not upset. I'm a scientist and like to state the facts simply."

By that point, I wasn't upset.

In fact, I was elated on some perverse level. I was *worse* than average. This meant that any future achievements could be almost completely attributed to training effect. It took a huge variable (genetics) largely out of the picture.

If I could do it, others stood a good chance—actually, a better chance—of doing the same.

That leads us back to our story.

18. See "From Geek to Freak".

I allocated four weeks to pre-training preparation, in addition to using ART[19] for the quads, hamstrings and hip flexors.

The following five movements and running prep were what I focused on. Stretches are held for at least 90 seconds and performed on both sides.

1. HIP FLEXOR (ILIOPSOAS) AND QUAD FLEXIBILITY

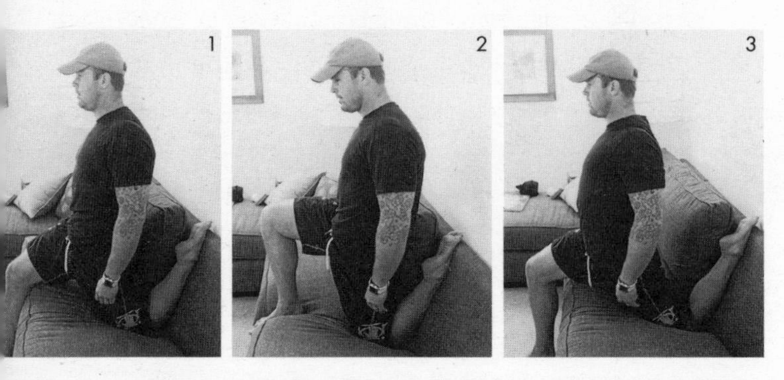

Here, Kelly demonstrates the "super quad" stretch on a sofa. Frame 1 is variation A, which is easier, and frame 2 is variation B. I prefer to use B on the floor in front of the sofa, with my rear foot resting (ankle bent) on top of the sitting cushions.

It's critical to keep your spine neutral. Slightly contracting your abs, as seen in frame 2, helps. Kelly illustrates **bad form in frame 3:** back arched and abs protruding forward.

2. PELVIC SYMMETRY AND GLUTE FLEXIBILITY

This is similar to "pigeon pose" in yoga, but using a table makes it easier to perform and harder to cheat. Place the leg as seen in frame 1 on a table top, knee bent 90 degrees. Lean directly forward (12 o'clock) for 90 seconds, then to both 10:00 A.M. (frame 2) and 2:00 P.M. for 90 seconds each. Notice that one hand is placed on the foot itself for support.

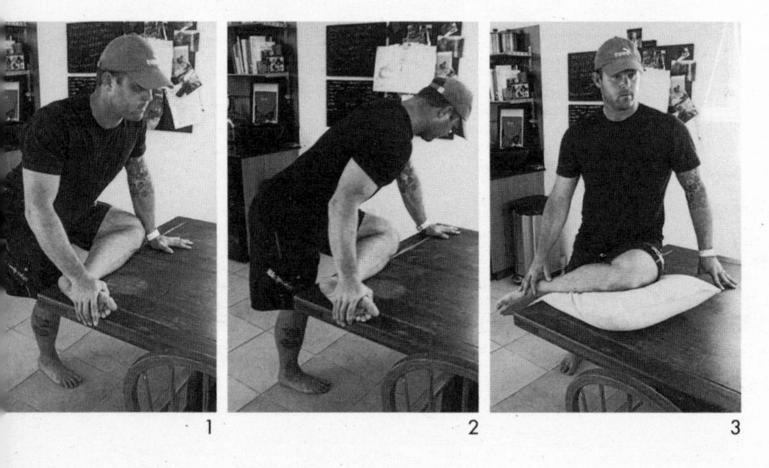

If your knee bothers you, you can rotate and slide the ankle off the table (frame 3), which is what I do.

19. See "Reversing Permanent Injuries".

In this case, you place one hand on the ankle for support. If you work at a computer for long periods of time, this ankle-off version can even be used in coffee shops without making much of a fuss. Use a pillow or books to elevate the knee if it's still strained.

Once you've finished the table "pigeon pose" on both sides, place your foot on top of the table (less coffee-shop friendly) and lean directly forward for 90 seconds (frame 4). Then place your hand on the inside of the knee (frame 5) and extend your arm as you lean away from your leg (frame 6) for 90 seconds. The foot on the table will naturally roll to its outer edge. Repeat on the opposite side.

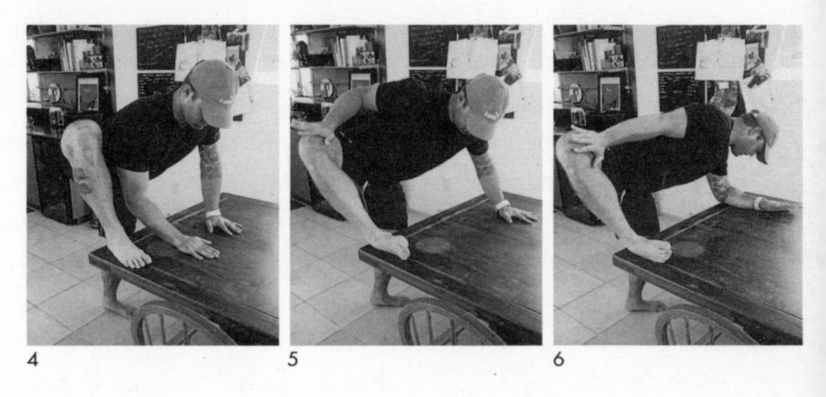

4 5 6

3. REPOSITIONING THE PELVIS

This is designed to put the head of the femur (thigh bone) in the back of the hip capsule. Extended periods of time in the seated position can move this ball into the front of the socket, causing all sorts of mechanical mayhem and pain.

Get on all fours, knees under the hips and remove all weight from one knee for 90 seconds to two minutes. Next, shift your weight about 10cm (4in) to the outside of your support knee (frame 2) and rotate the foot in

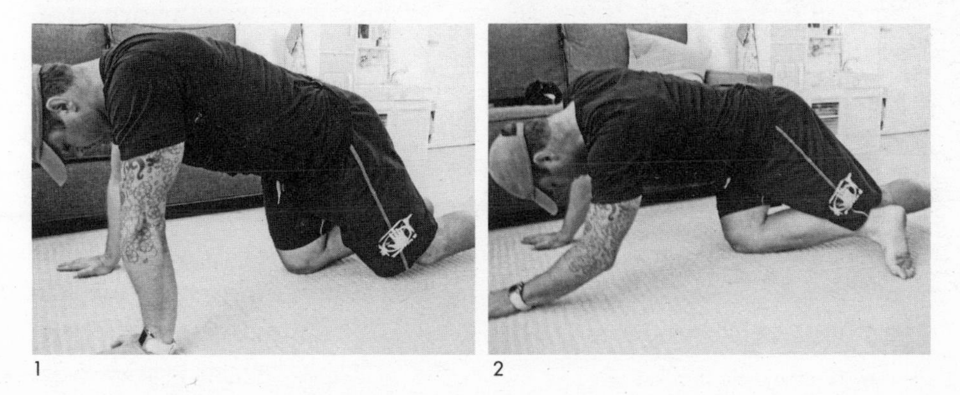

1 2

slightly as shown. In frame 2, no weight is on the left leg. Hold again for 90 seconds to two minutes.

Repeat on the opposite side.

4. PRE-WORKOUT (WEIGHTS AND OTHERWISE) GLUTE ACTIVATION

Start with ten repetitions of the double-leg glute activation seen in "Perfect Posterior". Be sure your feet are approximately 30cm (12in) forward of your glutes, and make a note of how high you're able to lift your hips.

Then perform 15 repetitions of the single-leg variation (shown here) on each side, pausing for one second at the top of each rep. It's important to hold your non-support thigh as close to your chest as possible with laced fingers, while pushing hard into your hands with your shin. This non-lifting leg should be under a hard isometric (non-moving) contraction for the entire set. Be sure to keep the toes of the support foot up in the air, and drive from the heels.

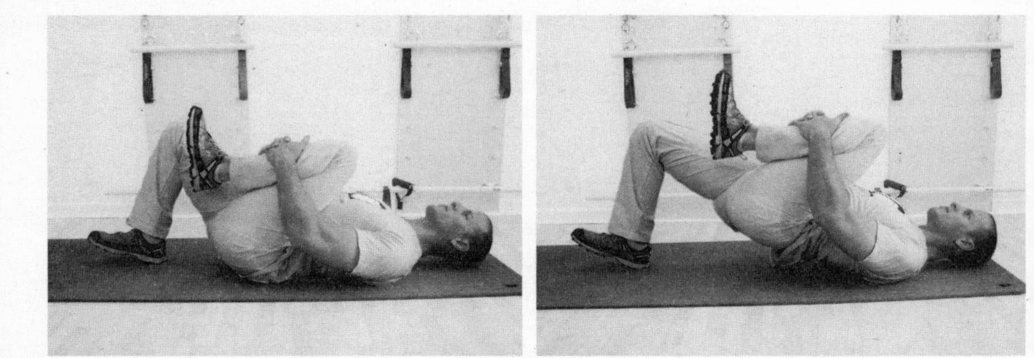

Once finished, test the double-leg lift again. There should be a clear gain in hip height. If not, repeat the single-leg variety but contract harder at the top of the movement.

5. STRENGTHENING THE FEET AND ANKLES

Jog barefoot on grass for 30 minutes, three times per week.

This is the advice of Gerard Hartmann PhD, an Irish PT trusted by many of the world's top distance runners, including Haile Gebrselassie, who's broken 27 world records.[20] Legendary Stanford running coach Vin Lananna, who has produced five NCAA team championships in track and

20. *Born to Run.*

cross-country, also has his runners perform a portion of their workouts barefoot on the track's infield.

But how do you run properly in the first place?

That's where the Russian doctor comes in.

Becoming Biomechanically Efficient Technique (Form and Tempo)

> Motion is created by the destruction of balance.
> —*Leonardo da Vinci*

There *is* a right way to run.

That, at least, is the contention of not only Brian MacKenzie, but also seven-time Western States champion and three-time "Ultramarathoner of the Year" Scott Jurek.

For Brian, the right way is one way: *Pose.*

Nicolas S. Romanov PhD, creator of the Pose Method, was born in 1951 in the unforgiving climes of Siberia. It makes sense on some level that he would become Internet-famous in 2005 for running on ice.[21] How the hell can you run on ice?

According to Romanov, by applying the same principles you should use on dry ground:

1. **Use gravity (via forward lean) for forward motion** instead of push-off and muscular effort.
2. **Land on the balls of the feet** and aim to have the feet land under your centre of gravity instead of in front of you.
3. **Never fully straighten your legs.** Keep a slight bend in your legs at all times to prevent push-off.
4. **Pull each foot off the ground and towards your buttocks** (rather than pushing off) using the hamstrings as soon as it passes under your centre of gravity.
5. **Maintain at least a 180 step per minute rate,** which means at least 90 steps per minute with each leg. This will use muscle elasticity to your advantage. Michael Johnson, who held the 200-metre world record for an astonishing 12 years, and also won four

21. www.fourhourbody.com/ice-run

Olympic gold medals at different distances, was known for eschewing a high knee lift in favour of short steps. His per-minute step rate? Around 300.

Brian suggests training tempo using a Seiko DM50L Metronome, and I found it easiest to use 90 beats per minute for one leg and count when that heel was highest (near the buttocks) as opposed to tapping the ground.

RUNNING BY THE NUMBERS: USING VIDEO TO CAPTURE THREE SNAPSHOTS

Brian explains running as a four-step process: lean, fall, catch and pull.

Forget pushing off: "The *support phase*, the foot hitting the ground, should be thought of as catching you from falling, not a push." He videotapes all trainees at 30 frames per second with a Casio High-Speed Exilim EX-FC100 camera. He believes, as do I, that you can learn more in one hour of video analysis than you can in a year of self-correction without video.

Looking at my third 400-metre repeat to get an accurate picture of semi-fatigued form, Brian reviewed the following numbers:

1. Frames from ground contact to under General Centre of Mass (GCM)
2. Frames on the ground
3. Frames in the air

The "Figure 4" or "Fig. 4" indicates the Pose position, in which the bent leg crosses the support leg and looks like a number 4.

Bear with me. This gets geeky (but cool).

Trial 1—Uncorrected

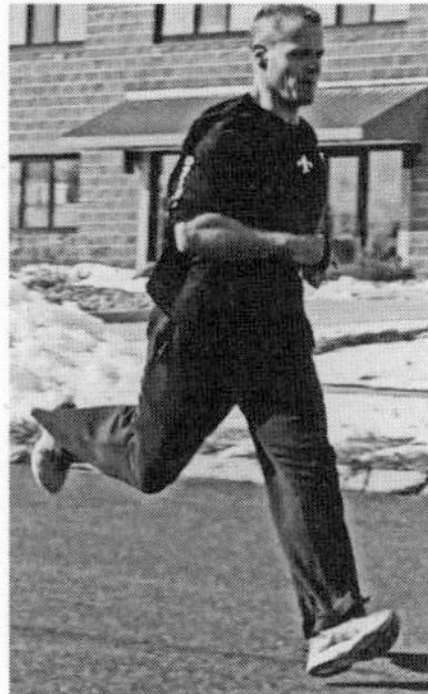
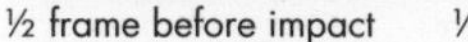

½ frame before impact

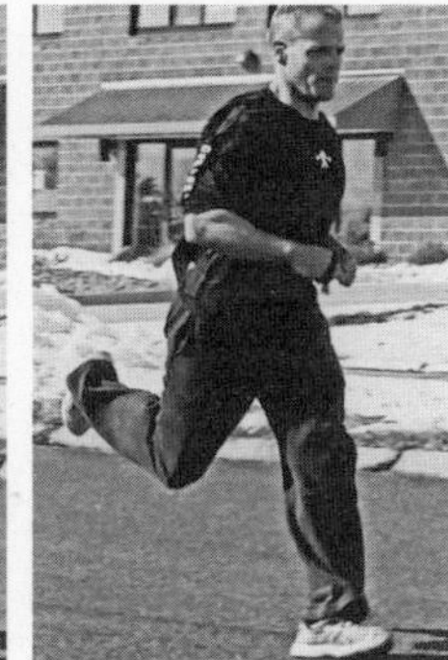

½ frame

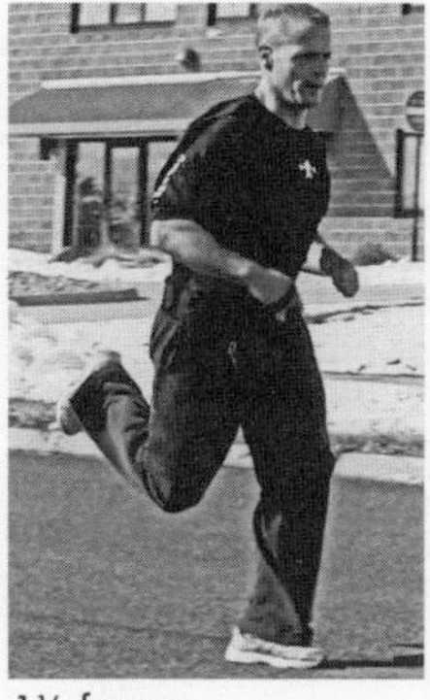

1½ frames

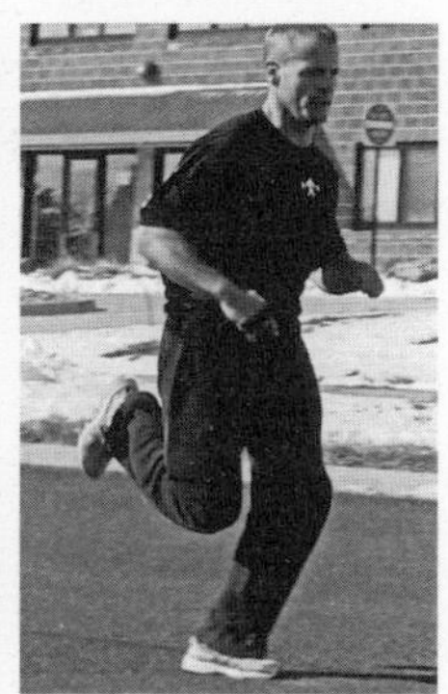

2½ frames

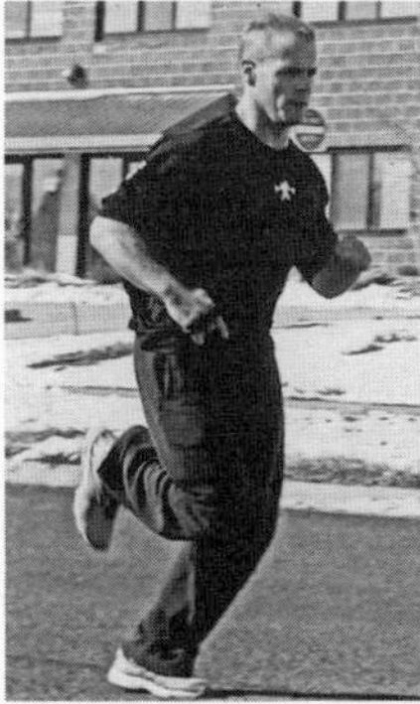

3½ frames—GCM (figure 4)

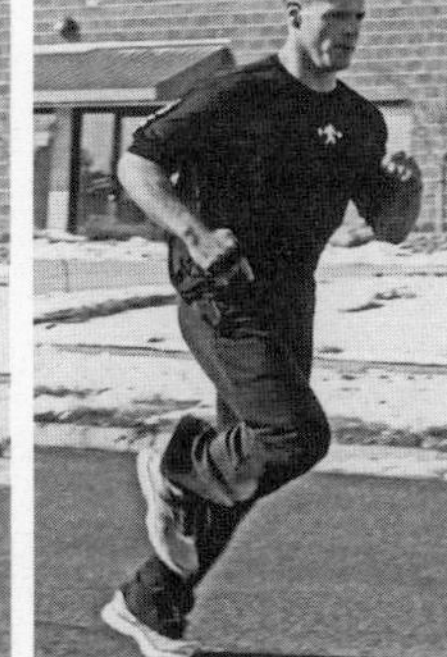

4½ frames

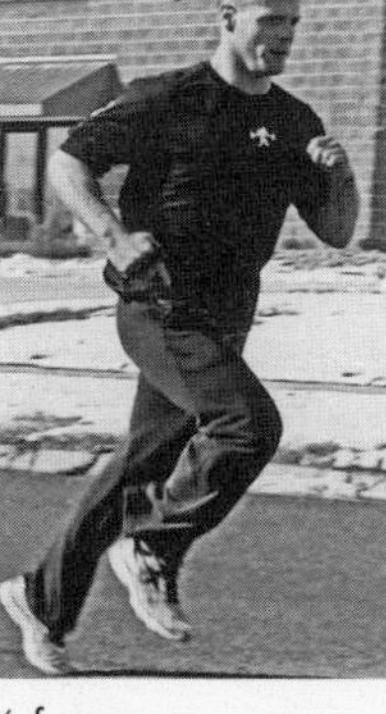

5½ frames

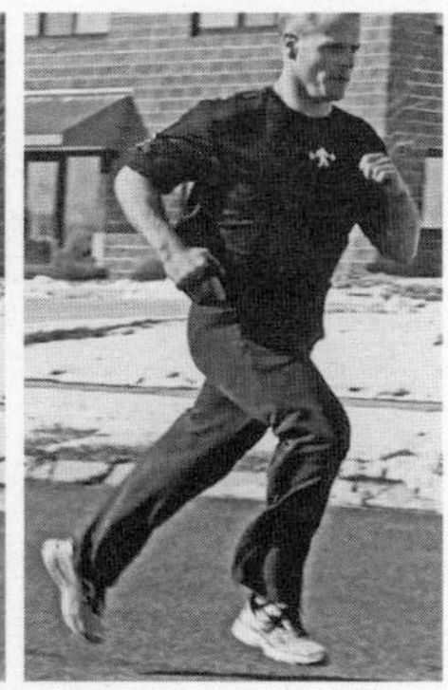

6½ frames

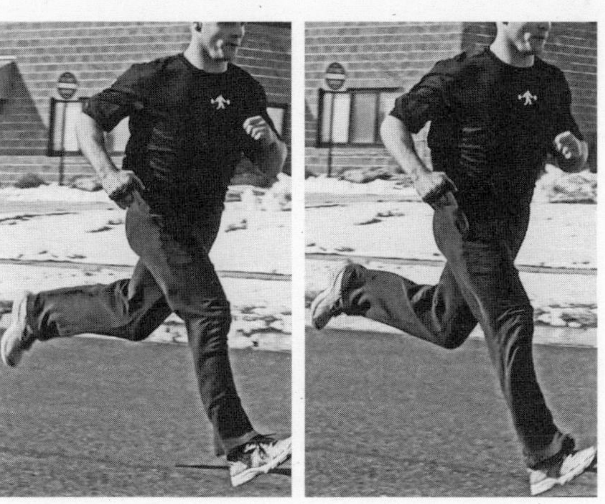

1½ frames in air

2½ frames in air (which means in ½–½ frame I make impact again)

Frames from ground contact to under General Centre of Mass (GCM): **3.5** (goal: ¾ of one frame).

Frames on the ground: **6** (goal: less than 3).

Frames in the air: **3** (goal: 5).

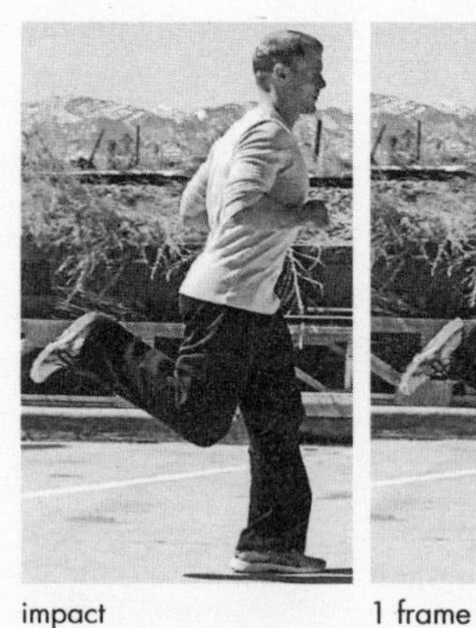
impact

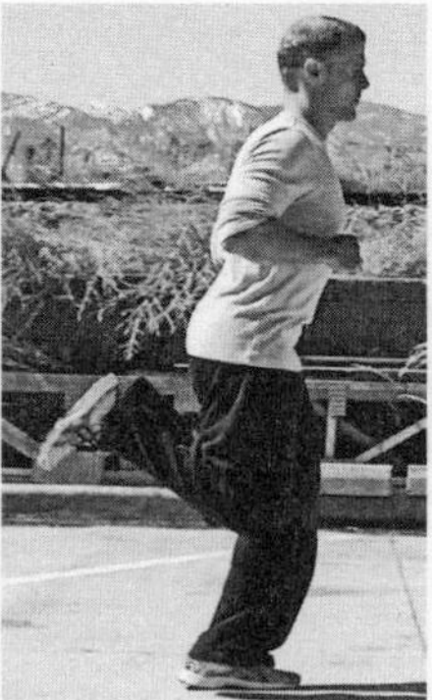
1 frame

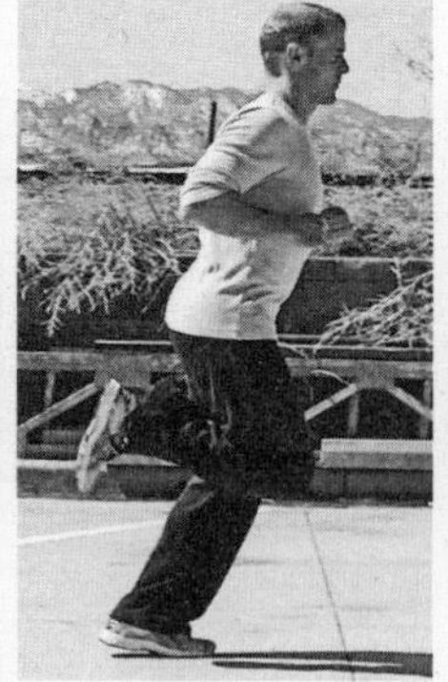
2 frames (Fig. 4)—GCM

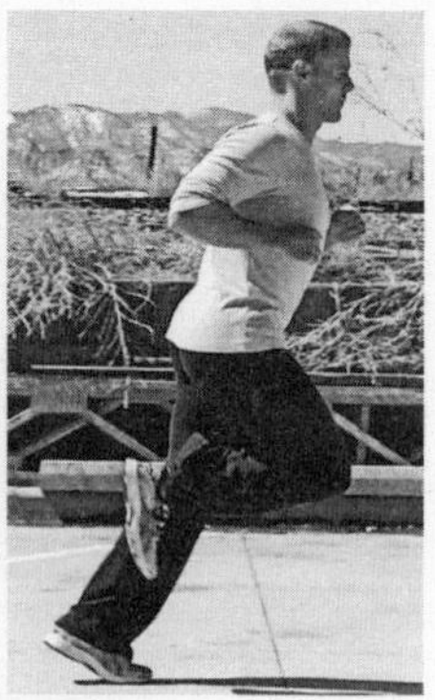
3 frames

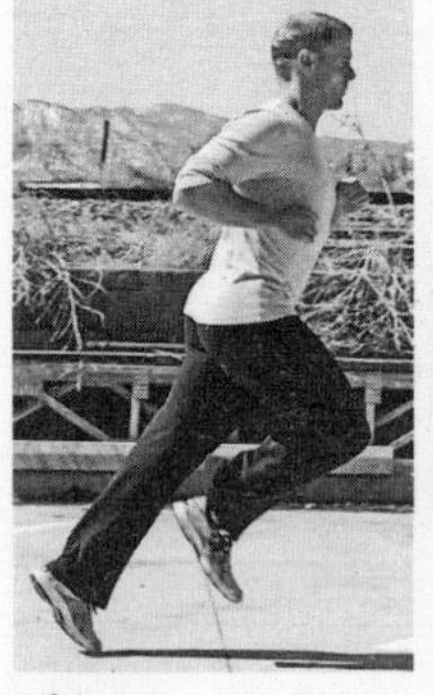
4 frames

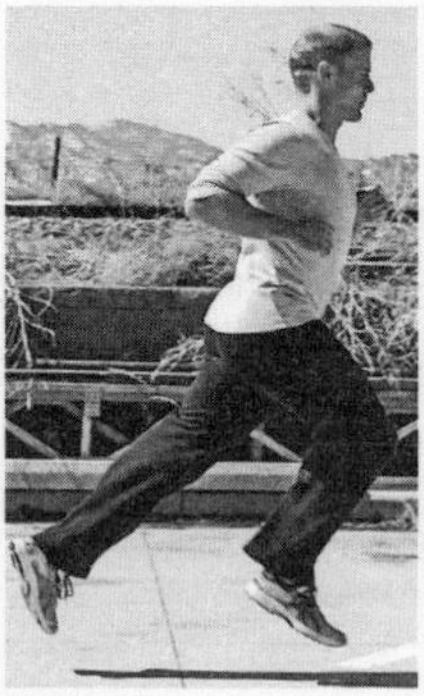

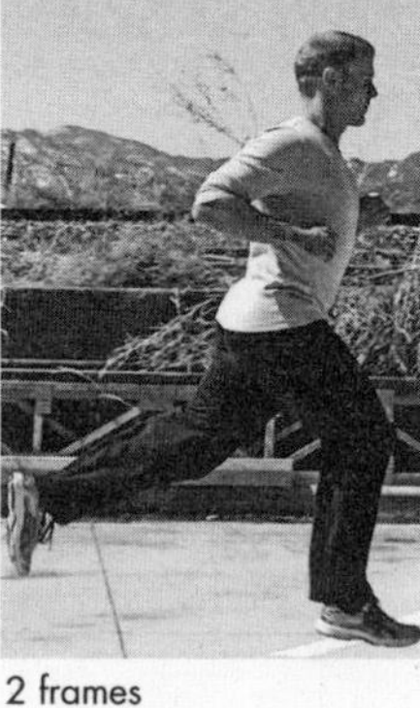
1 frame air

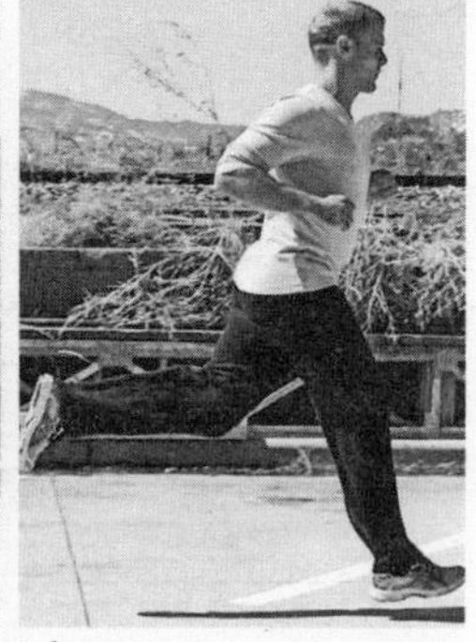
2 frames

3 frames

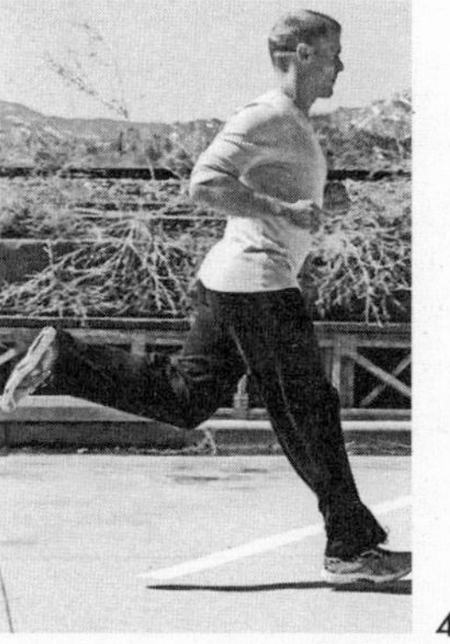
4 frames

TRIAL 2—24 HOURS LATER

Frames from ground contact to under General Centre of Mass (GCM): **2** (goal: ¾ of one frame).

Frames on the ground: **4** (goal: less than 3).

Frames in the air: **4** (goal: 5).

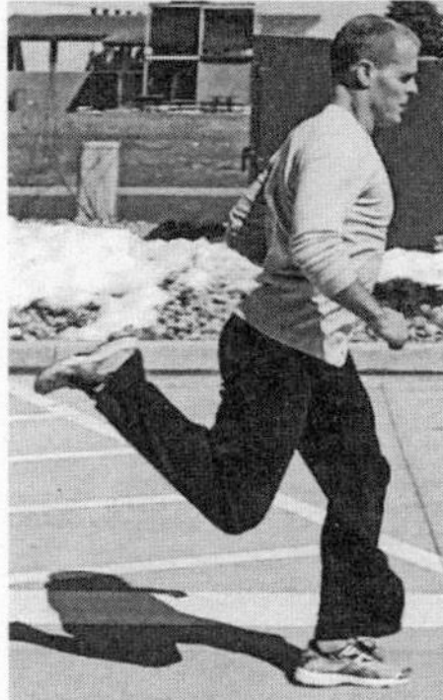
Impact

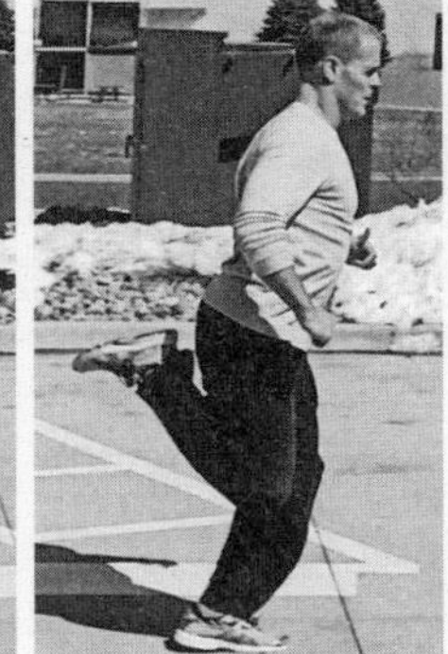
1 frame—almost GCM

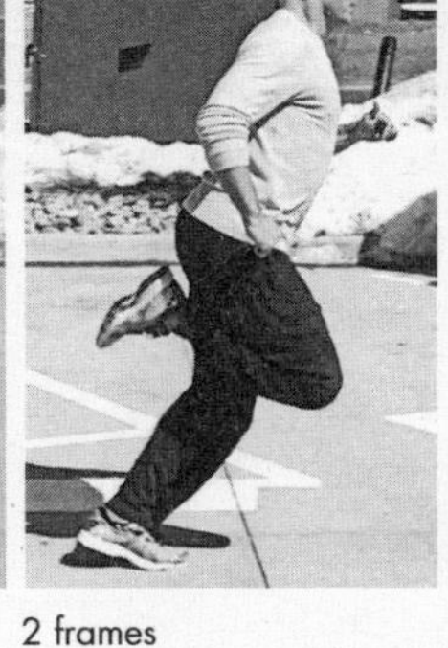
2 frames

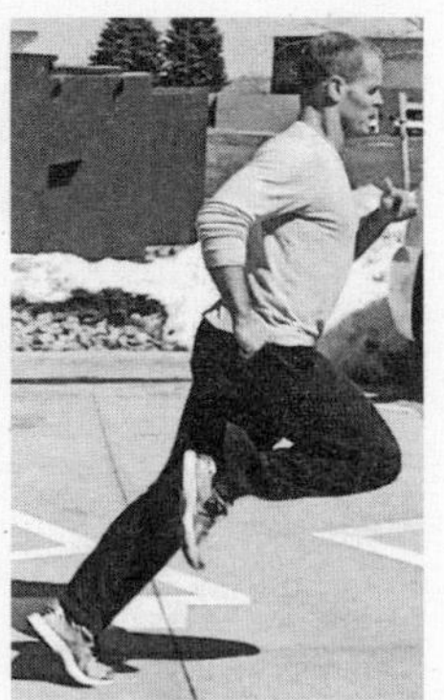
3 frames

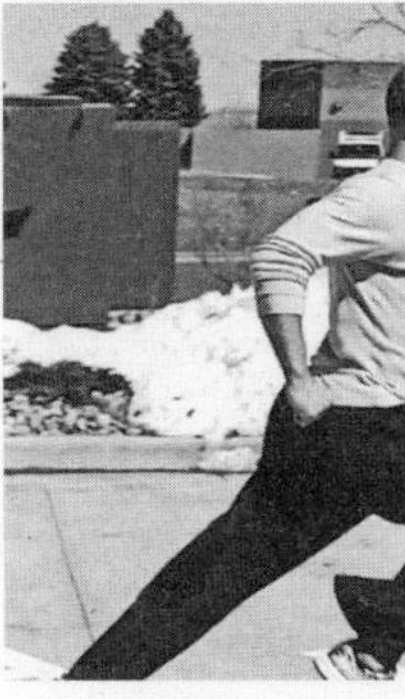
1 frame air

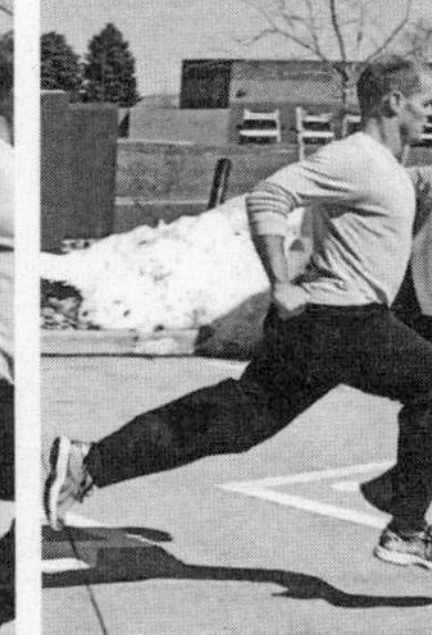
2 frames

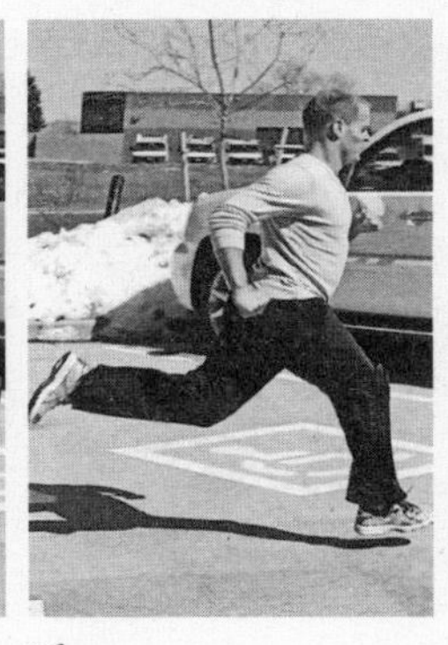
3 frames

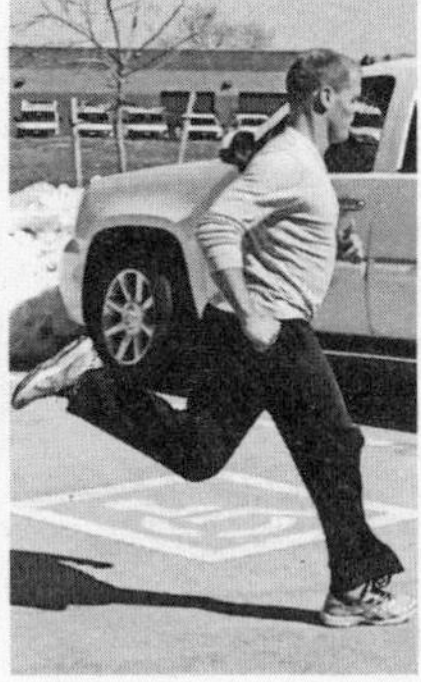
4 frames

TRIAL 3—2 HOURS AFTER TRIAL 2

Frames from ground contact to under General Centre of Mass (GCM): **1.5** (goal: ¾ of one frame).

Frames on the ground: **3** (goal: less than 3).

Frames in the air: **4** (goal: 5).

In less than 36 hours, based on the metrics used, I improved my running economy[22] 100% in the first two phases (3→1.5, 6→3) and improved desirable air time 33%.

Over the full two days of the certification, we covered more than six hours of whiteboard mechanics and hundreds of details. In practice, four things helped me most:

1. **Focus on at least 90 steps per minute with each leg.** Particularly if fatigued, focus on this stride rate, which automatically produces the other characteristics of good running mechanics (landing on the balls of the feet, fast pull, etc.). Scott Jurek reinforced this: "If you focus on higher stride rate, much of the rest corrects itself."

This, to me, is the crucial insight. Ken Mierke, a world-champion triathlete and exercise physiologist, studied Kenyan runners frame-by-frame and now trains his athletes to mimic this "running on hot coals" approach of smaller steps and higher cadence. The result? Some of them—like Alan Melvin, who was a world-class triathlete to begin with—do the seemingly impossible, as described in the book *Born to Run.* After five months of training at 180+ beats per minute, Melvin ran four 1.6km (1-mile, repeats, and every lap time was better than his previous best in the 400 metres.

2. **Lean, but fall like a tree instead of bending at the hips.** There should be no sitting back. Think of falling forward from the pelvis rather than from the head.
3. **For the pull off the ground (see the first three frames of Trial 3), imagine pulling the heel up to your buttocks at a 45-degree forward angle instead of straight up off the ground.** This visualization is what allowed me to go from Trial 2 to Trial 3 in two hours. If I thought of pulling the leg straight up off the ground, I subconsciously leaned less, which was self-defeating. Lean at an angle, and envision pulling the heel up at an angle.
4. **Use minimal arm movement and consider keeping your wrists near your nipples the entire time.** During the initial 100-metre repeats, I purposefully ran directly behind the best

22. *Not* defined here as L O_2/min.

ultra-distance runner in our group, matching his tempo and form. He ran with the shortest, most contained arm movements of all. I noticed it was infinitely easier to maintain a high stride rate when mimicking this. Reflecting afterwards, it made perfect sense: we are contra-lateral in motion. If one leg moves forward, the opposite arm must move backwards, which means you have to maintain the same "stride" rate with both the arms and legs. If your arm movements are too large, your lower-body stride rate has to drop to match them. Solution: bend the arms at least 90 degrees and use small movements.

POSE AS PANACEA: CAREFUL WITH THE ANKLES

The Pose method isn't all rainbows and kittens. It's very useful, but it doesn't, despite confusing claims, rewrite physics. It's hard to make forces disappear.

The Pose marketing machine points to one particular study as evidence of the method's ability to reduce landing forces on the knee: "Reduced eccentric loading of the knee with the pose running method", published in 2004.

This isn't the problem. The problem is that they fail to point out another finding in the study: two weeks with the Pose method also increased the eccentric work of the ankles. This, in theory, increases risk of Achilles tendon injuries and calf muscle problems. Ross Tucker PhD, a friend and Pose Level I certified instructor who was involved with this study, helped supervise an attempted follow-up study. Runners were split into supervised and unsupervised groups, and the objective was to observe retention of the Pose technique. The study couldn't be finished because almost every runner in the unobserved group (all of whom had been trained in the Pose method) and about half of the supervised runners (who'd been trained by Romanov himself) developed Achilles tendon and calf muscle problems.

In an e-mail to me, Ross concluded:

"In some, the technique might stick and work. But in many others, the technique will stick and destroy their calves, ankles and tendons." The moral of the story? Take it slow. Make changing your running a gradual process and stop if it hurts.

Pose has devotees with religious fanaticism for a reason: it can work spectacularly well. But that doesn't mean it's a cure-all. For some, the drills will help more than strict adherence to the gospel while running. For others, like me, the focus on increased stride rate will make the exposure to Pose extremely valuable, even if the other "rules" aren't followed to the letter.

Find your own path. One-size-fits-all, taken to extremes, results in pain.

We run, not because we think it is doing us good, but because we enjoy it and cannot help ourselves. . . . The more restricted our society and work become, the more necessary it will be to find some outlet for this craving for freedom. No one can say, "You must not run faster than this, or jump higher than that." The human spirit is indomitable.

—Sir Roger Bannister, first runner to break the 4-minute mile

ULTRA-ENDURANCE II

Going from 5K (3 miles) to 50K (31 miles) in 12 Weeks—Phase II

To get to 50K (31 miles) in 12 weeks, you first need to understand some normal limitations of the human body. Only then can you overcome them.

The liver and muscles can only store 1,800–2,200 calories of carbohydrates in the form of glycogen. In simple terms, if your running becomes an *anaerobic* process (literally, without oxygen) you have to pull from these limited stores. Remember what happened to Brian's 43-year-old female runner at the outset of training? She "had no gears" because she became anaerobic as soon as she attempted to increase her per-mile speed.

Even if you refuel 200–600 calories per hour, all the stomach can handle, it's likely you will run out of glycogen before the finish line of an ultra marathon. This is called "bonking" and usually means game over.

Force feeding during the race is one option, but it pays to flip another switch.

450g (1lb) of fat, used during long-state aerobic exercise, contains roughly 4,000 food calories, the same energy density as petrol. Even if you're a lean 5% body fat at 10.7st (68kg), your available 3.4kg (7.5lb) of fat can keep you humming for several hundred miles.

The trick is, of course, that you have to remain aerobic at higher speeds, which is the fundamental goal of all of Brian's training. Incredibly, some of his athletes are able to remain aerobic throughout eight rounds of sprints at a 12% incline with just 10 seconds of rest.

His athletes are using a near-endless supply of fat calories, when you or I would be choking on carb-based fumes.

The training used to get them there is predicated on two assumptions:

1. The muscle soreness runners feel after long distances is primarily from a weak sodium-potassium pump. Strength training is what improves the sodium-potassium pump, and what allows Brian's athletes to walk around the day after an ultra instead of lying in bed: "If I can get a runner's back squat up, I see their marathon time drop. It's crazy, but it works." Maximal strength training will improve endurance recovery.
2. If you can run a decent 10K (6.2 miles), you already have a sufficient aerobic base to run a 50K (31 miles). The training should therefore focus on getting you to move at faster speeds while remaining aerobic.

Point 2 is called "moving the aerobic line". It sounds more pleasant than it is.

Moving Your Aerobic Line

Brian produces fast-recovering 161km (100-mile) runners on less than 48km (30 miles) of total running per week, including the intervals and sprints.

His recipe is deceptive in its simplicity: focus on improving all of the energetic pathways, performing no runs over 21km (13.1 miles) and seldom doing more than 10K (6.21 miles).

The lactic acid system is one of several pathways that Brian aims to conquer. According to Brian, becoming "competent" in all these systems takes six to eight weeks for a lower-calibre runner:[23]

23. This substrate-based training approach is not universally accepted. Proponents of the Central-Governor theory, for instance, posit that the altered metabolism is the effect, not the cause, of the improved exercise performance, which is brain-regulated. To learn more about the Central-Governor, *The Lore of Running* and *Brain Training for Runners* are good sources.

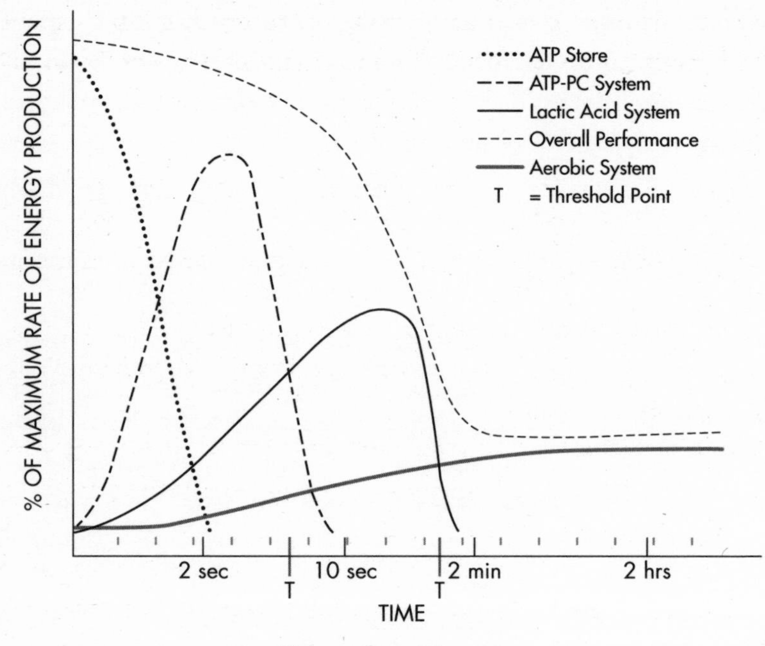

Diagram of energetic systems

In simplest terms, an energetically comprehensive programme might take the following form, with at least three hours between A.M. and P.M. work-

	Mon	Tues	Wed	Thurs	Fri	Sat	Sunday
A.M.	Int	Rest	Rest	Int	Rest	Rest	Rest
P.M.	CF	CF	CF	CF	CF	Rest	TT

outs:

Int = "Interval" training is often in a total that equals 1,600 metres, such as: 8 × 200m (90 secs rest between), 4 × 400m (90 secs rest), or 2 × 800 m (2–3 min rest).[24]

CF = "CrossFit" (2–10 minutes of metabolic conditioning; examples are provided later in my 12-week schedule).

TT = "Time Trial", used to test progress in a distance such as 1.6km (1 mile), 5K (3 miles) or 10K (6.21 miles).

24. In a given interval workout, the "rep" duration shouldn't deviate more than 2–3 seconds. For example, if running 4 × 400, times of 1:27, 1:29, 1:30, 1:28 would be better than 1:20, 1:25, 1:30, 1:33. Learning to pace precisely is part of the training.

Alternatively, you might use the popular "three-on-one-off" schedule for CrossFit, making sure to include two to three intervals and one time trial per week:

Day	1	2	3	4	5	6	7	8	9	10	11
A.M.	Rest	INT	Rest	Rest	Rest	Rest	INT	Rest	Rest	INT	Rest
P.M.	CF	CF	CF	TT	CF	CF	CF	TT	CF	CF	CF

If you don't have a track nearby for measuring distances, use GMaps Pedometre online[25] or a Keson RR112 Roadrunner 1 Measuring Wheel from a DIY Store or Amazon.

Expect your run times (Time Trials) to worsen in the first three weeks of training. This is normal, and your body will quickly return to baseline and then exceed previous bests.

In each interval, hill, or Tabata workout, if you can't recover to a heart rate of 120 in less than two minutes, the workout is ended. You haven't recovered and adding more stress would just impede progress. Call it quits if needed and come back stronger the next workout. In the first four weeks, if you are unconditioned, this rest period can be increased to three minutes.[26]

25. Go to http://www.gmap-pedometre.com/ and double-click to set start and finish points.

26. For the OCD runners: Alternatively, and this is Brian's preference, you can slow your speed slightly. In intervals, as a hypothetical example, this could be done by aiming to hit 200-metre repeats in 40 seconds each, as opposed to an original 37-second target.

In generic terms, the *taper*—a reduction in volume—the last week prior to competition might look like the chart below.

The key to the Tabata sprints in this schedule is maintaining a very high per foot strike rate (110+ per foot). If using a treadmill and unsure of speed, set the per-mile time to 30 seconds less than your average 5K per-mile time.

Taper Schedule

	Sun	Mon	Tues	Wed	Thurs	Fri	Sat
A.M.	45–60 minute recreational run/ride	10 sets × 2 reps (10 × 2) or 7 × 3 "on minute"[1] back squat (50–60% 1RM) or 8 × 1 deadlift on minute (70–90% 1RM)	8 × 200m (90s recovery) using original time at beginning of 12-week programme	REST	Tabata × 6–8 (20 sec sprint, 10 sec rest) at 80–90% of previous best[2]	REST	Race day!
P.M.	REST	CF (not a killer; something like a 10-minute "Cindy")	REST	REST	REST	REST	Eat pizza and enjoy beer, if you're done

1. "On minute" means once you start the count up on your stop watch, you do a set at 1:00, 2:00, 3:00, etc. Rest will depend on how quickly you finish each set. "On two minutes" would mean sets at 2:00, 4:00, 6:00, etc.
2. For example, if your previous best Tabata was completing 6–8 "reps" at 16kph (10mph) on a 12% incline, use the same incline but lower the speed to 13 or 14kmh (8 or 9mph). If you're running on flat ground, just reduce the distance you normally run by 20% (e.g., 100m→80m).

12 WEEKS TO 50K (31 MILES)

Pages 392–397 represent the exact 12-week programme Brian designed to take me from 5K (3 miles) to 50K (31 miles). I also wanted to target a 24-minute 5K (3 miles) time, which would (if sustained) approximate a 3:50 marathon.[27]

The 12-week programme is based on my following stats, which he requested:

27. If I wanted to then get aggressive, I could target a 19:29 5K, which would extrapolate to a 3:10 marathon, qualifying me for the Boston Marathon. To determine how your times at one distance translate to another, Google "McMillan Running Calculator."

400m times, with 90 seconds of rest between: 1:20, 1:30, 1:34 and 1:39.

Military press with barbell: 65.7kg (145lb) × 4 reps.

1-repetition max deadlift (DL): 204kg (450lb).

CrossFit (CF) routines for comparison: I didn't have this, so I indicated I could do 50 shoulder-level swings with a 40kg (99lb) kettlebell.

5K time and back squat poundages: I had neither, the latter due to shoulder surgery in 2004. I asked him to include front squatting if squatting were required.

Some additional notes on the three-month programme:

If there is only one workout prescribed for the day, it is possible to do an A.M. workout in the P.M. or vice versa.

Unless indicated otherwise, assume no rest between exercises. "AMRAP" means "as many reps (or rounds) as possible" within a given time. If it's a single exercise, it's reps; if it's a circuit of exercises, it's rounds. Doing something "for time" (e.g. "seven rounds of *ABC* for time") means completing the prescribed workout as quickly as possible and recording the total time.

"10 × 2" would mean 10 sets of 2 repetitions, for example (sets × reps).

Reread the "on minute" footnote on page 390.

DL = deadlift and BS = back squat.

Instructionals and videos of almost all CrossFit exercises, routines (often named after people, like "Cindy"), and unfamiliar exercises can be found at **www.fourhourbody.com/crossfit**. Common tools include rowing machines, pull-up bars and barbells. If you ask yourself "What the hell is that?" in the schedule, it's probably a CrossFit exercise.

Weeks 1–2

Week		Mon	Tues	Wed	Thurs	Fri	Sat	Sun
Week 1	A.M.	Good mornings: 2 x 8 w/ 180 sec rest	8 x 200m "on 2 min" not slowing more than 2–3 sec	Row 1500m[1] (sprint) + power clean 75% max for 30 reps		2 x 800m on 3 min not slowing more than 4–5 sec	Bench Press/Floor Press (50–60% 1RM) 8 sets of 3 on min Rest 10 min Tabata row 20:10 x 8	15, 12, 9 Thrusters @ 52kg (115lb) alternated with (e.g. 15 thrusters, 30 box jumps, 12 thrusters): 30, 20, 10 box jumps 24
	P.M.	Double Unders[2] + Sit-ups (superset): 50 reps of each, 40, 30, 20, 10 (no rest between)	3+ hrs later . . . 21, 15, 9 reps for time of Push Press (75% max press) + kipping pull-ups		5K TT	3+ hrs later . . . 3 rounds of max rep (no time limit on any) push-ups, rest 1 min, pull-ups, rest 1 min, air squats (no weight), rest 1 min		
Week 2	A.M.	Day off	Box Back Squat: 10 x 2 on min w/ 80% 1RM Rest 10 min Deadlift 8 x 1 on min w/ 90% 1RM	7 rounds for time of: Snatch[3] 3 reps @ 135 (use 8RM weight) + pull-ups 10	"Kelly": 5 rounds for time of 400m run 30 "wall ball" @ 9kg (20lb) + 30 box jumps @ 20"	10K (6.21 miles) @ 80% of 5K (3 miles) TT pace[4]	Press: 5, 5, 5. Push Press (no more than 4" drop in height): 3, 3, 3. Push Jerk: 1, 1, 1 Rough guideline: Increase weight 30% from each exercise to next 2–3 min rest between sets	3 x 800m on 2:30, holding same paces as last week or better
	P.M.			3+ hrs later . . . 10 x 200m on 2 min, not slowing more than 2–3 sec			3+ hrs later. . . strict chin-ups: 5, 5, 3, 3, 1, 1 Rest 2–3 min btw sets Maxing out—record weights used, if added to bodyweight	3+ hrs later . . . "The Bear": 5 rounds of 7 sets, rest as needed between rounds, increase weight each round. . . 1 pwr cln, 1 front squat, 1 press, back squat, 1 press = 1 set 3–5 min rest between sets day off

1. Unless otherwise noted, all distances are "all out" sprints.

Week 3

	Mon	Tues	Wed	Thurs	Fri	Sat	Sun
A.M.	Strength and Conditioning Recovery . . . (20 min) This can and should be done the day of races, after long runs, or on Sundays after interval work. Glute Ham Developer sit-ups (make sure you are extending knees aggressively to come up. . . your quads should also burn on this) 3 x 15, Glute Ham Developer hip extensions (hamstrings and buttocks should burn), Kettlebell/Dumbbell swings 3 x 15, Bench Press, Pull-ups. All exercises with light to medium weight. 3 sets! Reps are until you feel burn in target area or prescribed amount. This is not a timed WOD. Perform one set of each in circuit fashion. Take 1 min rest between sets. Should not be seriously debilitating workout. If you have not performed GHD sit-ups, start at 5–10 reps. If no GHD machine, can use physio/Swiss ball or BOSU and anchor legs. Use soft knees (slight bend) on way down, hard extension on way up.	10 x 200m on 90 sec rest, not slowing more than 2 sec per 200	Row:45 on/:45 rest + 1:30 on/1:30 rest + 3:00 on/3:00 off (repeat sequence total of 3x)	Row: 3 rounds of:45 on/:45 rest + 1:30 on/1:30 rest + 3:00 on/3:00 off	Diane: 21, 15, 9 reps for time of 102kg (225lb) Deadlift + handstand push-ups (no rest between sets)	4 x 800m on 2:00, holding within 4 sec of each other	
P.M.		2 Good mornings on the min for 10 min @ 50% 1RM BS weight	10 min "Cindy": AMRAP in 10 min of 5 pull-ups, 10 push-ups, 15 squats			Grace: 30 Clean and Jerks at 61.2 kg (135 lbs.) for time	

3. If you cannot perform snatches safely, you can substitute power cleans with 70kg (155lb)
4. Take 5K (3 miles) per mile time x 1.2 = target 10K (6.21 miles) per mile time; then use mile markers or GPS (like Garmin) to determine if you need to slow down or speed up.

Weeks 4–6

Week		Mon	Tues	Wed	Thurs	Fri	Sat	Sun
Week 4	A.M.	5 x 400m w/ 2 min rest, holding within 3 sec of each other. . .		5 miles @ 85% RPE (rate perceived exertion)[5]	Work up to a 1 rep max press within 15 min (more of a testing day)	2 x 1.6km (1 mile) all out with 10 min recovery between km/miles	Deadlift 1.5 times bodyweight, Bench Press bodyweight, clean 3/4 bodyweight for 10, 9, 8, 7. . . down to 1 rep	
	P.M.	5 front squats @ 75% 1RM, front squat on the minute for 5 min . . . Rest 10 min . . . DL 8 x 1 on min at 90%	7 Rounds For Time: 7 unbroken[6] hang squat cleans @ 43kg (95lb) + 7 unbroken handstand push-ups		Tabata Run on treadmill @ 12% Grade and current 5K (3 miles) pace	6 Rounds: Power snatch 135 lbs. 5 reps + 200m row		Helen: 3 x Run 400m + 21 kettlebell swings @ 24kg (53lb) (1.5 pood) + 12 pull-ups
Week 5	A.M.	Back Squat 3 × 5, rest 3 min between sets . . . 21/15/9 of 84kg (185lb) front squat, Chest-To-Bar (CTB) pull-ups	5 rounds of 100 double unders, 25 burpees. Rest 3 min after each round		5 rounds for time: 10 hang power snatches @ 52kg (115lb), 30 box jumps @ 24 inches	6,5,4 . . . 1 rep of each: Deadlift @ 315, muscle-ups, Handstand push-ups (no rest between cycles)	7 rounds: 30 sec max thrusters @ 95 lbs., rest 30 sec, 60 sec of max 10m line touches, rest 60 sec	
	P.M.	10 x 200m. Rest time is 3x your run time		10K TT		Tabata 20:10 x 8		
Week 6	A.M.	Bench Press 3 x 5, rest 180 sec between sets, then 15 min AMRAP of: 10 clapping push-ups, 20 GHD sit-ups, 30 KB Swings @ 55 lbs.	Back Squat 3 x 5, rest 3 min btw sets and increase weight from last week. 21/15/9 of: 70kg (155lb) power clean, burpees (e.g. 21 clean, 21 burpees, 15 clean, 15 burpees, etc.)	10 x 100m repeats, rest 1:30 between sets and don't deviate more than 2 sec either way		Split Jerk 3 x 3, rest 180 sec between sets. 5 rounds of: 40 wall balls, 30 pull-ups	Deadlift[7] 3 x 3 (3RM), rest 4 min between sets. Sumo Deadlift High Pull: 5 sets of 10 unbroken reps @ max weight. Rest 3 min between sets	
	P.M.		1 min on 3 min x 5		3 x 5K repeats on trail, rest 10 min between sets		Tabata-esque 30:20 x 8	

5. See the RPE scale here for percentages: http://su.pr/2JlHro.
6. "Unbroken" means that you, if you cannot complete seven reps one after another, rest as needed but do not stop the exercise. For hang cleans, you'd rest at top deadlift position, and for handstand push-ups, you'd rest at fully extended position.
7. Sumo or conventional style.

Weeks 7–8

Week		Mon	Tues	Wed	Thurs	Fri	Sat	Sun
Week 7	A.M.	Clean 3 x 1, rest 2 min between sets Then 16 min AMRAP: Top of every min do 6 KB swings at 31.7kg (70lb), then 4 clean and jerks at 60% of your 1 RM Clean	6 x 800m repeats with 3 min rest between sets. Keep within 4 sec of slowest 800m	Bench Press 3 x 3, increase by 4.5kg (10lb) from previous week. Then 7 rounds of 7 HSPU (handstand push-ups), 12 reps deadlift at 225		Shoulder Press 3 x 3, at 85% of your 1 RM. Push Press 3 x 3, rest 180 sec between sets	Deadlift 3 x 3, increase 2.3kg (5lb) from previous week. Rest 4 min between sets. 4 rounds of: 7 front squats at 185, 100m run, 21 pull-ups. Rest 2 min after each round	
	P.M.		1.6km (1 mile) TT then 3 x 400m repeats at your km/mile pace. Rest 90 sec between sets		90 min trail run at 85% RPE		Tabata	
Week 8	A.M.	20 min AMRAP: 1 power clean @ 225, 3 weighted pull-ups @ 22.7kg (50 lb), 5 "parallel" hand HSPU,[8] Row for 7 calories	Back squat 3 x 1, rest 3 min (95–97% 1RM). 4 rounds of 50 unbroken double unders, 30 unbroken wall balls	3 rounds of: 10 power snatches @ 135, 20 ring dips		5 rounds of: 30 sec AMRAP Body Weight Bench Press, rest 30 sec; 45 sec AMRAP Russian KB swing @ 80 lbs., rest 15 sec	7 rounds. Start 2:30 countdown: run 400m, then AMRAP pull-ups. Once 2:30 min alarm goes off, rest 60 sec and repeat	
	P.M.		5 x 800, rest 2:30 and maintain same splits as previous week		3 x 1.6km (1 mile). Rest 5 min between sets		10 x 200 with 2 min rest	

8. Handstand push-ups. Can use push-up grippers or mounted PVC pipe to lessen wrist strain.

Weeks 9–10

Week		Mon	Tues	Wed	Thurs	Fri	Sat	Sun
Week 9	A.M.	"Snatch Balance"—7 min to build up to a heavy set of 1. Snatch—7 min to build up to a heavy set of 1. 4 sets of: 12 Hang Power Snatches @ 115, 5 muscle-ups, 250m run.	Shoulder Press 3,3,1,1 (95% of max for each). Rest 120 sec after each set Then: 5 rounds of 20 pull-ups, 30 push-ups, 40 sit-ups, 50 squats. Rest 3 min after each round	Deadlift 3 x 1, rest 3 min between sets Then Row 30 sec on for max calories (displayed on machine) x 10 sets. Rest 1:30 after each set		Back Squat 3 x 3. Then 5 rounds of 7 reps with 70kg (155lb) hang power clean, 7 reps 70kg (155lb) push press, 7 reps 70kg (155lb) front squat	20 min AMRAP of 12 handstand push-ups, 20 SDHP (sumo deadlift high pull) @ 34kg (75lb), 20 Knees to elbows	
	P.M.		Sprinting (track or outside)—goal is to cover as much distance as possible: 1 min on, 60 sec off, 1 min on, 50 sec off, 1 min on 40 sec off . . . down to 1 min on, 10 sec off, then back up to 1 min on, 50 sec off		4 x 2K (1.24 miles) repeats. Rest 3 min between sets. Perform on hilly trail		8 x 100m hill repeats (aim for 6 percent grade) on trail. Rest 2 min between sets	
Week 10	A.M.	5 x 3 touch-and-go cleans. Rest 3 min between sets		7 sets of 10 push presses @ 135, 15 box jumps @ 30 inches	10 sets of 10 thrusters at 43kg (95lb), 10 CTB pull-ups. Rest 60 sec after each set	Bench Press 3 x 1, rest 120 sec between sets On the top every min, for 3 min, run 400m then max overhead squats @ 43kg (95lb) for 5 rounds	60 min trail run at 95% RPE	
	P.M.	5 sets of 1 min AMRAP burpees. Rest 3 min between sets		Trail or flat ground: 10 x 30-sec repeats	Hang Power Clean 3 x 1, rest 120 secs. Ring Push-ups AMRAP x 3 (3 min rest between)			

Weeks 11–12

Week		Mon	Tues	Wed	Thurs	Fri	Sat	Sun
Week 11	A.M.	Back Squat 5,5,5 rest 3 min. "Cindy" 5 pull-ups, 10 push-ups, 15 squats. AMRAP in 20 min, no rest between	5 rounds of 50 double unders, 15 ring dips, 7 power cleans @ 175. Rest 2 min after each round	Push Jerk @ 85% of your 1 RM. 1 rep every 45 sec for 12 rounds. Then 3 rounds of 800m run, 5 bar muscle-ups, 15 push press @ 43kg (95lb)		Snatch, 20 min to determine a new 1 RM. Clean, 20 min to determine a new 1 RM	60 min EZ Jog	
	P.M.		4 x 5 min intervals with 3 min recovery on trail. Goal: cover as much distance as possible. Remember to measure using Google Maps or GPS		6 x 800m repeats with 1:30 rest and a 6 sec buffer			
Week 12	A.M.	Back Squat 5 x 5	5 rounds of 5 reps deadlift (65% 1RM), 20 ring dips. Rest 45 sec after each set		Tabata 20:10 x 8, scaled back to 75% of last Tabata km/mph speed		Race Day!!	Strength and Recovery
	P.M.		8 x 200s @ 90% with 2 min rest					

FAQ WITH BRIAN

What type of shoes should I wear?

I suggest the Inov-8 X-Talon 212 or Inov-8 F-Lite 230 for trail running. For tarmac and other hard surfaces, I suggest the Inov-8 F-Lite 220, but the F-Lite 230 can be used as well.

What not to use: I've seen more problems with Newton shoes than any other. Avoid them.

Don't fall for the barefoot myth, either. There is a misguided belief that you can go barefoot and immediately fix all of your problems. If you have been wearing shoes with heels for years and start barefoot running with no transition, expect problems with your Achilles tendons. One year of stretching might get an additional 5mm (¼in) range of motion out of them, so if you remove a 1cm (½in) heel and go pound the pavement, you're asking for major issues. Removing the heel will not automatically fix your form. Most of the grandfathers of barefoot running still run with their hip flexors.

Take, for instance, the Copper Canyon Ultramarathon. It's held in the Mexican backyard of the near-mythical Tarahumara Indians, who are world-famous for running in sandals called huaraches. The soles consist of little more than one layer of old tyre rubber.

It sounds romantic, but the top three runners in 2010 were all wearing shoes. Running barefoot alone does not make you a better runner.

The front of my shins kills me after running. How can I prevent this?

Don't "dorsiflex", or pull the toes up towards the knees, while running.

Just imagine doing 21,600 toe raises on each side while sitting down. That's what will happen if you run 180 total steps per minute for a 4-hour marathon and dorsiflex the entire time.

If this is a habit, pre-fatigue the muscle involved (your tibialis anterior) before training by pushing down on your toes with your hands and dorsiflexing slowly on both sides 30 times.

Is there a simple indicator of bad form I can monitor while running?

If you hear a loud stomp, which is clear during video analysis, you are over-engaging your quads and therefore your hip flexors. Aim to be as quiet as possible.

If you watch the end of a 10K (6.2 miles) and listen to the loudness of footfalls, you'll find that the first finishers are the quietest, then you have louder runners, followed by the loudest runners, followed by the walkers. The better the runner, the quieter they are.

What should I do if I get fatigued during intervals and my form starts to fail?

If you find your form deteriorating, focus on keeping turn-over (stride rate) high.

What type of diet do you follow while in training?

The biggest problem in endurance sports is, hands down, nutrition. I've seen people finish the 217km (135-mile) Badwater Ultra in the top 10 who had no business being in the top 10. One of my runners PR'd (set a personal record) in nine hours off of nutrition alone. Most runners subsist on drinking Gatorade and eating gels. The high-carb diet is crap. You need to replenish glycogen, but that doesn't mean you need to eat pizza and pasta, or cereal and bread, during training.

I follow, and suggest my athletes follow, a Paleolithic or "paleo" diet, which omits starches, grains and beans. It consists of lean protein, vegetables, a little fruit, a sh** ton of fat and nothing else. The most critical thing a runner or athlete can do is record three days of food logs, which includes weighing their food. This will give you a clear idea of baseline.

Do you take anything in particular post-workout?

This time window is a paleo exception.

I consume GENr8 Vitargo S2, a carbohydrate supplement, which allows me to replenish glycogen faster than any other product I've used. Some athletes can consume 1,100 calories an hour of Vitargo, if needed, versus 200–600 calories of carbs from whole foods.

If I'm able to consume Vitargo within ten minutes of my workout, I usually take 70 grams. If more than ten minutes have passed, 35 grams. I'll also consume Vitargo for the first 3–4 hours of a race, after which I move to whole food.

FORCED EVOLUTION

Brian's protocol, 12 weeks of murderous intent (but not volume), has worked for nearly everyone who's done it to the letter.

Did it work for me? Enzymes notwithstanding, was I able to create a 50K (31 miles) ultrarunner out of a huffing and puffing mess?

RACE FEEDING: TIPS FROM SCOTT JUREK

"It's important to train the body to process food during movement, and you should practise this during your longer training runs. Aim to consume one gram of carbohydrate (CHO) per hour, per kilogram body weight. For example, if you weigh 7.8st (50kg), you would aim for 50 grams of CHO per hour. . . . Most bananas are approximately 25g of CHO, so, in this example, you could eat two bananas per hour. But don't eat all your carbs at once. Consume 25g, in this bodyweight example, every 20–30 minutes and gulp water at the same time. Why gulping? Gulping, and the subsequent pressure in the stomach, is an important trigger for gastric emptying. Sipping doesn't have the same effect."

THE DEAN'S LIST

4:00 A.I., Daly City, California

Dean Karnazes didn't know how long he'd been running. In fact, he wasn't sure where he was. The tequila was wearing off and he came to three realizations all at once:

1. He had just turned 30, which explained the tequila the night before. Normal.
2. He was not wearing trousers and was running in his underwear. Not normal.
3. He felt more alive than he had in 15 years, when he last ran in high school.

So he kept going.

He later called his wife from a 7-Eleven car park in Santa Cruz, 48km (30 miles) south of where he'd started: on his porch in San Francisco, grabbing old plimsolls he'd used for mowing the lawn. She was a bit confused, especially by the underwear part. Dean, on the other hand, had achieved ultimate lucidity. The corporate life, even with the new Lexus and the perks of indoor servitude, was not for him. Things needed to change.

Change they did.

From cubicle dweller, he transformed into a mainstream demigod in the world of ultramarathoning. If running 217km (135 miles) non-stop in the 48°C (120°F) heat of Death Valley[28] weren't enough, he also decided running 42km (26.2 miles) at –40° around the South Pole would be a challenge. (It was, especially in tennis shoes; he was the only one to spurn snowshoes.) To bring national media attention to childhood obesity and exercise, he then ran 50 marathons in 50 consecutive days in all 50 states.

28. The aforementioned Badwater ultramarathon.

In other words, Dean sees more marathons in a year than most will see in a lifetime. He competes almost every weekend.

Here are Dean's top-5 lists of must-run and must-experience marathons for newbies and pros alike.

In his words:

FAVOURITE 5 U.S. MARATHONS

New York City (www.ingnycmarathon.org): The most culturally and ethnically diverse marathon in the world.

Portland (www.portlandmarathon.org): The lore of Oregon running pervades this marathon.

Marine Corps Marathon (www.marinemarathon.com): Running through the nation's capital will give you the chills.

Rock 'n' Roll San Diego (www.rnrmarathon.com): Who needs an iPod when there's a live band every mile?

Boston (www.bostonmarathon.org): Hey, it's Boston. 'Nough said.

TOP 5 PICKS FOR FIRST-TIMERS

Napa Valley (www.napavalleymarathon.org): Flat course, cool temperatures, wine waiting at the finish!

Hartford (www.hartfordmarathon.com): Perfect big-city marathon for first-timers.

Fargo (www.fargomarathon.com): Great aid-stations along the course and terrific crowd support.

Dallas White Rock (www.runtherock.com): The Texan hospitality doesn't get much better.

Disney (http://bit.ly/3chiv): No denying it, the Disney people do a great job in creating a wonderful marathon experience.

5 MOST BEAUTIFUL U.S. MARATHONS

Big Sur (www.bsim.org): Unparalleled coastal scenery.

Boulder Backroads (www.bouldermarathon.com): If you're lucky, there'll already be snow covering the nearby mountain peaks.

Myrtle Beach (www.mbmarathon.com): The course runs along the beach almost the entire way. Surf's up!

St. George (www.stgeorgemarathon.com): The bonfires at the start are unforgettable.

Kauai (www.thekauaimarathon.com): The Aloha Spirit shines through all the way.

MARATHON SEARCH ENGINES

www.fourhourbody.com/marathon
www.fourhourbody.com/race-finder

TRIATHLON SEARCH ENGINE

http://www.trifind.com

CAN SIX MINUTES OF EFFORT IMPROVE AN 30KM (18.6-MILE) TEST?

On 6 June 2005, Martin Gibala of McMaster University appeared on CNN with news that seemed too good to be true:

"Six minutes of pure, hard exercise three times a week could be just as effective as an hour of daily moderate activity."

Changes that were thought to require hours per week were achieved with just four to seven 30-second bursts of all-out (250% VO2 Max) stationary biking, with four minutes of recovery time between bursts. These bursts were performed 3x a week for just two weeks. Total on-bike time for the two weeks was a mere 15 minutes. Endurance capacity for this "sprint" group almost doubled, from 26 to 51 minutes, and their leg muscles showed a significant 38% increase of our friend citrate synthase (CS), one of the desirable endurance enzymes. The control group, which was active (jogging, cycling or aerobics) showed no changes.

It seemed like a fluke.

It had to be repeated, and it was. This time with an even higher bar for evaluation: a 30km (18.6-mile) cycling test.

The sprint group followed the 30-second burst protocol. The control group performed more traditional moderate-intensity cycling for 60–90 minutes at 60% VO2 Max. Both groups worked out 3x a week and were evaluated before and after with a 30km (18.6-mile) cycling test. The improvements were almost identical, as were the increases in muscle oxidative capacity.

Recognize that working long in the gym is often a form of laziness, an avoidance of hard thinking. Three to four hours per week or less than 15 minutes per week? The choice is yours—work long or work hard—but the results appear to be the same. Trust data instead of the masses.

That's where we have a cliffhanger. This chapter was a last-minute addition, and dead-tree publishing being what it is there wasn't time to update before hitting the shelves.

Find the outcome here: www.fourhourbody.com/ultra.

Will it reflect my self-realization or self-destruction? Only time, or distance, will tell.

TOOLS AND TRICKS

CrossFit Endurance (http://www.crossfitendurance.com/) Brian MacKenzie's homebase and house of pain, replete with workouts and forums. If you don't want to suffer or celebrate alone, there is a full listing of nationwide teams that train and compete together.

"The Marathon Monks of Mount Hiei" (http://der.org/films/marathon-monks.html) Check out this documentary about the incredible Hiei monks from Japan, and their path to enlightenment. The DVD shows their death-defying fasts, their vegetarian training diet, their handmade straw running shoes, and more. You can visit the following link for an 11-minute preview: www.fourhourbody.com/monks.

ENDURANCE WORKOUT TOOLS

Gmap Pedometre (www.gmap-pedometre.com) As nice as fancy gadgets can be for tracking your runs or bike routes, a Google Maps hack gives you the same data with no added equipment. Gmap Pedometre lets you superimpose your route over Google's map data, generating the distance travelled. The site lets you save your favourite routes and share them with friends.

Keson RR112 Roadrunner 1 Measuring Wheel (www.fourhourbody.com/roadrunner) This lightweight wheel is primarily used by real estate agents appraising houses, but you can use it to quickly measure short distances for sprints, whether around the block or on the track.

Seiko DM50L Metronome (www.fourhourbody.com/metronome) Brian suggests training your step per minute tempo with the help of this metronome. I found it easiest to use 90 beats per minute for one leg.

Casio High-Speed Exilim EX-FC100 (www.fourhourbody.com/exilim) Brian uses this camera to videotape all his trainees at 30 frames per second. As he says, "You can learn more in one hour of video analysis than you can in a year of self-correction without video." Casio claims it can record slow-motion videos at up to 1,000 frames per second.

"Pose Method of Running" by Dr. Nicholas Romanov (www.fourhourbody.com/pose-method) This book teaches running as a skill with its own theory, concepts and exercises. Just mind the ankles.

CrossFit Exercises (www.fourhourbody.com/crossfit) Instructional videos of almost every single CrossFit exercise and routine.

GENr8 Vitargo S2 (www.fourhourbody.com/genr8) This is the carbohydrate supplement that Brian uses to rapidly replenish glycogen. He can consume up to 1,100 calories an hour of Vitargo. Don't try that with Gatorade.

***Trail Runner* (www.trailrunnermag.com)** The only magazine dedicated to off-road running, written by trail runners who have races and runs from 5K (3 miles) to 322-plus-kilometres (200-plus miles). *Trail Runner*'s annual race directory features 1,100 trail races worldwide.

***Born to Run* (www.fourhourbody.com/borntorun)** This book, authored by Christopher McDougall, introduces most readers to the incredible Tarahumara Indians, a tribe of superathletes hidden in the mountainous deserts of Mexico, and details a once-in-a-lifetime foot race pitting them against US ultrarunning legends like Scott Jurek. It's a wonderful read that made a non-runner—me—finally get off my arse and on the grass 3 times a week barefoot.

Running Barefoot: Training Tips (www.fourhourbody.com/harvard-barefoot) Harvard's Running Barefoot project is one of the key drivers of the barefoot movement. This article provides basic forefoot striking and training tips for those who are just getting started.

ULTRA-ENDURANCE SHOES FOR TRAIL RUNNING

Inov-8 X-Talon 212 (www.fourhourbody.com/talon212) Of all the shoes Brian recommended, these are my favourite.

Inov-8 F-Lite 230 (www.fourhourbody.com/f-Lite230) Inov-8 is a small manufacturer and will likely run out of stock, but there are other mainstream options: for trail running, get a low-profile shoe like the La Sportiva Crosslite.

ULTRA-ENDURANCE SHOES FOR TARMAC AND HARD SURFACES

Inov-8 F-Lite 220 (www.fourhourbody.com/talon220)

Inov-8 F-Lite 230 (www.fourhourbody.com/f-lite230) These shoes appear above and are multi-purpose.

GETTING STRONGER

EFFORTLESS SUPERHUMAN

Breaking World Records with Barry Ross

Do as little as needed, not as much as possible.

—Henk Kraaijenhof, coach of Merlene Joyce "Queen of the Track" Ottey, who won 20 combined medals at the Olympic Games and World Championships

SAN JOSE, CALIFORNIA KORET ATHLETIC TRAINING FACILITY

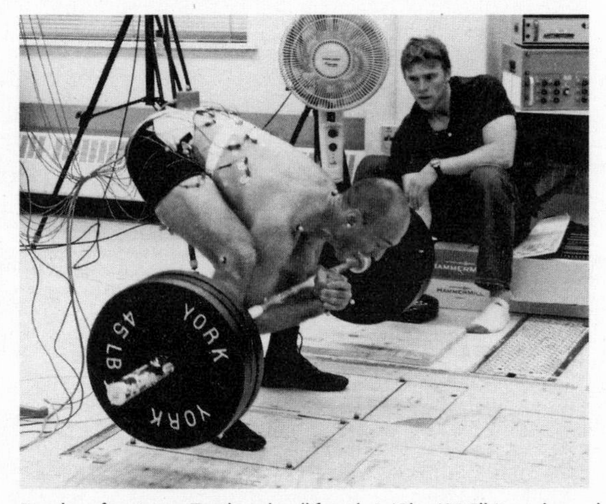

Pavel performing a Zercher deadlift with 143kg (315lb) as electrodes measure muscular activity. (Photo courtesy Prof. Stuart McGill PhD and Spine Biomechanics Lab, University of Waterloo, Canada)

Pavel Tsatsouline was punching me in the bottom. It's not every day that you have a former Soviet Special Forces instructor punch you in the buttocks. But it was the second day of Russian Kettlebell Certification (RKC), and we were practising constant tension, one of several techniques intended to increase strength output. In this case, we spot-checked each other with punches. Pavel, now a U.S. citizen and subject matter expert to the U.S. Secret Service Counter Assault Team, wandered the ranks, contributing jabs where needed.

Two hours earlier, Pavel had asked the attendees for someone stuck at a 1-rep maximum in the one-arm overhead press. He then proceeded to take the volunteer from 24kg (53lb) to 33kg (72lb) in less than five minutes: a 26% strength increase. Translated into more familiar terms, this would represent a jump in one-repetition max from 48kg (106lb) to 65kg (144lb) in the barbell military press.

There were dozens of such demonstrations throughout the weekend, and each was intended to reinforce a point: **strength is a skill**.

Not only is strength a skill, but it can be learnt quickly.

I didn't realize how quickly until several months later, when Pavel introduced me to a curious sprint coach: Barry Ross.

Reducing the Irreducible

In 2003, Allyson Felix was a 17-year-old high school student.

In the space of 12 months, she broke all of Marion Jones's high school records in the 200 metres, went on to run the fastest 200 metres in the world, and then became the first high school athlete to go directly into professional track.

Her coach was Barry Ross.

Ross has spent the last 20 years looking for the most elegant answer to one of the biggest questions in all of sports: how do you make humans as fast as possible?

His solution has been to reduce the irreducible, beyond even what I thought possible. As I write this over fried calamari and cioppino at Fisherman's Wharf in San Francisco (it's Saturday), I still can't believe that I've gained more than 54kg (120lb) on my maximum deadlift in less than two months, with less than 4.5kg (10lb) of weight gain. It's easily the fastest strength increase I've ever experienced.

In Barry's world, it's nothing special.

Here is a quick look at three of his athletes that you might find surprising:

His best female multi-event athlete has deadlifted 184kg (405lb) at a bodyweight of 9.4st (59.8kg). (See her photo in this chapter.)
His best female distance runner has deadlifted 172kg (380lb) at a bodyweight of 10st (63kg).
His youngest male lifter, 11 years old, has lifted 102kg (225lb) at a bodyweight of 7.9st (50kg).

Nearly all of his athletes, including women, can lift more than twice their bodyweight without wrist straps, and all have gained less than 10% of additional bodyweight to get there.

The kicker: these results were achieved with less than 15 minutes of actual lifting time (time under tension) per week.

From Pac 10 titles in shot put, to gold medals in the 4x100-metre relay, Barry's unusual methods are redefining what is possible. In this chapter, I'll explain how he does it in sprinting, and how you can do the same in the gym or in your sport.

The Effortless Superhuman Protocol

The training protocol for Allyson Felix in 2003 consisted of the following, three times per week:

1. **Dynamic stretching before each session ("over-unders", detailed later).**
2. **One of the following, five minutes rest between sets:**
    a. Bench press:[1] 2–3 sets of 2–3 reps or
    b. Push-ups: 10–12 reps[2]
3. **Conventional deadlift to knees, 2–3 sets of 2–3 reps at 85–95% of 1-repetition max (1RM).** Bar does NOT go higher than the knee and is dropped from that height rather than returned to

1. To avoid shoulder problems, do not lower the bar to the chest, but to approximately 10–12.7cm (4–5in) (the width of your fist) above the chest. Use a power rack if needed, and set the pins at this point. Doing competition-standard lifts is of no interest, as his athletes are training for sports performance, not powerlifting competition.

2. Once athletes can complete 12 standard push-ups, Barry has them elevate their legs to increase resistance. The legs aren't elevated above 50 degrees (relative to the floor) because it would involve the shoulders more than the pectorals. For pure runners, the exercise is for general pectoral work, rather than for the purpose of the sport. The pectorals are just about the only muscle group not stimulated by the deadlift, which follows.

the ground by the athlete. Dropping, and therefore avoiding the eccentric lowering portion, is critical for reducing hamstring injuries when also doing sprint training. Time under tension should be less than 10 seconds per set. For deadlift sets:

- Plyometrics are performed immediately after the end of each set (box jumps[3] of various heights × 4–6 reps)
- Take five minutes rest in between sets, with the five-minute countdown starting after plyometrics

4. Core exercise, 3–5 sets of 3–5 reps (isometric holds)

5. Static stretching

GA

The workout Allyson used was predicated on research that suggested greater ground force support (applying force to the ground at landing), rather than shorter leg swing times,[4] enabled runners to reach faster top speeds. The amount of support force needed to increase speed by one metre per second is equal to one-tenth the bodyweight. Skeletal muscle is a very effective generator of force. One kilogram can produce enough force to support 44 kilograms of mass.

Previously, coaches believed that a reduction in fuel supply to the muscle was the cause of speed drops. Research has since shown that the real cause of speed loss is the inability of the fibres to supply sufficient tension.

If you need more tension, you need more strength.

An elite athlete will impact the ground with approximately two times their mass while receiving an equal amount of push back from the ground. Mass-specific support force—the force muscles generate in response to impact—can exceed five times the bodyweight of the elite athlete and is delivered to the ground in approximately 0.05 seconds. Keep in mind that this is on one leg at a time. All other things equal, the stronger runner will win.

3. The idea is to keep ground contact as short as possible on each landing, six landings maximum. In Barry's training sessions, these jumps are sometimes onto a box, sometimes over a box, and standing triple jump or broad jump can also be substituted. Personally, to keep it simple, I used a standard flat bench and tapped both feet on the top (rather than landing) before returning to the ground, repeating six times.
4. Also referred to as "turnover".

HOW TO PERFORM THE CONVENTIONAL DEADLIFT

The following sequence of photographs, courtesy of Mike Lambert, editor of *Powerlifting USA* magazine, shows the incredible Lamar Gant. Lamar, a member of the International Powerlifting Federation Hall of Fame, was the first person to deadlift *five times* his bodyweight in competition: 300kg (661lb) at a bodyweight of 9.4st (60kg).

Here's how he does it:

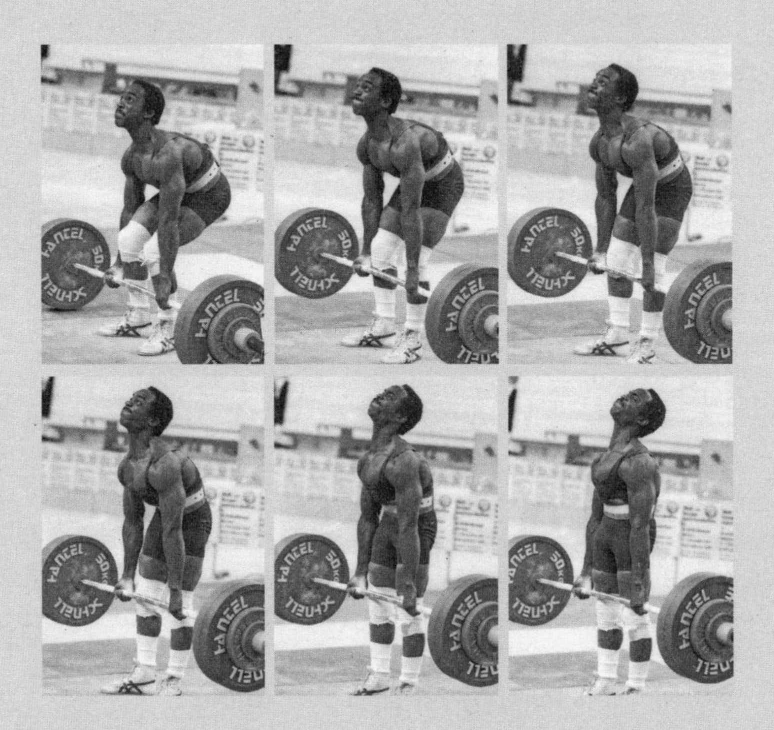

Barry has his athletes drop the weight at the top of the kneecaps (fourth photo in the series) to avoid hamstring injuries, which is also illustrated in the below pictures:

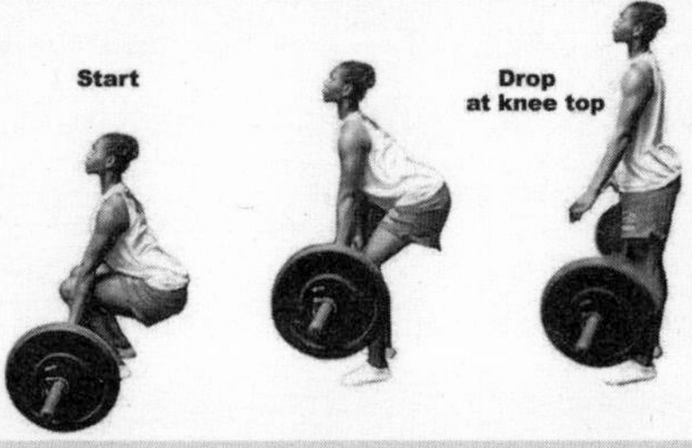

His athletes are taught to avoid straightening the legs prematurely and to also maintain a perfectly straight back,[5] as if pinching a wallet between their shoulder blades.

This strength training protocol allows running immediately after strength training,[6] eliminating the need for a time-consuming split training. No lifts are done to failure.

Besides "over-unders" performed prior to the first exercise, there are no warm-ups in the workout.[7] Over-unders are executed as follows:

Using a power rack or hurdles, set one pin/hurdle to approximately 76–81cm (30–32in) and the other at waist height. Squat low enough to step sideways under the lower pin/hurdle, then immediately step over the higher one.[8] That is one repetition. Do not use your hands or put them on your legs. Repeat six to seven times. Then move directly into work sets. Barry has his athletes lift the heaviest load of an exercise first, followed by sets with lighter loads, if needed.

To estimate your 1-rep max (1RM) in a given exercise, just multiply your 5-rep max weight x 1.2.

The Basic Rule: Less Than 10 Seconds

As a general guideline, we don't want time under tension for exercise sets to exceed 10 seconds, as we want to minimize lactic acid production.

Though lactic acid (often felt as muscle "burn") can be helpful in some circumstances, it can also delay recovery. In cases where athletes need to hit benchmarks in short periods of time, Barry wants to retain their ability to do the same workout for five straight days.

This approach is not limited to sprinting.[9]

5. Lamar appears to be slightly rounding his back in his photos, but it's his thoracic (upper back) spine and not his lumbar (lower back) that's rounded. This upper rounding is common in the conventional deadlift when handling world-class weights. Mere mortals should maintain a flat back until deadlifting well more than two times bodyweight.

6. Note that the opposite is not true. Lifting before running is fine, but running before lifting is asking for injuries.

7. This is one place where I diverged from instructions and performed warm-up sets of 1–2 reps leading up to my heaviest work weight. If I have an unidentified injury, I'd prefer it to blow out with 45kg (100lb) instead of 181kg (400lb). This is a topic that Barry and I agree to disagree on.

8. This format wasn't practical at my closest gym, which is crowded and only has one rack. I opted instead to simply step sideways over a bench with knees as high as possible, which I followed with an immediate parallel squat and sidestep that increased in width with each repetition. The lateral "unders" are particularly important for increasing hip mobility before heavy "sumo" style deadlifts, which both Barry and Pavel recommend when possible.

9. It's not limited to 15–30-year-olds either. Take a look at Professor Arthur DeVany and his version of alactic training. Art, a professor emeritus of the University of California Irvine in economics and mathematical behavioral sciences, is 72 years young, 185.42cm (6ft 1in), and 14.6st (93kg) at 8% body fat.

One non-runner example is Skyler McKnight, who needed to bench 102kg (225lb) 20 times to be a starter for the San Jose State football team. There was just one problem: he could only complete three reps and had three weeks until the test. He had only 15 workout days to make the mark. Five days a week, he did five sets of two repetitions with five minutes' rest between sets. He increased the weight but did not increase the repetition range.

On test day, he completed 18 reps and, yes, the coach was shocked enough to give him a starting position.

Consider another set of results from Greg Almon, strength consultant to the Chinese national speed skating team:

> Dear Barry,
>
> I would just like to give you an update as to how my skaters have performed this year from switching to a Deadlift based protocol;
>
> The Chinese women's team has won more than 10 gold medals in the sprint categories (500, 1000m), as well as 10 more silver and bronze combined. We now have 5 skaters that skate 44 seconds or better in the 500m and broke the world record in the last competition.
>
> It was tough to convince the coach to switch, but after several days of conversation, she agreed to try it. Our women skaters have increased their deadlift by an average of 52kg (115lb) over the last 3.5 months and the results speak for themselves. . . .
>
> Thanks again,
>
> Greg

The New and Improved Trinity

What has Barry refined and improved since Allyson's record-breaking performances in 2003?

Based on the latest research, he has narrowed his sprint-specific programme to three simple and sequential training goals:

1. Competition conditioning
2. Maximal strength
3. Maximal speed

For each, Barry relies on the core philosophy of coach Henk Kraaijenhof: "Do as little as needed, not as much as possible." All three objectives require (that is, demand) less workload than commonly thought necessary.

COMPETITION CONDITIONING

Training for the first goal, conditioning, draws heavily from a study titled "Energetics of High-Speed Running: Integrating Classical Theory and Contemporary Observations", first published in 2004.

This study provides the ASR speed algorithm, a mathematical formula patented by Rice University that claims to predict running times for any individual (not just a trained athlete but *any* individual) for distances ranging from a few metres up to a mile. Incredibly, it's proven more than 97% accurate for every runner Barry has tested. The algorithm also shows the level of a runner's condition.

The minimum baseline conditioning for athletes engaged in runs of less than a mile is approximately 4.2 metres per second. This equates to a 100-metre run time of no more than 23.8 seconds.

How do you get athletes to this baseline? Believe it or not, by walking. The prescription is simple: **walk as fast as possible for 15 minutes, three sessions per week.** The walk is seven and a half minutes out and the same time back. This doesn't sound difficult, and it isn't . . . at first. The challenge is that the athlete must walk further out at each session and still return in the same seven and a half minutes.

"Walk as fast as possible" means that the athlete should strongly and persistently want to jog. He or she is experiencing extreme inefficiency in locomotion, and that's the point.

If you don't have enough flat ground (a track is ideal) to walk seven and a half minutes straight out and back, just use a set distance (five blocks, for example) and match the number of lengths in the second seven and a half minutes.

After four weeks of this timed walking (three sessions of 15 minutes per week) the athlete has accomplished the first goal: reaching baseline conditioning for competition.

It seems impossible, but reserve judgement until you see some of their results, described later in this chapter.

MAXIMAL STRENGTH

Next, Barry gets his athletes strong. Really, really strong.

His current protocol is similar to what Allyson used in 2003, but the exercises have been further refined and limited. Notice that "2–3 sets of 2–3" has been replaced with "1 set of 2–3 @ 95% 1RM, followed by 1 set of 5 @ 85% 1RM" for both the bench press and deadlift.

Reminder: take five-minute rest periods between sets, and the countdown starts *after* completion of plyometrics.

The following general workout template would be performed three times per week for most athletes (e.g., Monday, Wednesday and Friday):

1. **Dynamic stretch** before each session: over-and-unders × 6–7 reps, no more than 5 minutes. No static stretching.
2. *One* of the following at each session (time under tension should be less than *15* seconds per set):
   Bench press: 1 set of 2–3 @ 95% 1RM, followed by 1 set of 5 @ 85% 1RM *or*
   Push-ups: 10–12 reps (same as in earlier programme)

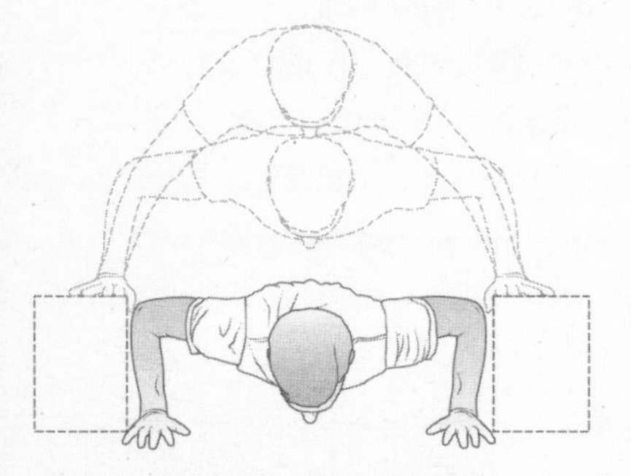
BENCH-PRESS PLYOMETRICS

If you choose bench press and if equipment permits, perform plyometrics (four to five reps) immediately after bench-press sets.

Place two 15–30cm (6–12in) high boxes just outside of shoulder width. From the fully lowered position between the boxes (chest on the floor), jump up onto the boxes by fully extending your arms as quickly as possible, extend your arms fully again on top of the boxes, then drop back down inside the boxes into the fully down position. Just as with box jumps, it is critical to keep ground contact as short as possible.

If the plyometrics hurt your shoulders (as they did mine) or are too inconvenient, the programme still works well without them.

3. **Deadlift,**[10] 1 set of 2–3 @ 95% 1RM, followed by 1 set of 5 @ 85% 1RM. Same rules as before: lift to the knees and then drop. If you're not practising high-speed running, lowering is fine. Plyo-

10. Felix used the conventional stance with her legs inside her arms, but Barry suggests sumo-style for those who can perform it.

metrics are performed within one minute after each set of deadlifts: box jumps of varying heights, jumping rope, or even a few short, fast 10-metre runs if space is available. First choice is two to four 10–15-metre sprints. This provides at least two times bodyweight borne by each leg upon impact. Second choice is five to seven 30–46-cm (12–18-in) box jumps.

4. **Core exercise:** the Torture Twist, 3–5 sets of 3–5 reps (30 seconds between sets).

For the core, Barry now only uses one exercise: the Torture Twist. Every single trainee who uses it hates it. To perform the Torture Twist, set yourself perpendicular on a bench so that you look like a cross from above. Hold your feet under a pole in a power rack or, worst case, under another bench.[11]

Remain parallel to the ground for each set and come up to sitting position for 30 seconds of rest between sets. Start with three sets × three reps of three seconds on each side. Your first session would look like the following:

SET 1

Turn fully to the right side and hold for three seconds.
Turn to the left side and hold for three seconds.
Repeat two more times for a total of 3x three-second holds *per side.*
Sit up and rest 30 seconds.
Repeat for two more sets.

The Torture Twist

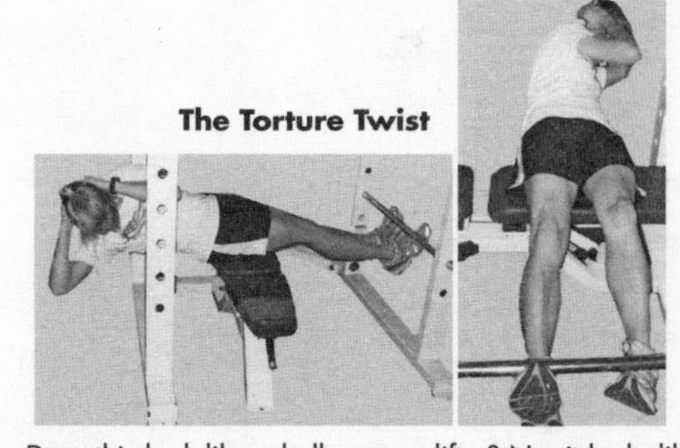

Does this look like a bulky powerlifter? No, it looks like a normal high school girl. Normal, except that she's 9.4st (132lb) and can deadlift 184kg (405lb)! Holy emasculation, Batman!

Progression: In future workouts, gradually increase up to five sets of three-second holds, then increase time, one second at a time, up to a maximum of 15-second holds for five sets (each set = 3 holds per side).

This concludes the workout.

Total workout time, including rest: less than 60 minutes.
Total time under tension per workout: less than 5 minutes.
Feeling at workout conclusion: exhilarated instead of exhausted.

11. This was also inconvenient to set up at my gym, so I either used a decline bench press bench, where I could hook in my feet with bent legs; or I simply sat on a BOSU ball at home with my feet hooked under the sofa (be sure to weigh down the sofa; I used a 24kg/60lb kettlebell).

THE SUMO DEADLIFT

Barry suggests the sumo deadlift instead of the conventional deadlift whenever possible. The pull distance is shorter and the lower-back position is safer.

The following sequence of photographs, also courtesy of Mike Lambert from *Powerlifting USA*, show the incredible Mike Bridges, who was considered by many to be the best weight-for-weight powerlifter in the world during his prime. He dominated three different weight classes, and even now, in his fifties, he regularly deadlifts more than 272kg (600lb).

Keep in mind that Barry's athletes drop the weight when the bar reaches the top of the kneecaps (here the fourth photo). Notice that, like Lamar, Mike is looking up at almost exactly 45 degrees the entire time, until completion.

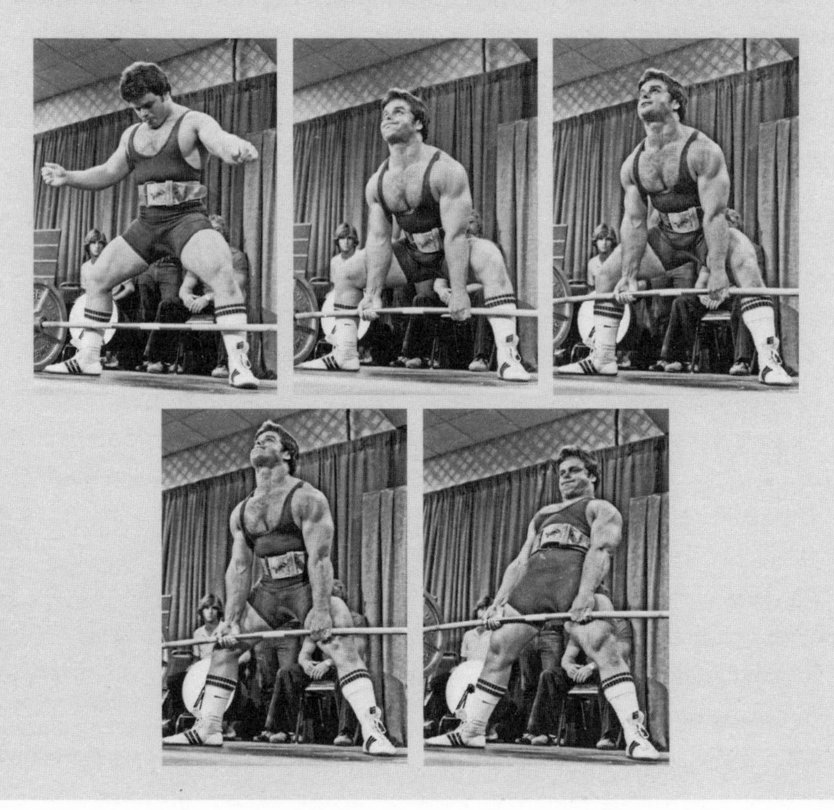

MAXIMAL SPEED

Finally, once Barry's athletes are strong, he makes them faster.

If you have no interest in running, you can skip this section and just read the sidebars. But, if nothing else, the competition anecdote at the end is fun to read. Now back to our story . . .

Each athlete runs two time trials to start. The short trial (T1) is a "fly-in" 20-metre run and the long trial (T2) is a run of 300 metres. For T1, the athlete runs a 40-metre dash, but only the second 20 metres are timed. For T2, the athlete has a five-metre run up to the line, and then a timed 300 metres. In both cases, the runners should already be close to top speed when they cross the *start* line.

Once he has these two times, Barry plugs the numbers into the ASR algorithm, which gives him a precise distance and time to run for each runner. This distance/time will form the basis for their speed workout. **For events of 400 metres or less, Barry's athletes do no training runs longer than 70 metres.**

The determined "X distance performed under time Y" can be thought of as one "repetition", and reps are performed until the runner cannot complete the distance in the time allotted, or cannot complete 10 repetitions under a predetermined total time (a timed "set" of 10 repetitions). Exceeding time in either case marks the end of the workout.

Here is a real-world example from a runner named Scott:

20-metre fly-in	1.88 seconds
300-metre fly-in	36.00 seconds

The workout distances are then randomized between 15 metres and 55 metres, such as 55 metres < 5.57 seconds. This means that Scott's workout is a series of 10 runs of 55 metres that must not exceed 5.57 seconds each. Four-minute rests are taken in between runs.

If Scott does not run under 5.57 in his first attempt, he is given one more opportunity to make it on a second run. If he exceeds his time on this second run, or any "rep" before his 10th, his workout is finished for that day.

This is a sharp contrast to conventional methods.

Sprint coaches usually tell their runners to run "repeats" at a particular distance and at a particular speed. A typical workout prescription might be "10 × 100-metre runs at 80% of top speed". Unfortunately, no one knows when he or she is running at 80%, or any other per cent for that matter.

Coaches also prescribe so-called "over-distance" runs to improve "speed endurance". This is another added stress that Barry does not incorporate.

But how does his approach measure up in competition?

Keep in mind that his athletes' average repeat running distance is under 40 metres, and that he's completely eliminated training runs of over 70 metres for events of 400 metres or less. This is sacrilege in many corners of the track and field world. Despite this minimalism—or more accurately, because of it—the results speak for themselves.

One of his high school female athletes cut two seconds off her 400 metre, one and a half seconds off her 300 intermediate hurdles (IM), and dropped her 100 metre from 13.35 to 12.75 seconds. Though it's hard for non-sprinters to appreciate, dropping from 13.35 to 12.75 is a huge improvement for such a short anaerobic event, where milliseconds matter.

Her average repeat distance (her "rep" distance) was a mere 33 metres, and she is by no means a novice. She had been running for six years.

Her pre-track season conditioning was just 15 minutes of fast walking three days per week. Her goal was to increase the distance covered (but never the time) each session. She, her dad and her team coach doubted she'd ever be able to run a competitive 400-metre or 300-metre hurdle. The low volume almost drove her to panic.

The outcome: the first meet of the year, she beat two runners in the 300 hurdles she had not bested in the previous two track seasons.

After watching her against the competition, her track coach told her dad, "Never again will I make my sprinters practise over 70 metres!"

She also weighs 8.5st (54kg) and deadlifts 154kg (340lb).

The paradigm is shifting and the writing is on the wall: working smarter beats working longer, whether in the weight room or on the track.

THE RULE OF 10 REPS

by Pavel Tsatsouline

Athletes often miss the point of strength training.

Some confuse it with conditioning. Others confuse themselves with powerlifters. The barbell is not there to make you a better man (or woman) by testing your mettle. That is what the court, the field or the mat is for. The barbell is there to give you a strength advantage over an opponent of equal skill.

Strength training cannot interfere with the practice of your sport. This is the point—the most important point—that many strength and conditioning coaches somehow miss.

The crucial principle is to **lift heavy but not hard**. This is where the "rule of 10 reps" can be applied:

1. Use two to three "global" compound exercises (e.g., the deadlift and the bench press).
2. Lift three times a week (e.g., Monday, Wednesday and Friday).[12] Do your conditioning and supplementary work on separate days, practise your sport skills six days a week, and take one day off completely.
3. Focus on sets of two or three reps. Two reps is the most preferred rep choice of the Russian National Weight Lifting Team.
4. In all cases, complete approximately 10 reps per lift per workout (e.g., three sets of three, five sets of two, etc.).
5. Never train to failure, and always leave at least one to two reps "in the bank".
6. Rest for five minutes between sets.
7. Finish your workout feeling stronger than when you started.

The goal is to build as much strength as possible while staying as fresh as possible for your sport.

When I worked with Maria Sharapova, I had her do a few singles, doubles and triples of pull-ups, pistols,[13] hard push-ups, Janda sit-ups and nothing else. The future Wimbledon star had plenty of conditioning from her daily tennis practice, and the last thing she needed was fatigue and injuries from her strength regimen.

But what about less frequent training?

Less frequent training than Monday, Wednesday and Friday (i.e., once a week) is not ideal for an athlete, even if it builds strength and consumes less time. U.S. powerlifting records in the 1980s and 1990s leave no doubt that you can achieve

12. If unable to recover, the deadlift can be reduced to Monday and Friday.
13. One-legged squats with the unused leg extended straight in front of you.

a world-class squat by trashing yourself once a week. But you will not walk well afterward. Every time you lift, you will get as sore as a newbie. This isn't a big deal for a powerlifter, but it's very bad news for a boxer or someone who needs to train in the subsequent 48 hours.

Can more volume build strength?

Of course. The iconic Smolov squat cycle, a 13-week nightmare, calls for a gruesome 136 reps per week during the first month! The cycle delivers beyond anyone's wildest dreams. One man I knew added 47.6kg (105lb) to his squat in 13 weeks of Smolov and peaked in the mid-600s, drug-free. His gains are not atypical. But it takes its toll. You will be so sore and exhausted that the only "sport" you could practise at the same time is chess. The Smolov is a specialized programme for an athlete who does not have any skills to practise outside of the gym. An exception would be an athlete who must gain a lot of muscle mass in the off-season, such as a football lineman.

Canadian track coach Charlie Francis's approach to strength training the infamous sprinter Ben Johnson is very illuminating. The sprinter stayed with low reps and low volume, e.g., to 600×2/6[14] (sets/reps) in the below parallel box squat and 385×3/2 in the bench press. The 12.4st (78kg) Johnson eventually benched over 181kg (400lb), and Francis was convinced he was good for 200kg (440lb). But—pay attention!—to avoid injury, the sharp coach never maxed his athlete. This obviously did not prevent Johnson from breaking his personal records. Without maxing.

Francis's in-season strength training was in line with the Russian school. Nikolay Ozolin, one of the founding fathers of Soviet sport science, recommends cutting back in-season lifting volume to 2/3 of off-season lifting volume without reducing weight. Francis downshifted Johnson from two sets of six with 600 in the squat to two sets of doubles or triples, a 1/2 to 2/3 reduction of the already low volume. This reduction allowed Johnson to get extra fresh for the season without losing his strength. Francis quipped that "Ben was never far from strength and speed." Indeed, he was not pushing as hard, but he was still handling 272kg (600lb).

Francis did the opposite of most coaches: "Ninety percent of my time is spent holding athletes back to prevent overtraining, and only 10 per cent is spent motivating them to do more work."

2–3 is a great rep range to emphasize throughout an athlete's programme. 4–5 is where neural training and muscle-building meet, which means you could end up with some hypertrophy. This is out of the question in weight-class-based sports like boxing.

Steve Baccari, strength coach extraordinaire to top fighters like the UFC's Joe Lauzon, agrees with the heavy but not hard approach:

14. Note from Tim: Coincidentally, I've made my greatest strength gains outside of the deadlift using two work sets of six, two exercises per workout.

"In my opinion, 'easy' strength training is the only productive way a competitive fighter can strength train. . . . But most people think if you don't break a sweat, it must not work. This used to bother me a lot, but not any more, because I think it is one reason why my fighters win so much."

Concludes Baccari:

"Strength training is like putting the money in the bank to take it out on the fight day."

Save the fatigue for your sport.

THE SHARAPOVA SIT-UP: JANDA

If you're looking for an abdominal exercise well-suited to power development without bulk, look no further than the Janda sit-up.

Pavel has been able to register contractions in excess of 175% MVC (maximal voluntary isometric contraction) for the rectus abdominis at Dr. Stuart McGill's laboratory performing the Janda sit-up with a device called, appropriately enough, the Ab Pavelizer. Some scientists theorize that the downward contraction of the hamstrings forces the hip flexors to relax, which largely prevents them from helping with the movement. Ergo, more than 100% MVC of the remaining workhorse: the rectus abdominis.

To perform the Janda sit-up without any equipment, do the following:

1. • Loop a towel around your calves and have a training partner pull on it lightly at a 45-degree upward angle, trying to lift your feet.

Or, less ideal but practical for solo use:

• Wrap a resistance band around the knob of an open door and wrap the band around your calves, ensuring a downward 45-degree angle.

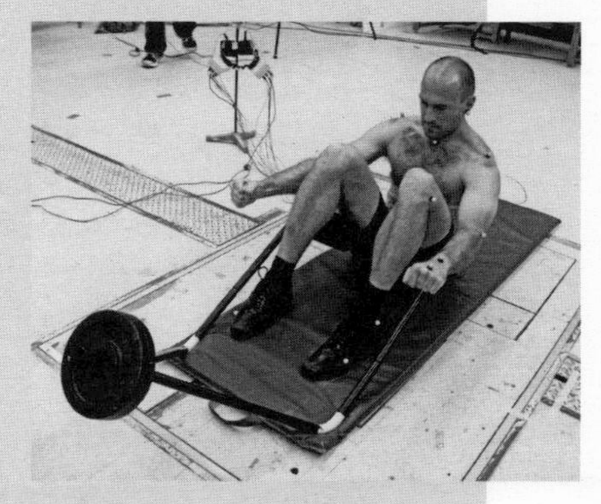

Then:

2. • Bring your tailbone and your navel together, and slowly sit up without allowing your feet to lift up or to slide towards you.

It's much harder than it looks: even if you can do 50 normal sit-ups, don't be surprised if you can't complete a single proper Janda sit-up in the beginning.

In this case, start with lowering from the top position (negatives) only.

The "rule of 10 reps" can be applied here. For instance, you might start with five sets of two (5 × 2) negatives and then progress through the following rep schemes as you get stronger: 2323 ("2323" means four sets total: 2 reps, 3 reps, 2 reps and 3 reps), then 343, then 235, and then 2 × 5. Once you can do these negatives under control, you can start doing full reps using the same progression or another "rule of 10" combination.

Remember to maintain a continual speed for negatives: don't stay in one spot forever and then free fall to the floor. Hold on to something with your hands if necessary, such as a table leg or a resistance band around a door knob.

TIMING WORKOUTS: USING CHRONOBIOLOGY FOR FASTER GAINS

"Chronobiology" is the science of investigating time-dependent changes in physiology.

Muscle strength and short-term power output peak in the early evening (4:00–6:00 P.G.), which coincides with daily maximum body temperature.[15] Pain tolerance, at least for arthritis and fibromyalgia, is also highest between 4:00 and 5:00 p.m.

But 4:00–6:00 P.G. workouts never produced the best results for me. I believe this is because the ideal window depends on circadian rhythm and therefore wake time. These variables are almost never accounted for in studies.

If we assume an average wake time of 8:00 A.G. for most subjects who have work or classes beginning at 9:00 A.G., and if peak power output and pain tolerance is between 4:00 and 6:00 P.G. in their studies, this corresponds to 8–10 hours after waking.

I am a night owl, and my average wake time is 11:00 A.G. Using this average,[16] 8–10 hours after waking would put my ideal window between 7:00 and 9:00 P.G.

That's how I arrived at an optimal workout time of 7:00 to 9:00 P.G., which has allowed me to add two to three repetitions to most exercises when using less than 85% of a one-repetition maximum (usually a set of six reps or more).

This doesn't mean you have to train at night, but you should keep training times consistent so you can accurately gauge progress.

15. Heart-rate-based tests of work capacity appear to peak in the morning because the heart rate responses to exercise are minimal at this time of day.
16. It's important to use an average, not just the wake time on a scheduled workout day.

TOOLS AND TRICKS

Over-unders Dynamic Warm-Up (www.fourhourbody.com/over-under) This is a demo of the hip mobility movements using a single bar. Focus on the side hurdle (0:30) and under-the-hurdle side squat (1:30), which, when alternated, constitute the over-unders Barry recommends as a dynamic warm-up.

***Underground Secrets to Faster Running* by Barry Ross (www.fourhourbody.com/underground)** Allyson Felix used this strength training system right before she ran the fastest 200 metres in the world back in 2003.

"High-Speed Running Performance: A New Approach to Assessment and Prediction" by Matthew W. Bundle, Reed W. Hoyt, and Peter G. Weyand (www.fourhourbody.com/hsrp) This is the original study from Rice University that developed the ASR speed algorithm. In Barry Ross's words, "What they found was the Holy Grail to faster running speed."

ASRspeed (www.fourhourbody.com/asr) The actual sprinting programme that Barry Ross discussed in this chapter. Any athlete who plays a sport requiring sudden bursts of forward speed (sprints, basketball, baseball, football, soccer, etc.) can benefit tremendously by using this programme. It will largely eliminate the need for hill runs, sled towing, parachutes and all the other tricks and toys people use to get faster.

"How to Add 100 Pounds to Your Squat in 13 Weeks with the Smolov Cycle" (www.fourhourbody.com/smolov) The Smolov Cycle is a Russian strength training routine designed by Master of Sports S. Y. Smolov. This cycle, though complex and very brutal, can easily add 27–45kg (60–100lb) to your squat. You can also download an Excel spreadsheet that's designed to help you keep track of your progress during the Smolov programme (www.fourhourbody.com/smolov-excel).

Fat Gripz (www.fourhourbody.com/fatgripz) Thick-bar training increases grip strength fast. The problem is that thick bars cost $200 (£125) or more. The solution is Fat Gripz, each the size of a Red Bull can (easy for travel), which slide onto normal bars in ten seconds. Take a week after every four weeks of heavy training to use Fat Gripz with lighter weights (I do stiff-legged deadlifts). Trust me, it will be harder than you think.

EATING THE ELEPHANT

How to Add 45kg (100lb) to Your Bench Press

Just remember: somewhere in China, a little girl is warming up with your max.

—Jim Conroy, Olympic weightlifting coach

"If you get to 315, you can change the music on the iPod."

I laughed again, not getting the joke. But it wasn't a joke. DeFranco pointed a finger at the wall, where a large piece of paper was taped:

Bench 315?
Squat 405?
Play on ESPN?
If not, don't touch the iPod!

There was some distance to go before I benched 315lb.[17] I would have to wait to put Disco Duck on the loudspeakers.

DeFranco's boys, on the other hand, had

17. I had, however, just set a personal record. It wasn't technical improvement, nor was it from training—it was from doing max vertical jumps beforehand. This hyperclocking of the nervous system was precisely why DeFranco had me jump first. See "Hacking the NFL Combine".

no problem with 315. His cadre of beasts included freaks of nature like Rich Demers, who could bench-press 96kg (215lb) for 39 reps. That impressed me.

It impressed me, but it didn't stun me.

Stunning was Joe Ceklovsky, who has bench-pressed 272kg (600lb) in competition at 148lb bodyweight.

Stunning was Scot Mendelson, who has bench-pressed 468kg (1,031lb) in competition at 275lb bodyweight.

To put 468kg (1,031lb) in perspective, imagine loading a standard gym barbell with 20.4kg (45lb) plates until no more can fit. That is a measly 401kg (885lb). Scot has to use 45kg (100lb) plates, and the tempered-steel bar literally bends around his hands. He wears a mouth guard so he doesn't shatter his teeth with jaw tension, and his vision gets pulled out horizontally when the bar pauses at his chest.

These are unusual people. But that's a compliment. You can learn a lot from the extremes.

Background on the Bench: My Achilles' Heel

The bench press has always been my weakest exercise. Few sports require much of the chest, and my principal sport of wrestling practically made a point of neglecting it.

Even on a steady diet of doubles (sets of two) on Barry's programme, my maximum bench wouldn't budge. In this, I was an exception.

So I called one of the sages of powerlifting to settle the issue.

Marty Gallagher stays out of the limelight, but has long been in the record books. He has coached some of the most legendary powerlifters of all time, including Ed Coan, Kirk Karwoski, Doug Furness, Mike Hall and Dan Austin. Coan alone set more than 70 world records. Kirk "Captain Kirk" Karwoski increased the International Powerlifting Federation (IPF) world record for the squat an astonishing 45kg (100lb) during his reign, from 410 to 455kg (903 to 1,003lb), and this world record still stands *16 years* later.

Marty is also a three-time master powerlifting world champion and six-time master national powerlifting champion, not to mention that he coached the U.S. powerlifting squad to the IPF world team title in 1991.

Suffice to say, he understands the subtleties of the iron game.

In his words, what follows was his weight-by-weight, workout-by-workout presciption for me, or anyone who wants to add 45kg (100lb) to their current max in six months.

Enter Marty Gallagher

Is it possible for a regular fellow with a 91kg (200lb) bench press to add 45kg (100lb) to his bench press in six months? The answer is that, while improbable, it is not impossible. It requires eating the elephant one bite at a time.

There are three requirements:

Requirement #1: A periodized tactical game plan. Periodization is another word for progressive resistance pre-planning. Elite powerlifters, Olympic weightlifters and professional athletes use periodization to stair-step their way upwards to ever greater strength levels over a specified time period, usually 12–16 weeks. By expropriating a periodization strategy and applying it to the bench press, the impossible becomes plausible.

Towards the end of his career, Kirk Karwoski never missed a rep in any lift over an entire 12-week cycle. Can you imagine? A man sits down with a pad and pencil 12 weeks prior to a National or World Championship, writes out the projected weights, reps and sets for every single session for every workout for the next three months, then never misses a single predetermined rep. Ed Coan and Doug Furness could do the same.

Precision is critical.

Requirement #2: No missed workouts.

Requirement #3: Adding a *significant* amount of muscular bodyweight.

Let us assume our hypothetical athlete is a fairly serious fitness buff who has several years of progressive resistance under his belt and can already bench-press 91kg (200lb) using proper technique. Regardless if he is 185cm (6ft 1in) and weighs 14.3st (91kg) with a 14% body fat percentile or he's 168cm (5ft 6in) and weighs 14.3st (91kg) with a 30% body fat percentile, in order to increase his bench press from 91kg (200lb) to 136kg (300lb) it is *critical* to increase lean muscle mass. Our man will need more muscular firepower.

Any "fitness expert" who tells the uninformed that they can add 50% to their bench press in short order with no weight gain by using (or more likely purchasing) some utopian bench-press routine is either delusional or a shyster. There is no magical, mythical exercise routine that will miraculously add 50% to the bench press without a concurrent gain in muscle mass. It takes a 10% increase in lean muscle mass to net a 50% increase in strength, and that's being optimistic. Period.

Our hypothetical athlete starts off weighing 14.3st (91kg) and will need to push his lean muscle mass up 15–20lb (6.8–9kg) over a 26-week period.

Bench press will be trained once per week, and in each session, you will train three grips: competitive grip, the most powerful grip; wide grip, which builds starting power; and narrow grip, which builds finishing power.

WEEK	POWER GRIP (71cm/28in)	WIDE GRIP (81cm/32in)	NARROW GRIP (56cm/22in)	BODY WEIGHT
1	140 (70%)×8, 1 set	120 (60%)×10, 2 sets	110 (55%)×10, 2 sets	14.3st (91kg)
2	150 (75%)×8, 1 set	130 (65%)×10, 2 sets	120 (60%)×10, 2 sets	14.4st (91.2kg)
3	160 (80%)×8, 1 set	140 (70%)×10, 2 sets	130 (65%)×10, 2 sets	14.43st (91.6kg)
4	170 (85%)×8, 1 set	150 (75%)×10, 2 sets	140 (70%)×10, 2 sets	14.5st (92kg)
5	185 (93%)×5, 1 set	165 (83%)×8, 2 sets	145 (73%)×8, 2 sets	14.6st (92.5kg)
6	195 (98%)×5, 1 set	175 (88%)×8, 2 sets	155 (78%)×8, 2 sets	14.64st (93kg)
7	205 (103%)×5, 1 set	185 (93%)×8, 2 sets	165 (83%)×8, 2 sets	14.7st (93.4kg)
8	215 (108%)×5, 1 set	195 (98%)×8, 2 sets	175 (88%)×8, 2 sets	14.8st (93.9kg)
9	225 (113%)×3, 1 set	205 (103%)×5, 2 sets	185 (93%)×5, 2 sets	14.9st (94.3kg)
10	235 (118%)×3, 1 set	215 (108%)×5, 2 sets	195 (98%)×5, 2 sets	14.92st (94.8kg)
11	245 (123%)×2, 1 set	225 (113%)×5, 2 sets	205 (103%)×5, 2 sets	15st (95.3kg)
12	260 (130%)×1	—	—	15st (95.7kg)

PHASE I: 12-WEEK BENCH-PRESS CYCLE[18]

It's possible to estimate the grip widths without bringing a tape measure to the gym. Here are several guidelines, keeping in mind that the narrow smooth bands on a standard Olympic barbell are 81cm (32in) apart:

If you are 178–183cm (5ft 10in–6ft), the power grip will have the edge of your pinkies just inside the rings.

For someone 168–175cm (5ft 6in–5ft 9in), the power grip will have your hands one hand-width in from the rings.

If in doubt, the power grip is simply the placement that allows you to lift the most weight. Experiment.

For all heights, from the power grip, the wide grip would be one hand-width out in both directions, and the narrow grip would be one hand-width in for both hands.

In this phase I, the athlete jumps his lean muscle mass upward bys 11%, resulting in a 30% increase in the bench press. Calories are methodically increased each week, keeping the individual anabolic. How many calories? As many as necessary to provoke the requisite weekly weight gain. How much weight gain? If you weigh less than 14.2st (91kg), aim for 1lb (450g) per week of gain. If you weigh 14.2+st (91+kg), 2lb (900g) per week. There is no hard number of calories—you just need to move the scale up.

Protein must be kept high: 200+g (7+oz) per day each and every day.

Now What? Alike Yet Different

Experience has shown time and time again that after an athlete has completed a successful 12-week cycle, gains need to be solidified. Engaging in yet another power cycle immediately after a successful initial cycle is doomed to failure. The natural inclination is to be greedy and continue down the same path—that, however, is biological suicide.

Science and empirical data have shown that the body needs 4–6 weeks to reset and regain its physiological bearings. The hypothalamus gland controls bodyweight, body temperature, hunger, thirst, fatigue and circadian cycles. The interim phase allows the hypothalamus gland to recalibrate and

18. Tim: The percentages are provided to help you personalize the programme. Take "140 (70%)×8, 1 set", for example. 140 is 70% of my starting 91-kg (200-lb). 1-rep max (1RM). But if your individual 1RM is 68kg (150lb) when starting the programme, you would simply multiply 150×0.7 to arrive at 105 lbs. Later in the programme, if you see "133%", it means you multiply 150×1.33 and use the resulting 90kg (199.5lb) for that set.

readjust. It is equally important to "get away" from the three bench-press versions used in phase I. We also kick the reps upwards.

The ideal interim phase retains bench power by substituting heavy dumbbell pressing for barbell bench pressing. Allowing the body to "forget" the three exercises (competitive grip bench, wide grip bench and narrow grip bench) makes these movements feel fresh and new when they are reinstituted in phase III, and the training effect is profound.

The paused flat dumbbell bench press and the paused incline dumbbell bench press are the phase II workhorses and are performed together in each workout, once per week. Maintain tension for a one-second pause at the chest; do not relax and rest the weight *on* the chest.

WEEK	DUMBBELL BENCH PAUSED	DUMBBELL INCLINE BENCH PAUSED	BODYWEIGHT
1	27kg (60lb) (60%)—3 sets × 10	22.7kg (50lb) (50%)—3 sets × 10	15st (95.3kg)
2	29kg (65lb) (65%)—3 sets × 10	25kg (55lb) (55%)—3 sets × 10	15st (95.3kg)
3	36kg (80lb) (80%)—2 sets × 6	32kg (70lb) (70%)—2 sets × 6	15st (95.3kg)
4	38.5kg (85lb) (85%)—2 sets × 6	34kg (75lb) (75%)—2 sets × 6	15st (95.3kg)
5	43kg (95lb) (95%)—2 sets × 4	36kg (80lb) (80%)—2 sets × 4	15st (95.3kg)
6	45kg (100lb) (100%)—1 set × 4	39kg (85lb) (85%)—1 set × 4	15st (95.3kg)

PHASE II: RE-ESTABLISH HOMEOSTASIS[19]

After the six-week interim phase, all initial gains have been solidified: the athlete's bodyweight regulation thermostat has been reset, while pushing strength has been retained. The body has "forgotten" flat barbell benching, and when we reinstitute our classical regular/wide/narrow flat bench strategy, the training effect is achieved. Chest, arms and shoulders are (once again) shocked into growth. More muscle means a bigger bench.

WEEK	POWER GRIP (71cm/28in)	WIDE GRIP (81cm/32in)	NARROW GRIP (56cm/22in)	BODY WEIGHT
1	215 (108%)×5, 4 sets	185 (93%)×5, 2 sets	175 (88%)×5, 2 sets	15st (95.7kg)
2	225 (113%)×5, 3 sets	195 (98%)×5, 2 sets	185 (93%)×5, 2 sets	15.1st (96.1kg)
3	235 (118%)×5, 2 sets	205 (103%)×5, 2 sets	195 (98%)×5, 2 sets	15.2st (96.6kg)
4	245 (123%)×5, 1 set	215 (108%)×5, 2 sets	205 (103%)×5, 2 sets	15.3st (97kg)

19. Please note that all weights are per dumbbell. For example, "27kg/60lb (60%)" represents 2 x 27-kg (60-lb) dumbbells, which total 54kg (120lb), or 60% of the starting 1RM.

PHASE III: ASSAULT ON 300

WEEK	POWER GRIP (71cm/28in)	WIDE GRIP (81cm/32in)	NARROW GRIP (56cm/22in)	BODYWEIGHT
5	255 (128%)×3, 4 sets	225 (113%)×3, 2 sets	215 (108%)×3, 2 sets	15.4st (97.5kg)
6	265 (133%)×3, 3 sets	235 (118%)×3, 2 sets	225 (113%)×3, 2 sets	15.42st (98kg)
7	275 (138%)×2, 2 sets	245 (123%)×2, 2 sets	235 (118%)×2, 2 sets	15.5st (98.4kg)
8	285 (143%)×2, 1 set	255 (128%)×2, 2 sets	245 (123%)×2, 2 sets	15.6st (99kg)
9	300 (150%)×1	—	—	15.7st (99.7kg)

This is how you can, if you don't miss a thing, add 45kg (100lb) to your bench press in six months.

TOOLS AND TRICKS

The Bench Press Interviews (www.fourhourbody.com/bench) What separates the 1x bodyweight bencher from the 2x? The 2x bencher from the 3x? If you could add one thing to most training programmes, what would it be? I asked all of the above questions and more of some of the best in the power business, including Dave Tate, Jason Ferruggia and Mike Robertson. Unfortunately, due to space constraints, we couldn't include them in the book, but you can find them here.

***The Purposeful Primitive* by Marty Gallagher (www.fourhourbody.com/primitive)** Perhaps the single best book on bodybuilding, powerlifting and fat loss that I've read in the last five years. This diverse tour of elite physique enhancement covers training, diet and otherworldly anecdotes from a wide cast of characters, including Dorian Yates, Ed Coan and Kirk Karwoski.

***Powerlifting USA* Magazine (www.powerliftingusa.com)** If you want to get serious about the sport of powerlifting—where bench, squat, and deadlift maxes are totalled in competition—*Powerlifting USA* is the oldest and most trusted source for training and gym recommendations. If you have any delusions of strength grandeur, find an upcoming meet in "coming events" and observe world-class powerlifters live. Stop puffing out your chest before you walk in.

BENCH PRESSING 387KG (854LB): SET-UP AND TECHNIQUE

Mark Bell, owner of Supertraining Gym in Sacramento, California, can bench press 387kg (854lb) at 19.6st (124.7kg) bodyweight.

Some world-class bench pressers use near-contortionist form to compete: a full back arch with the feet under the hips (or even closer to the head). This shortens the distance you need to press—a good thing for adding weight—but it can produce injuries in novices and intermediates.

Mark uses a stable slight bridge and places his feet flat on the floor. He uses this form to bench 387kg (854lb), so there's no reason you can't use it to bench 227kg (500lb) or less.

Here is the process:

Set-up

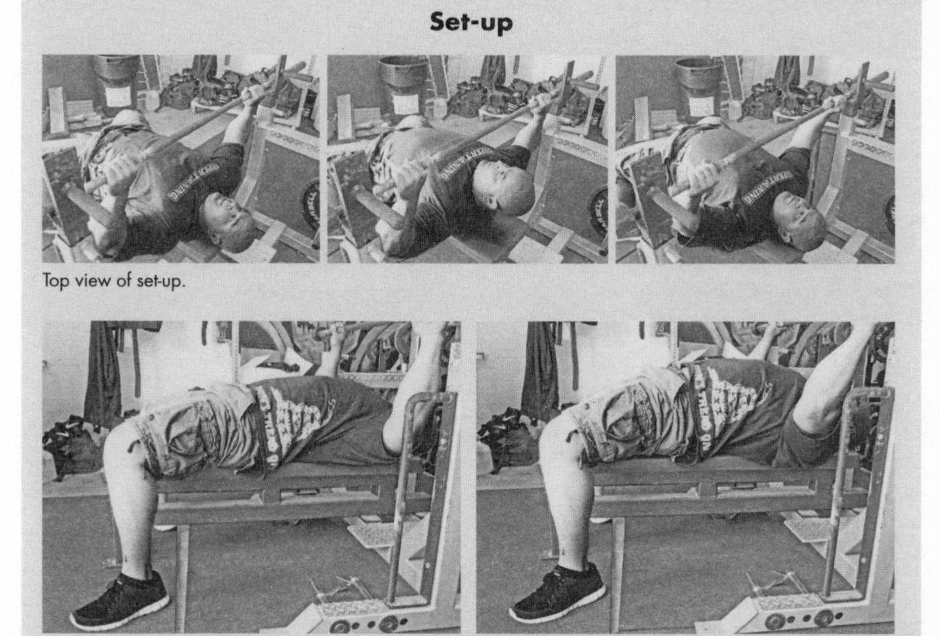

Top view of set-up.

Side view of before and after set-up. Notice that his heels are approximately under his knees.

1. Lie on the bench with your head half off of the edge.
2. Take your power grip (Mark has his ring fingers on the smooth bands), lift your chest to the bar and pinch your shoulder blades together as if holding a penny between them.
3. Keeping your bottom in place and your shoulders pinched, arch your back and push your shoulders down towards your hips.[20]

20. The movement is like an upright row, as if you were pulling the bar up to the top of your forehead.

4. Reset your back on the bench and aim to have the top of your head aligned with the edge of the bench. Mark is the size of a truck and can't quite manage. Most of you will not have that as an excuse.
5. Now your shoulders are protected. This position will be quite uncomfortable, and it should be.
6. Your legs and glutes should be fully tensed, and your toes should be pushed into the front of your shoes. If your legs and glutes wouldn't be fatigued after 20 seconds, you're not contracting them hard enough.
7. Now you're ready for the hand-off from a spotter. Never bench alone if using free weights.[21]
8. The spotter should, using an alternating grip like in the deadlift (see Lamar's photos in the last chapter), lift the bar off the supports and help move it to just over your nipples.
9. Now that you're supporting the weight over your nipples, depress your shoulders fully—as if you were starting a rowing movement—before bending your arms. The less you have to bend your arms to get to the bottom of the movement, the safer it will be and the more weight you will be able to lift.

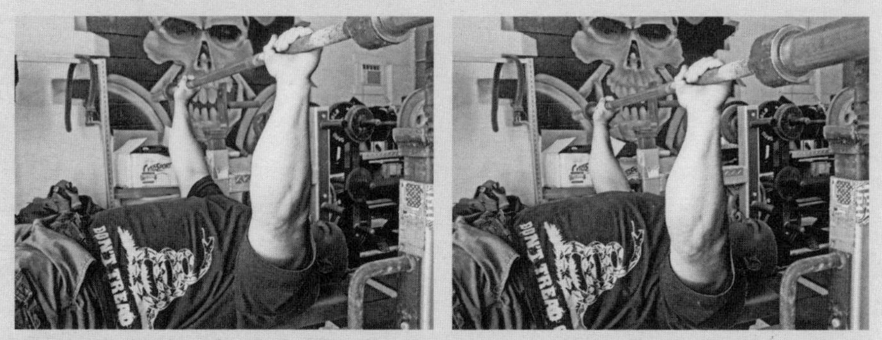

Depressing the shoulders before bending the arms. Compare the height of Mark's elbows in both photographs. He's lowered the weight 7.5–10cm (3–4in) and his arms are still straight.

10. Crush the bar with your grip and lower it to the sternum or highest point on your abdomen, tucking the elbows a little closer to your sides in the lowest 1/2 of the movement.
11. Press straight up in the shortest line possible. If struggling with the weight, you can flare your elbows slightly outwards in the top 1/2 of the movement to bring the weight towards the rack, which will help with full extension.

21. I know some of you will do this anyway. If you do, DO NOT use collars. This allows you to dump the weight, one side at a time, if you get trapped under it.

FROM SWIMMING TO SWINGING

HOW I LEARNT TO SWIM EFFORTLESSLY IN 10 DAYS

I always wanted to be Peter Pan, the boy who never grows up. I can't fly, but swimming is the next best thing. It's harmony and balance. The water is my sky.

—Clayton Jones, president and CEO of Rockwell Collins

Swimming had always scared the hell out of me. Despite national titles in other sports, I could barely keep afloat for 30 seconds. This inability to swim well was one of my greatest insecurities and embarrassments.

I'd tried to learn to swim almost a dozen times, and each time my heart jumped to 180+ beats per minute after one or two pool lengths. It was indescribably exhausting and unpleasant.

No more.

In the span of less than 10 days, I went from a two-length (2 × 18.39 metres/20 yards) maximum to swimming more than 40 lengths per workout in sets of two and four. From there, I moved to one kilometre in the open ocean, then onward to 1.6–3.2km (1–2 miles). The entire progression took less than two months.

This chapter will explain how I did it after everything else failed, and how you can do the same.

At the end of January 2008, a good friend issued a New Year's resolution challenge: he would go all of 2008 without coffee or stimulants if I trained and finished an open-water one-kilometre race in 2008.

He had grown up a competitive swimmer and convinced me that, unlike my other self-destructive habits masquerading as exercise, swimming was a life skill. Not only that, it was a pleasure I needed to share with my future children. In other words, of all the potential skills you could learn, swimming was one of the most fundamental.

I agreed to the challenge.

Then I tried everything, read the "best" books, and . . . still failed.

Kick boards? Tried them. I barely moved at all and, as someone who is usually good at most sports, felt humiliated and left.

Hand paddles? Tried them. My shoulders will never forgive me. Isn't swimming supposed to be low-impact? Strike two.

It continued for months until I was prepared to concede defeat. Then I met Chris Sacca, formerly of Google fame and now an investor and triathlete in training, at a barbecue and told him of my plight. Before I had a chance to finish, he cut me off:

"I have the answer to your prayers. It revolutionized how I swim."

That was the turning point.

The Method

Chris introduced me to Total Immersion (TI), a method usually associated with American swim coach Terry Laughlin. I immediately ordered the book and freestyle DVD.

In the first workout, without a coach, I cut my drag and water resistance at least 50%, swimming more laps than ever before in my life. By the fourth workout, I had gone from 25+ strokes per 18m (20-yard) length to an average of 11 strokes per 18m (20-yard) length.

In other words, I was covering more than twice the distance with the same number of strokes (thus expending half the effort), and there was no panic or stress. In fact, I felt better after leaving the pool than before getting in. I couldn't, and still can't, believe it.

I recommend reading the Total Immersion book *after* watching the DVD, as the drills are nearly impossible to understand otherwise. I was unable to do the exercises from pages 110 to 150 (I cannot float horizontally and have a weak kick) and became frustrated until the DVD enabled me to test technique with propulsion.

My Eight Tips for Novices

Here are the principles that made the biggest difference for me, and pictures follow:

1. **To propel yourself forward with the least effort, focus on shoulder roll and keeping your body horizontal (least resistance), not pulling with your arms or kicking with your legs.** This is counterintuitive but important, as kicking harder is the most universal suggestion for fixing swimming issues.
2. **Keep yourself horizontal by keeping your head in line with your spine—you should be looking straight down.** Use the same head position that you maintain while walking, and drive your arm underwater v. attempting to swim on the surface. See Shinji Takeuchi's underwater shots at 0:49 seconds (www.fourhourbody.com/shinji-demo) and Natalie Coughlin's explanation at 0:26 seconds (www.fourhourbody.com/coughlin). Notice how little Shinji uses his legs. The small flick serves only to help him turn his hips and drive his next arm forward. This is the technique that allows me to conserve so much energy.
3. **In line with the aforementioned video of Shinji, think of swimming freestyle as swimming on alternating sides, not on your stomach.** From Wikipedia's TI page:[1]

"Actively streamline" the body throughout the stroke cycle through a focus on rhythmically alternating "streamlined right side" and "streamlined left side" positions and consciously keeping the bodyline longer and sleeker than is typical for human swimmers.

For those who have rock-climbed or bouldered, it's just like moving your hip closer to a wall to get more extension. To test this:

1. 13 August, 2008.

stand with your chest to a wall and reach as high as you can with your right arm. Then turn your right hip so it's touching the wall and reach again with your right arm. Making this small rotation, you'll gain 7.5–15cm (3–6in). Lengthen your vessel and you travel farther on each stroke. It adds up fast.

Below is what a full stroke should look like, demonstrated by TI founder Terry Loughlin. Notice the minimal flick of the legs used to rotate the hips and body. This sequence of photos should be your bible for efficient swimming:

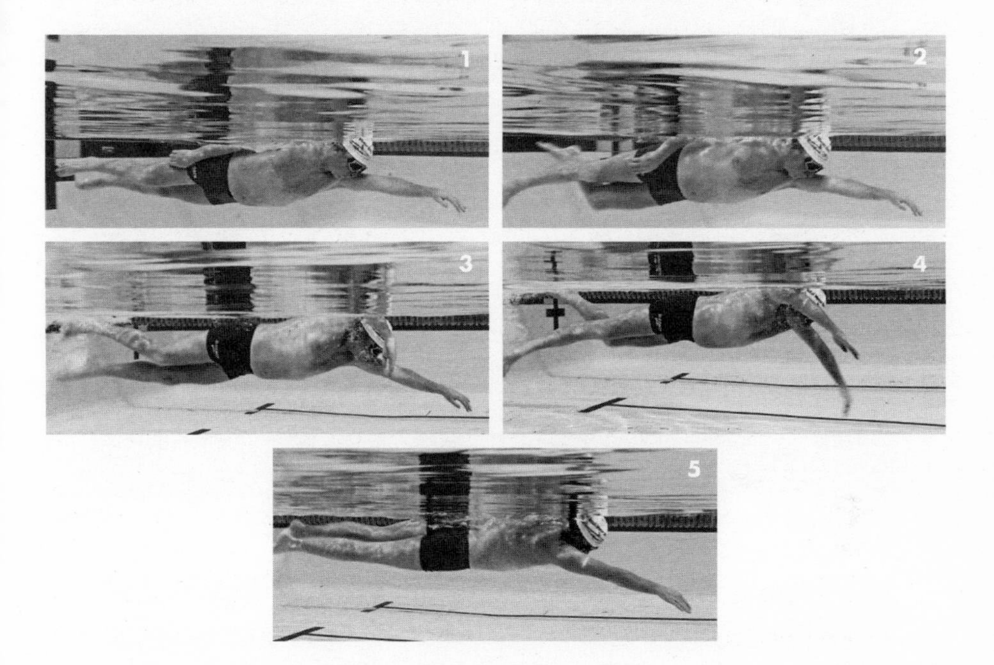

4. **Penetrate the water with your fingers angled down and fully extend your arm well beneath your head. Extend it lower and farther than you think you should.** This downward water pressure on the arms will bring your legs up and decrease drag. It will almost feel like you're swimming downhill.

The first photo on the next page illustrates the typical inefficient "reach", and the second illustrates the proper point of entrance, much closer to the head.

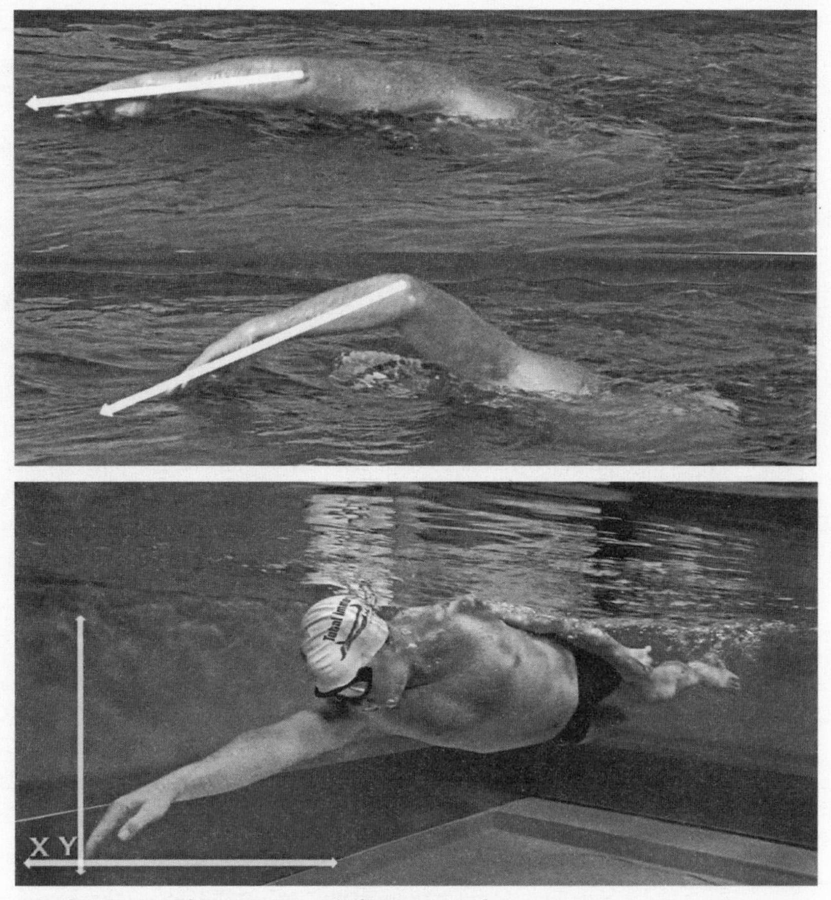

Once the arm enters the water, it extends down at an angle.

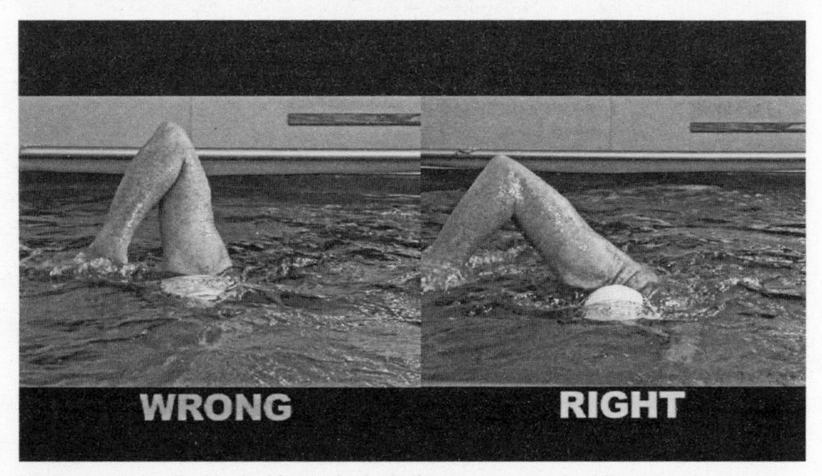

Don't impinge the shoulder by lifting it too high. If you rotate your shoulders properly, it's not necessary.

5. **Focus on increasing stroke length (SL) instead of stroke rate (SR).** Attempt to glide farther on each downstroke and decrease the number of strokes per lap.
6. **Stretch your extended underwater arm and turn your body (not just your head) to breathe.** For each breath, you should feel the stretch in your lats (back) on your lower side, as if you were reaching for a biscuit tin high on a shelf a few centimetres out of reach. This will bring your head closer to the surface and make it easier to breathe. Some triathletes turn almost to their backs and face skyward to avoid short gasps and oxygen debt (tip from Dave Scott, six-time Ironman world champion).

   In your first practices, breathe on every other stroke.[2] Once you become more comfortable breathing on your "weak" side, I encourage you to practise breathing every third stroke, which will force you to alternate sides.

   Remember to exhale fully and slowly while your face is underwater. If you don't, you'll need to exhale and inhale when you bring your head out, which will mean feeling rushed, swallowing water and exhausting yourself.

   Remember to exhale underwater, and "extend to air" (video: www.fourhourbody.com/extend-air).

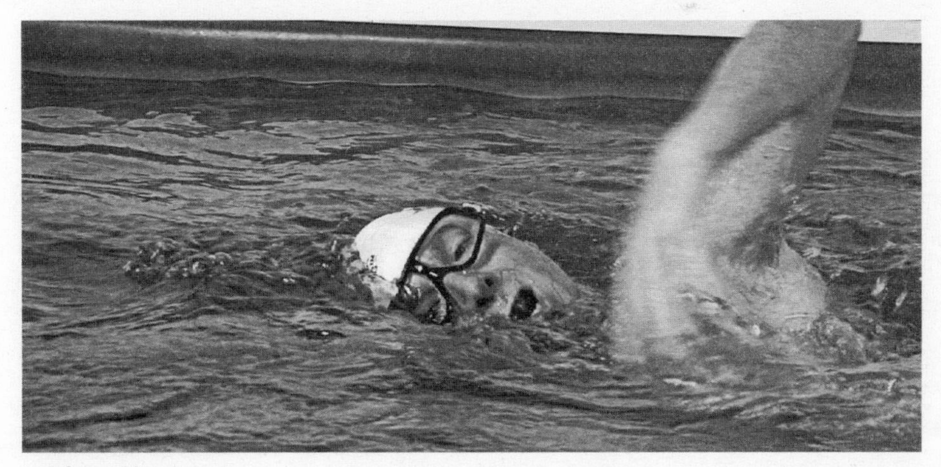

Look for your hand.

2. Tip: once turning to bring your face out of the water, look for your hand. Stop your inhale when it passes your goggles and rotate back into your stroke.

7. **Experiment with hand swapping as a drill.** It's difficult to remember all of the mechanical details while actually swimming. I short-circuited trying to follow half a dozen rules at once. The single drill that forced me to do most other things correctly is hand swapping.

   This is the visualization I found most useful: focus on keeping your lead arm fully extended until your other arm comes over and penetrates the water around the extended arm's forearm. This encourages you to swim on your sides, extends your stroke length, and forces you to engage in what is referred to as "front-quadrant" swimming. All good things. This one exercise cut an additional three to four strokes off each lap of freestyle.

8. **Forget about workouts and focus on "practice".** You are training your nervous system to perform counterintuitive movements, not training your aerobic system. If you feel strained, you're not using the proper technique. Stop and review rather than persist through the pain and develop bad habits.

Gear and Getting Started

Ready to give it a shot? If you have a phobia of swimming, you're almost there. Don't screw it up by choosing the wrong gear or the wrong pool. Some closing recommendations:

1. **Gents, don't swim in board shorts.** I tried this in Brazil and it's like swimming with a parachute behind you. Terrible. Get some Euro-style Speedos and streamline. Be cool on the beach and opt for efficiency in the water.
2. **Get good goggles.** I tried them all, from Speedo Vanquishers to Swedish swim goggles. In almost all tests, I needed to tighten the various straps every 329–410ft (100–125m) to prevent chlorinated water from blinding me.

   I now use nothing besides the much-acclaimed (and rightly so) Aqua Sphere Kaiman goggles, which are well sealed and can be tightened without removing them from your head. Leakage is non-existent. These are the only goggles I'll ever need.

3. **Start practising in a pool that is short and shallow.** Use a lane in the shallow end (1.2m/4ft or less in depth) and opt for a pool that is no longer than 18m (20 yards). It's easier to focus on technique in shorter pools. Once I adapted to 18m (20 yards), I moved to 23m (25 yards), and then (once I could do 10 × 91m /100 yards with 30–45 seconds of rest between sets) I moved to an Olympic-sized 50m (164ft) pool.

Hard to Believe

I never ever thought I'd say this but: I love swimming.

This is RIDICULOUS, as I have always HATED swimming. Now, whenever possible, I make time to do laps. It's like moving meditation.

I'll swim for two hours and sneak out later to get in an extra session. I still can't believe it.

What about the one-kilometre open-water race? Oh, I didn't forget about that. I wasn't able to find a practical race scheduled near me in the last quarter of 2008 (as much as I would have loved to visit Bonaire, it was a bit out of the way), but my friend excused it. For good reason. Four months before my December deadline, I had gone home to Long Island to spend my birthday with my family and closest friends.

One morning, I woke up early and went to the ocean. I was calm, despite the waves, and I stood on the damp sand at the edge of the whitewash looking out for a long time. Then I approached the lifeguard stand.

"How far away is that house?" I asked the lifeguard on duty, pointing far down the beach at a red rooftop.

"Almost exactly a mile."

"Great. Thanks."

With that, I started walking and, 20 minutes later, stopped in front of the red roof. I put on my Kaiman goggles, took a few deep breaths, said, "Fuck it," aloud, gave a sharp *kiai*-like yell, and got in the water.

I swam 1.6km (1 mile) alone in the ocean, parallel to the beach, about 329m (100ft) offshore. Alternating left and right breaths every third stroke, I entered a Zen-like state of almost supernatural confidence. It was odd.

I reached the lifeguard stand and passed it, continuing on another 183m (200 yards) or so, when I decided to get out of the water. There was no fatigue and no concern; I'd just proven my point. To myself. Walking up the sand, I have never been prouder or felt more alive. I looked around like a 21-year-old Mike Tyson after winning the heavyweight championship of the world. I was, for that moment, king of my universe. One of my deepest-seated lifelong insecurities was gone and would never return.

The elation was indescribable.

I encourage all of you, whether you want to overcome your fears or win the Ironman, to give TI training a test drive. It's the first instruction that's made sense to me and is 100% responsible for the fastest transformative experience I've ever had in the world of sports.

Enjoy.

Think it can't be that easy? Here are just two before-and-after responses from testers who used the above guidelines. Get your goggles ready:

From Rocky:

. . . I tried this in the gym and in 2 days have gone from 2 laps to 25 laps. I was telling friends yesterday that in my entire adult life if I had to pick 3 things that have held me in awe this would be amongst those three.

From Diego:

Tim,

. . . I had the biggest fear of water my entire life and finally stepped out of my comfort zone. Last month, just one (1) month ago, I was fighting water, trying to stay afloat. Definitely survival mode . . . I started learning [Total Immersion], read the TI book (it's literally in pieces now since I'd take it to the pool and leave it at the end of my lane soaking water each time I'd reference it) and watched several videos. I continually practiced . . .

It's been only a month . . . Last week I did a 1.5 mile swim in the pool nonstop . . .

Today I made it to a 2.5 mile swim and only stopped because the facility was closing. I'm graduating to open water now. It's been a lifelong dream of mine to perform in the Ironman, and my times, a month after learning, are below the cutoff times for the 2.4 mile swim.

Thank you so much! I hope to meet you some day.

Your friend in Florida,

Diego

TOOLS AND TRICKS

Total Immersion, *Freestyle Made Easy*, DVD (www.fourhourbody.com/immersion) This DVD was the reason I was able to completely overcome my fear of swimming, and actually learn to love it. In the span of less than 10 days, I went from a 2-length (2× 18m/20 yards) maximum to swimming more than 40 lengths per workout in sets of 2 and 4.

Aqua Sphere Kaiman Goggles (www.fourhourbody.com/kaiman) These leak-proof goggles were the last pair standing after I tested everything under the sun. I have three pairs and swim with nothing else, whether indoor or in open water. My favourites have orange-tinted lenses.

Total Immersion Swimming Freestyle Demo by Shinji Takeuchi (www.fourhourbody.com/shinji) If you want to see how effortlessly and tirelessly someone can swim, look no further than this video demo.

Swimmers Guide (www.swimmersguide.com) Find all the public swimming facilities in your area, or in 167 countries. Never leave home without your goggles.

THE ARCHITECTURE OF BABE RUTH

Only God can make a great hitter.

—Whitey Lockman, 60-year veteran player, manager, and Major League Baseball front-office executive

Discovery consists of seeing what everybody has seen and thinking what nobody has thought.

—Albert Szent-Gyorgyi, Nobel Prize-winning physiologist credited with discovering vitamin C

"Please tell me you're kidding."

We'd gone to the wrong hotel. Normally this wouldn't be a big deal, but we were in the middle of a blizzard. Getting a taxi was next to impossible, as all of them were either full, or covered in powder and spinning in place.

"Can't we just grab a taxi from here to the hotel?" Jaime, my coach for the day, had asked earlier. Taxis from Pier 40 on the water in Manhattan? Not on a Saturday night with a snowstorm crippling the city.

So we started walking. My date with Everlast would continue. Jogging through Times Square in slush with an a 36.3kg (80lb) boxing heavybag across my shoulders it was.

But I didn't mind. For the first time in my life, I felt like Babe Ruth.

Obsessive Batting Disorder

Jaime Cevallos isn't normal. Ever since he was a kid, when his classmates were off to prom or driving to house parties hooting and hollering, he was in his front garden, hitting baseballs through a tyre hung from a tree branch. He took notes, made changes and took more notes.

Now Major League Baseball players pay him to look at those notes, because Jaime has figured out how to improve some important numbers. One of them is "slugging percentage".

Slugging percentage,[3] the bread-and-butter of baseball hitter analysis, is the number of bases run, divided by the total number of appearances at the plate. The higher the percentage, the better. The Rain Man of slugging was Babe Ruth, and his 1921 record stood until Barry Bonds and his 51cm (20in) arms came along in 2001.

Tweaking this number is important.

In 303 plate appearances before working with Jaime, Ben Zobrist had three home runs and a .259 slugging percentage. In the 309 plate appearances after working with Jaime, Zobrist hit 17 home runs with a .520 slugging percentage. In 2009, Zobrist won the team MVP award for the Rays, finishing the season with a .297 batting average and 27 home runs.

Going from three home runs to 27 in approximately the same number of at-bats is astounding. In the majors, it's unheard of.

If only God can make a great hitter, does that make Jaime God?

Or was he just seeing something that other people weren't?

From God to Granularity

> Ted Williams once famously remarked, "Hitting a baseball is the hardest thing to do in sports."... Jaime Cevallos has made it his life's mission to conquer the unconquerable.
>
> —*Fort Worth Star-Telegram*

This leads us to the snowstorm.

I had invited Jaime to demonstrate his goods on a blank canvas: me. He had flown from Dallas, Texas, to land with a boatload of gear (including the heavybag) on the western edge of New York City.

Armed with a radar gun, video camera, laptop and a slew of baseball

3. Slugging percentage (SLG) = (1B) + (2B × 2) + (3B × 3) + (HR × 4)/AB. Walks are excluded from this calculation and were long undervalued in baseball, something Billy Beane and the Oakland Athletics capitalized on to create an incomprehensibly successful team on almost no budget, as described in *Moneyball*.

bats coated in pine tar, he then set out to turn me into a home run hitter in one session. The setting would be the sub-arctic batting cages of Pier 40, and each ball would be hit off a tee that put ball height at 89.53cm (35.25in) to eliminate the variability of pitches.

Perhaps it was the salsa music that pumped in from an adjacent room, where aspiring Dominican pros were playing cards, but after just 45 minutes of moulding and training, here were the ball speed results, measured with the radar gun off the bat:

Before instruction (km/h): 109, 111, 77, 80, 97, 76, 79, 103, 68, 109, 114, 108, 66
Before instruction (mph): 68, 69, 48, 50, 60, 47, 49, 64, 42, 68, 71, 67, 42
Before-training average: 92.22km/h (57.307mph)

After (km/h): 93, 98, 84, 101, 87, 105, 121, 122, 113, 126, 105, 98, 113
After (mph): 58, 61, 52, 63, 54, 65, 75, 76, 70, 78, 65, 61, 70
After-training (first round) average: 105km/h (65.23mph)

After After (after the second round with Mr. Miyagi, km/h): 117, 113, 106, 106, 117, 111, 126, 113, 95, 119, 109, 122, 111
After After (after the second round with Mr. Miyagi, mph): 73, 70, 66, 66, 73, 69, 78, 70, 59, 74, 68, 76, 69
After-training (second round) average: 112.77km/h (70.076 mph)

I was still no Mark McGwire, but jumping from 92km/h (57mph) to 113km/h (70mph) in off-bat ball speed translates into major distance gains. In terms of home run potential, what does this really mean?

Using a 45% angle incline on each hit, here's the difference:

For 92.23km/h (57.31mph) (84.05ft/sec), distance is 48m (158ft).
For 112.78km/h (70.08mph) (102.78ft/sec), distance is 65m (214ft) (a 35.4% increase)[4]

What follows are the fundamental principles and exercises we focused on in our 45 minutes.

4. I'm indebted to Professor Robert Adair, Sterling Professor Emeritus of physics at Yale University and author of the classic *The Physics of Baseball*, for this help with these numbers. His commentary: "The distances vary with the air temperature, wind velocity and backspin of the ball. Also, we don't have perfect values for the air resistance, which varies a little with the ball axis of rotation. . . . I took the backspins as 1,030 rpm and 1,260 rpm. The balls will go a little further at 40 degrees (57.31) and 35 degrees (70.08)." The projected distances varied for almost every PhD Jaime and I consulted, but the before-after differences were always large. Some physicists predicted slightly more significant increases approximating 50%, from roughly 55m (180ft) to roughly 76m (250ft) when accounting for air resistance.

Picking Your Angles

THE BIG THREE

The Cushion

The Cushion occurs when the front heel has landed, prior to the forward swing. In the Cushion, it is best to have optimal torque created between the shoulders and hips. Jaime calls this **Angle S**. A good Angle S measurement is 25 degrees.

Increasing Angle S is also one of the ways to "buy" time if the pitch is off-speed ("off-speed" means it's a curveball, changeup, knuckleball or any pitch that is significantly slower than a fastball). Off-speed pitches are meant to lure the hitter into opening up the front shoulder and losing the torque between his hips and shoulders. The battle between pitcher and hitter is really a fight for the hitter's form. The pitcher's job is to (1) throw strikes and (2) lure the hitter into weak hitting positions.

The "Slot" position of Babe Ruth.

The Slot

Two things define a proper Slot position: (1) the back elbow drops to the player's side, and (2) the spine angle stays vertical. The Slot is the kinetic link in action: the arms deferring to the more powerful legs and hips in order to work as a whip through the strike zone.

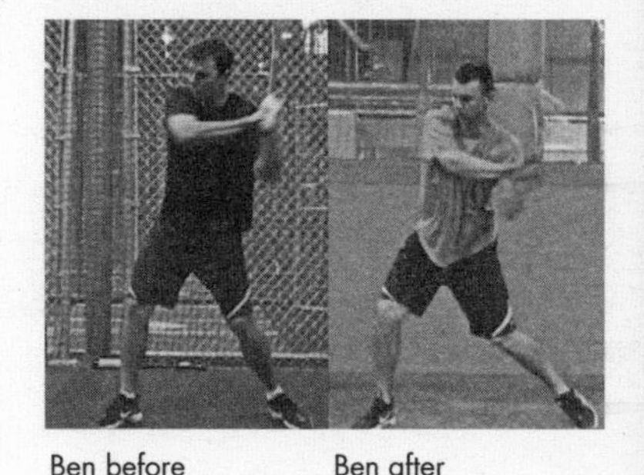
Ben before Ben after

See the picture of Ben Zobrist on the first day he filmed with Jaime in the winter of 2007. Next to it is Ben during the All-Star break mid-season in 2008. His much-improved Slot position is obvious. Zobrist went on a tear from that point in the season, averaging one home run every 18 at-bats (prior to that, it had been one home run for every 101 at-bats). He later made the 2009 All-Star team and was named Rays' team MVP.

Impact Position

The Impact position is the thumbprint of the swing. In this case, it tells you the ability of a hitter rather than their identity. There are two components to the Impact position: the E and W angles. E is the angle between the upper arm and forearm, which we want as small as possible (aim for 80 degrees), and W is the angle between the top wrist and the bat, which needs to be as large as possible (aim for 180 degrees). This one position paints the entire picture of a player's swing. The Impact position correlation to great hitting is extraordinary.

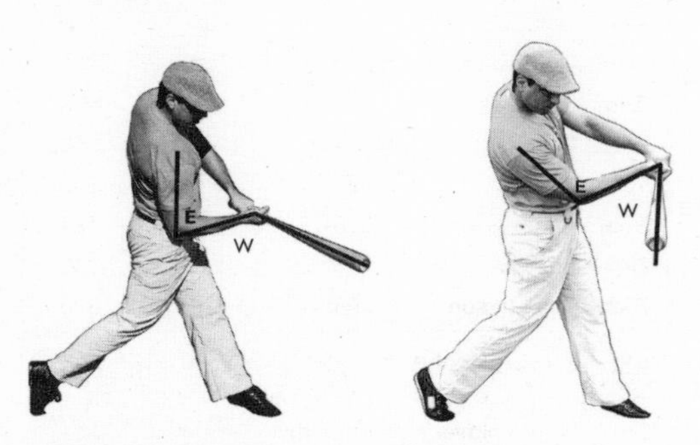

Good impact (left) and bad impact (right). We want E small and W big.

But Impact position becomes more actionable when we convert it to a number, the 80/20 metric to focus on: CSR.

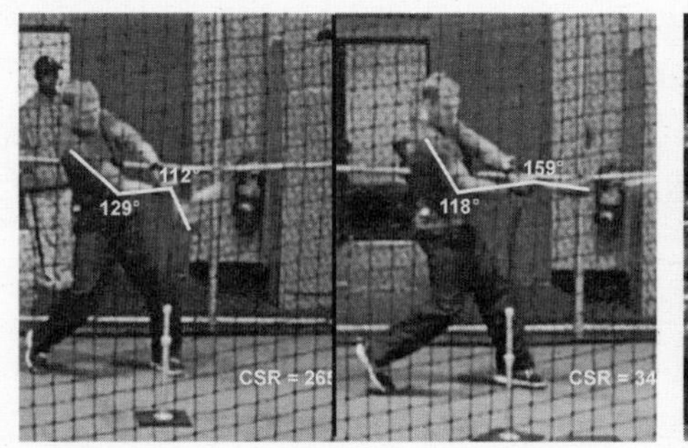

Before and after, with CSR overlaid: 265 before vs. 345 after.

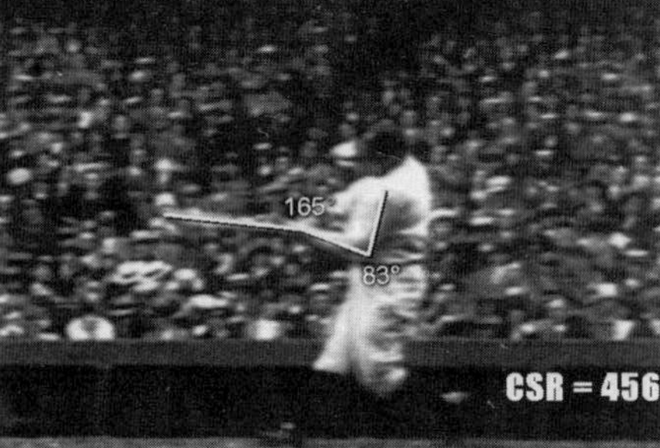

Babe Ruth, the reigning king of CSR.

CSR (Cevallos Swing Rating) = 3 (180 – E) + W. The CSR number contains unusual insight involving two simple-to-measure angles at the point of impact: the first at the elbow (E), and the second between the forearm and the bat itself (W). Here are just two benefits of a high CSR swing:

1. **A high CSR swing is naturally a tighter swing.** Since the swing is closer to the torso, thanks to the elbow-in Slot position, pitches that are too far outside of the strike zone are unreachable. The hitter with the tighter swing is forced into better pitch selection because he can't physically swing at pitches outside of the strike zone.

It's analogous to how novice boxers will sometimes practise proper chin position (down) by holding a wallet between their chin and chest. If the boxer keeps his chin down and makes this position instinctual, it will be hard to knock him out. If a batter doesn't let his elbow leave the Slot position through the strike zone, he can't reach for bad pitches, and it will be harder to strike him out.

	CSR	SLG	OPS
Babe Ruth	463	.690	1.1638
Ted Williams	429	.634	1.1155
Hank Aaron	422	.555	.928
Albert Belle	393	.564	.933
Harmon Killebrew	386	.509	.884
Bernie Williams	381	.477	.858
Wade Boggs	354	.443	.858
Tony Gwynn	321	.459	.847
Pete Rose	318	.409	.784
Don Mattingly	313	.471	.830
Rickey Henderson	296	.419	.820

Historical CSRs: Contrasted with CSR, SLG is essentially a measurement of a player's power and OPS is a measurement of both a player's power *and* consistency.

2. **In a high-CSR swing, contact with the ball is made further back, closer to the catcher.** This naturally gives the batter more time to assess the pitch before initiating the swing.

   Jaime elaborates:

"A high CSR is not just indicative of power (mass × acceleration). A high CSR is also a sign of consistency, as the back arm remains passive, allowing the body to whip the bat into the hitting zone early and keep it there for a long time, creating a long AOI [Area of Impact, covered next]."

AREA OF IMPACT (AOI)

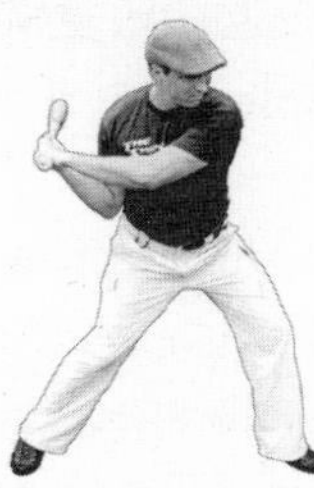
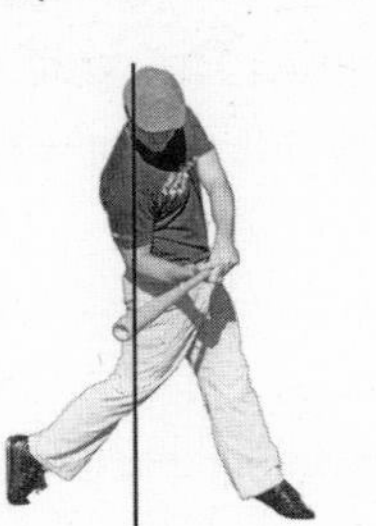
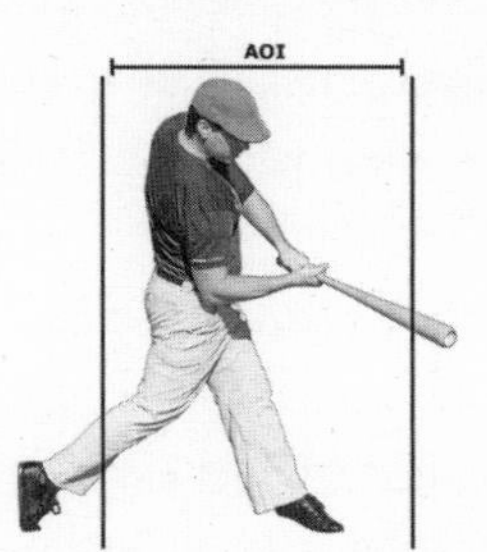

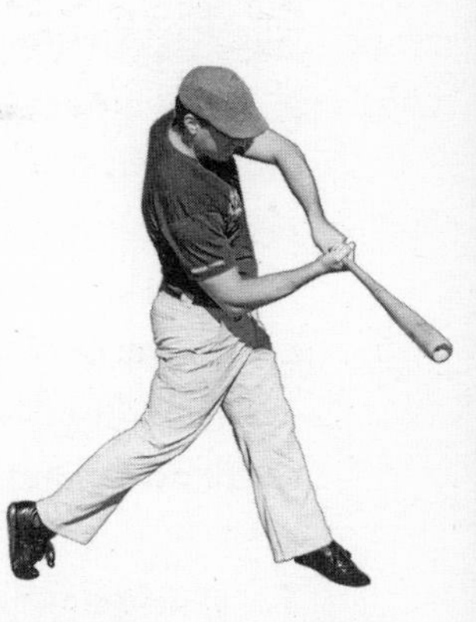

Big AOI—good.

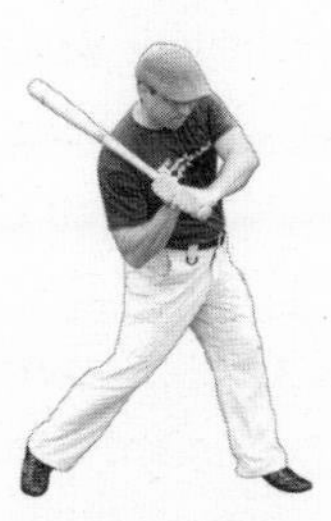
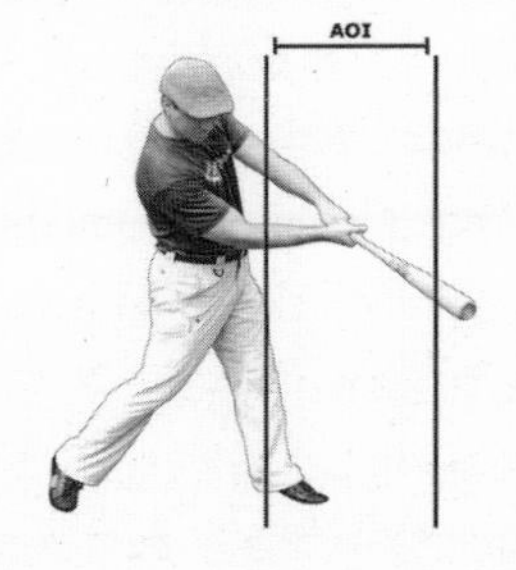

Small AOI—bad.

It is possible to achieve a high CSR while doing something that reduces power, such as having your front arm away from your chest (à la Derek Jeter). Much more mass, and therefore force, can be transferred to the ball if the front arm is tight to the chest, because the mass of the torso is transferred through the arm directly into the bat. It should be one unit.

Advanced Concepts (Important for live pitches)
See the illustrations of good and bad **Areas of Impact (AOI)** on the previous page. AOI is an indication of a hitter's level of consistency. It indicates how long the bat is square enough to the pitch to supply adequate force to the oncoming ball. You will notice that the Slot position and good CSR produce a long AOI. The longer the AOI, the higher the likelihood of hitting the ball, even if the hitter misjudges pitch speed.

Angle L measures bat-lag: how late your bat comes through the strike zone. Lag is achieved with a slight wrist "twitch" of the top of the bat towards your spine while the bat is still well behind you. The smaller the angle L, the more bat speed will ultimately be generated. The key is to achieve a small angle L early in the Slot position. If you achieve bat-lag too late in the swing, as the bat is travelling through the hitting zone, it will shrink your AOI.

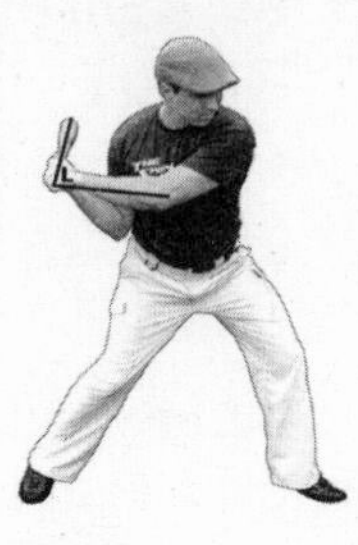
Angle L

Practising Your Angles

The best drill for honing a new Impact position is hitting the impact bag (usually a heavybag), pausing at impact, and checking your position. Do this for 10 minutes, then practise hitting balls off of a tee, duplicating the same movement.

This was the single exercise I performed while with Jaime. It works like gangbusters.

Hacking CSR and related biomechanics is a force multiplier (figuratively and literally) that can be used to transform mediocre hitters into MVP hitters.

God might create great hitters, but science also gives you the tools to build them.

The Exercise That Increased My Distance 35%

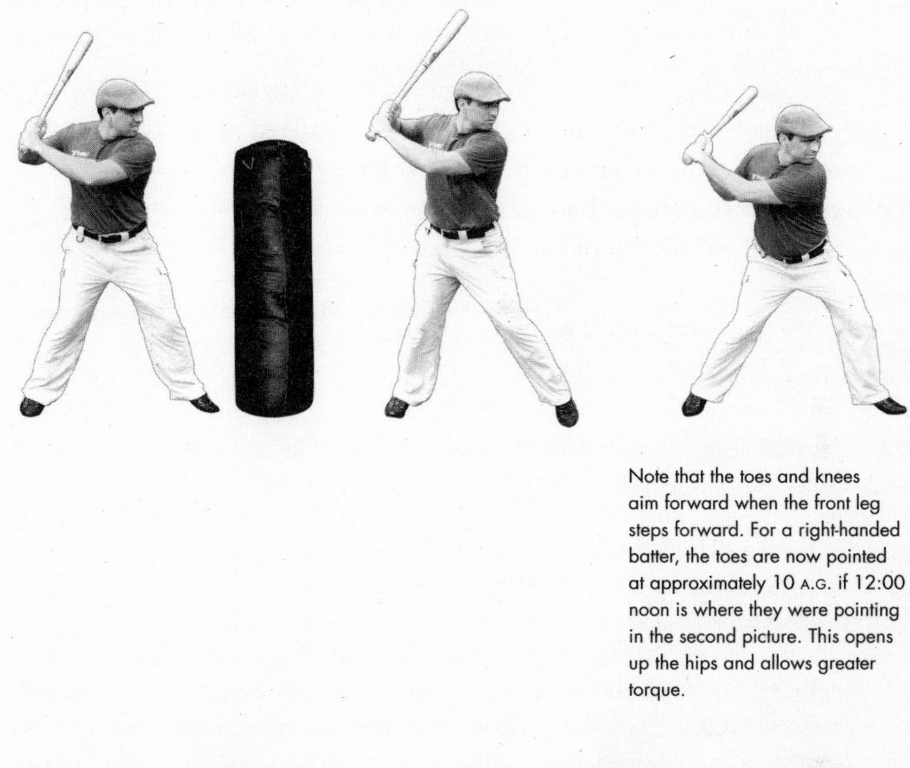

Note that the toes and knees aim forward when the front leg steps forward. For a right-handed batter, the toes are now pointed at approximately 10 A.G. if 12:00 noon is where they were pointing in the second picture. This opens up the hips and allows greater torque.

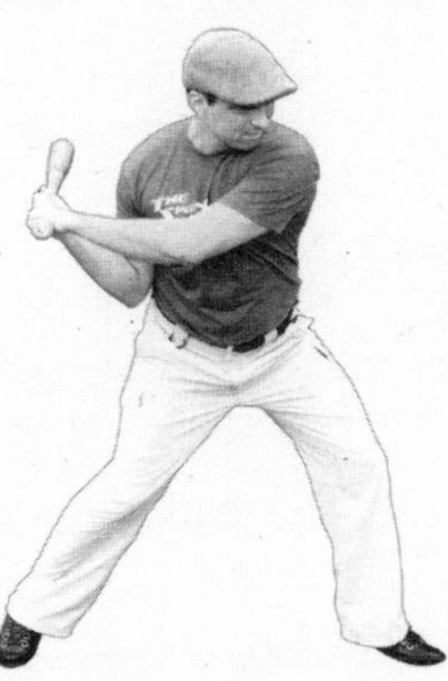

To prevent backward lean and ensure that my spine was perpendicular to the ground, I focused on keeping my left shoulder away from my left ear.

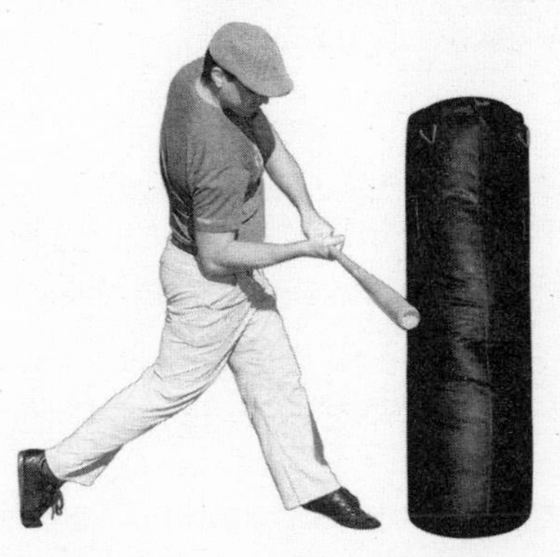

For the final impact, the largest speed increases (and sound increases) were achieved when I focused on driving the right hip forward by forcefully extending the front left leg. If you drill this forceful extension, expect better speeds—and intense soreness the next day—to follow.

TOOLS AND TRICKS

Impact Bag Drill in Motion (www.fourhourbody.com/impact) This is the actual training video of the Impact bag drill Jaime and I did together. The progress is clearly visible from start to finish, and Jaime's coaching is audible.

Jaime Cevallos Business Case (www.fourhourbody.com/cevallos) How did Jaime go from making $7 (£4) an hour to coaching MLB MVPs? He used *The 4-Hour Workweek* as a step-by-step manual. This blog post explains how he got access to the majors and landed in major media, including *ESPN: The Magazine*, among others.

The MP30 Training Bat (http://www.theswingmechanic.com/) Increasingly common in the majors, the MP30 Training Bat trains hitters to swing using the ideal Slot position to generate more power.

Sports Radar Gun (www.fourhourbody.com/radar) This radar gun will measure everything, whether pitches, swings or cars.

***Moneyball: The Art of Winning an Unfair Game* by Michael Lewis (www.fourhourbody.com/moneyball)** In *Moneyball*, master storyteller Michael Lewis describes how the Oakland Athletics achieved an astonishing winning record in 2002, despite the lowest player payroll of any major league baseball team. A's general manager Billy Beane believed that objective science could beat subjective scouts. He hired PhDs in statistics to help him acquire undervalued players based on neglected numbers, like ground-outs for pitchers. Even if you hate baseball, you will love this book.

ON LONGER AND BETTER LIFE

LIVING FOREVER

Vaccines, Bleeding and Other Fun

There is nothing in biology yet found that indicates the inevitability of death.

—Richard Feynman, co-recipient of 1965 Nobel Prize in Physics

Not life, but good life, is to be chiefly valued.

—Socrates

This will be the shortest chapter on life-extension ever written.

Let it begin, as all good short chapters do, with a story of two monkeys: Canto and Owen. Housed at the University of Wisconsin, these two rhesus monkeys are as close to identical as possible, with one exception. Canto is on a diet.

Specifically, his calories are restricted to 30% less than normal. He is part of a semi-fasting group of monkeys that has been on the animal equivalent of Weight Watchers® for two decades. Owen, in the feasting control group, is a stark contrast. He eats whatever the hell he wants. To date, in this 20+ year experiment, 37 per cent of the "eat, drink, and be merry" group have died due to causes related to old age. The calorie-counting group has a much lower death rate, **almost two-thirds lower**.

Cancel our reservations at the Cheesecake Factory! In fact, it's time to cancel dinner forever!

Or, wait a second, is that really all there is to the story? Roger Cohen, whose father, a doctor, studied baboons all his life, shared a less sensationalized perspective in a *New York Times* op-ed titled "The Meaning of Life", excerpted here:

Which brings me to low-cal Canto and high-cal Owen: Canto looks drawn, weary, ashen and miserable in his thinness, mouth slightly agape, features pinched, eyes blank, his expression screaming, "Please, no, not another plateful of seeds!"

Well-fed Owen, by contrast, is a happy camper with a wry smile, every inch the laid-back simian, plump, eyes twinkling, full mouth relaxed, skin glowing, exuding wisdom as if he's just read Kierkegaard and concluded that "Life must be lived forward, but can only be understood backward."

It's the difference between the guy who got the marbleized rib-eye and the guy who got the oh-so-lean fillet. Or between the guy who got a Château Grand Pontet St. Emilion with his brie and the guy who got water. As Edgar notes in King Lear, "Ripeness is all." You don't get to ripeness by eating apple peel for breakfast....

When life extension supplants life quality as a goal, you get the desolation of Canto the monkey. Living to 120 holds zero appeal for me. Canto looks like he's itching to be put out of his misery....

We don't understand what the mind secretes. The process of aging remains full of enigma. But I'd bet on jovial Owen outliving wretched Canto....

Laughter extends life. There's little of it in the low-cal world and little doubt pudgy Owen will have the last laugh.[1]

If your goal is to live as long as possible, there is a long list, an endless list, of things to avoid. The good news is that life-extension need not be complicated.

For the gents, it may be as simple as blocking a few websites and curbing a little maleness. The pro-ejaculation lobby slipped up in 1992, when the *New York Times* broke the story:

IN WORM, AT LEAST, MAKING SPERM IS FOUND TO SHORTEN A MALE'S LIFE

See, Dr. Wayne Van Voorhies of the University of Arizona had allowed nematodes, also called "roundworms", to kill themselves by copulating. In his research, nematodes prevented from mating lived an average of 11.1 days. Nematodes allowed to drop their drawers lived a scant 8.1

1. Roger Cohen, "The Meaning of Life", *New York Times*, 19 July 2009, sec. Opinion.

days. Never got to see the grandkids grow up, never got to play golf at St. Andrews.

It's a sad tale of weary scrotums (or whatever worms have as scrotums).

"The genes and biochemical processes nematodes use are the same as those that humans and other mammals use," elaborated Dr. Philip Anderson of the University of Wisconsin.

The *Times* connected the logical dots in their conclusion: "Ceaseless sperm production takes its toll on a male, perhaps requiring the use of complex enzymes or biochemical processes that have harmful metabolic effects . . . the difference in lifespan between men and women [women live an average of 6 years longer] just may be linked to sperm production."

Finally, no more ejaculating! It's like finding out that flossing is bad for you. No more tiring sex or aching wrists. Hassle removed. And you might live 37% longer!

In the quest for longer life, it pays dividends to err on the side of caution, to avoid any unnecessary risks or unknowns. To live, after all, you don't *need* much. Air, water, gruel with some protein and shelter will cover all the bases. One could therefore suggest no venturing outside the home, no driving or travelling, and certainly no exposure to other humans, who could be sick with cat flu or nappy rash.

Naturally, this level of risk-avoidance leads to what we all want: a long and shitty life.

But let's assume you're one of the few (billion) people who wants a degree of fun and freedom in life. The real question then becomes not "How can I extend life at all costs?" but rather "How can I increase the *length* of my life without severely decreasing my *quality* of life?"

The most basic approach would be to eat, drink and be merry, and believe that a few more laughs and tasty calories will beat most lab theories in the long run. I believe this to be true.

The second complementary approach, which can be followed right along with the first, is to consider therapies that are minimally inconvenient and that, based on the scientific literature, should work in humans.

The Short List

The short list of therapies should then be ethically filtered. "Ethics" can be nebulous, but here's an example:

If you're a woman and want to buy cancer insurance, you could opt to have a full-term pregnancy before age 20. Some scientists believe it could be "the most effective natural means of protecting against breast cancer" due to the hormone hCG.

Should you therefore have children before age 20? I suggest that life-extension is not a good enough reason, particularly since another life is involved. This option is therefore omitted from our list.

Separating the wheat from the chaff, we might consider four candidates that make the cut:

- Resveratrol
- Injections of the immunosuppressant drug rapamycin[2]
- Alzheimer's vaccines
- Stem cell therapies

These might just get you to 200 or beyond, especially if used in combination.

And I'm avoiding them.

But. . . why?

I believe, as do some scientists, that focusing on *global* therapies (drugs or treatments with broad molecular effects) without long-term human data is barking up the wrong tree, a tree fraught with unpredictable side effects.

Take resveratrol, for example, which is currently available over the counter. It is effective in extending lifespan in nearly all species tested, but it can also block or activate oestrogen receptors. Could this affect other metabolic or hormonal feedback loops, disrupting fertility if taken routinely? It's impossible to say, which is why I'll use resveratrol short-term at higher doses for endurance while tracking blood markers, but I won't use it indefinitely for life-extension. Telomerase activators like TA-65, another example, are purported to extend our chromosomal countdown clocks called "telomeres". TA-65 can cost up to $15,000 (£9,360) per year. Is it possible that, by amplifying cell replication, you increase the likelihood of dangerous cancerous growth? Perhaps. It's simply beyond our technology to guarantee one outcome or another, so I'm avoiding TA-65 as well.

But if not in global therapies, where is the promised land?

2. Rapamycin chemically induces autophagy, which protein cycling, mentioned later, achieves naturally.

Until we can go to a supermarket and get a *RoboCop* makeover with regenerative medicine, there are a few alternatives in a second short list.

These are the protocols I am currently using.

All of them are low-cost, low-tech and low-risk. Most of them also provide athletic or body composition benefits, even if their life-extension effects are later debunked:

1. CYCLES OF 5–10 GRAMS OF CREATINE MONOHYDRATE (COST: $20/MONTH / £12/MONTH)

Creatine monohydrate, popular among power athletes since its commercialization in 1993, has recently become a candidate for minimizing or preventing the development of Alzheimer's, Parkinson's and Huntington's diseases.

There are almost 20 years of published research involving human use of creatine monohydrate. Since my family has Alzheimer's and Parkinson's on both paternal and maternal sides, it is low-cost insurance: I'm ingesting 5–10 grams of creatine monohydrate powder per day for two consecutive weeks every two months. If you choose to use this protocol, I suggest tracking and trending hepatic enzymes, BUN, and all the usual blood testing suspects to ensure no kidney problems. Complications are rare, but an ounce of prevention is worth a pound of cure. Nowhere is this truer than in life-extension.

2. INTERMITTENT FASTING (IF) AND PROTEIN CYCLING (COST: FREE)

What if poor, hungry Canto only needed to fast on occasion to extend his life?

Constant caloric deprivation isn't without risks, after all. The decline in sex hormone production alone can cause amenorrhoea (cessation of menstruation) and bone thinning, among other problems.

It turns out that you can mimic, even exceed, the supposed life-extending effects of caloric restriction with intermittent fasting (IF). This can be true even if you consume twice as many calories as normal during your "on" times, resulting in no total decrease in weekly calories.

There are several versions of IF and semi-IF protocols popular among experimental subcultures:

Fast-5: Fast for 19 hours beginning at bedtime, followed by five hours of eating as much as necessary to satisfy hunger. This is popular for moderate weight loss, which typically appears starting in the third week and averages 450g (1lb) of loss per week thereafter.[3]

Some research suggests IF confers the same life-extension benefits as caloric restriction only when calories are consumed during daylight hours. This would, if accurate, make the Fast-5 better for fat loss than longevity.

ADCR: Alternate Day Caloric Restriction (ADCR) requires that calories be cut 50–80% every other day. It has been shown to improve insulin sensitivity, auto-immune disease and even asthma after just two weeks.

Protein cycling: Dr. Ron Mignery, author of the *Protein-Cycling Diet*, suggests that even a single day per week of restricting protein to no more than 5% of maintenance calories can produce effects similar to extended caloric restriction.

If the mechanism of IF or CR is a genetic self-preservation response,[4] protein cycling makes sense. There are no essential dietary carbohydrates. Simply reducing calories (or carbs) wouldn't necessarily qualify as a biological emergency. On the other hand, even brief absences of essential amino acids like lysine might be enough to flip the switch. The "switch" in our context is triggering a process of cellular housekeeping called *autophagy*, the purpose of which is, in Dr. Mignery's words, "to clear the cell of degraded and aggregated proteins that are not being handled by the other recycling mechanisms of the cell". In principle, if you clear the junk out faster than it builds up, you postpone or reverse ageing.

I'm currently experimenting with both 18-hour[5] and one-day protein cycling, which I believe (and it's pure conjecture) can also increase subsequent protein synthesis during overfeeding. For muscular growth phases, I have used the 18-hour protein cycling once per week precisely for this reason, usually ending between noon and 2 P.M. on my Saturday cheat day.

Below is a sample menu for one day of less than 5% protein, adapted from Dr. Mignery. It is distinctly non-slow-carb. Once you've cried a tear of dietary misery, I'll tell you what I do:

Miscellaneous breakfast—Breakfast can include wheat-based (lysine-deficient) products such as toast, muffins or bagels, pro-

3. http://www.Fast-5.com/content/summary.
4. Not entirely unlike hibernation in some species.
5. Following dinner until lunch the subsequent day.

vided that wheat is the only substantial source of protein, and its calories are heavily diluted with calories from non-protein sources (butter, sugar, juice, fruit, etc.).

Toast with mushrooms, onions and gravy—You can thicken the fat or drippings from meat with starch to make a gravy and drizzle it over the toast, mushrooms and onions.

Spinach with vinegar—Microwaved frozen spinach (less than 380g/13.4oz) can be flavoured with any kind of vinegar for a near-protein-free dish with the warmth and chew of meat.

Meat substitutes—A microwaved slice of aubergine can fill a sandwich and give something of the shape and texture of a lunch meat. Black olives can also provide something of the texture of meat without the protein.

Bean substitutes—Beans and peas are fairly high in protein and cannot be eaten in the restriction phase of protein cycling. But you can substitute spheres of cassava starch called tapioca pearls. They are a staple of tropical cuisine and are available in a wide range of sizes and colours. You may be familiar with them if you have ever had bubble tea.

So, here's what I do:

First, I drizzle fat gravy over a bowl of tapioca pearls.

Kidding. I fast following an early Friday dinner (6 P.M.) and then, around 10 A.M. the next morning (16 hours later), I eat 190g (6.7oz) spinach with vinegar and spices, one slice of sourdough toast with lots of butter, and enjoy it all with a large glass of grapefruit juice. Delish. Sometime after noon, I'll then head off to eat my usual chocolate croissants and continue cheat day as a binge monster.

3. THE LOST ART OF BLEEDING (COST: FREE)

Thought bloodletting went out of fashion around the time of the Salem witch trials? Not entirely.

I'm betting on a major resurgence, and it all has to do with excess iron.

More than oestrogen, it's thought to partially explain why post-menopausal (but not pre-menopausal) women have a similar incidence of heart attack to men. I've donated blood since 2001 to be on the safe side.

And I'm not alone. The New England Centenarian Study, conducted by Boston University's School of Medicine, is the world's largest and most comprehensive ongoing study of "centenarians", or people who live past 100. Dr. Tom Perls, director of the study and an associate professor of medicine, gives blood every eight weeks to mimic the loss of iron due to menstruation, which he believes will increase his longevity:

"Iron is a critical factor in our cells' ability to produce those nasty molecules called free radicals that play an important role in ageing . . . It may be as simple as having less iron in your body."

There is ample evidence that iron reduction through phlebotomy (bloodletting) can not only improve insulin sensitivity, but also reduce cancer-specific and all-cause deaths. High iron stores have been correlated to an increased number of heart attacks in otherwise symptom-free males, and blood donation has conversely been correlated to a decrease in "cardiovascular incidents".

Drs. Michael and Mary Dan Eades suggest aiming for blood ferritin levels of 50 mg/dl, which, if your levels aren't over 400, can usually be achieved with 1–4 whole blood donations spread two months apart.[6] No leeches required. If you'd like to increase the removal of pesticides and other environmental toxins normally stored in fat, you can do two things: schedule to donate a double portion of plasma, and drink a cup of caffeinated coffee about 60 minutes before going to the centre. Donated blood will always contain such toxins, so you are not being a bad citizen by temporarily increasing their excretion.

Though some scientists argue that iron *depletion* is necessary for full cardiac benefits, I see no harm in acting on the positive implications of dozens of other studies.

Consensus won't come any time soon, but even if you don't extend your own life, you might save someone else's.

Karma is what karma does.

A Little Flower, Please

The Danish writer Hans Christian Andersen, beloved for his fairy tales, including "The Little Mermaid" and "The Emperor's New Clothes", perhaps put it best: "Just living is not enough. One must have sunshine, freedom, and a little flower".

6. From *The Protein Power Life Plan.*

Extending lifespan at the expense of quality of life makes little sense. It's easier (and lazier) to focus on subtraction and avoidance, but a life of constant denial is not a life of freedom.

The greatest rewards come from a good life, not just a long life. This probably includes a bit of red wine and a few cheesecakes.

Perhaps even an ejaculation or two.

TOOLS AND TRICKS

Donating Blood If you have high iron levels (as I did after adding orange juice to my diet), an easy and karmically positive way to lower those levels is by donating blood. Any of the following sites can help you find a local centre, schedule an appointment, and save lives.

National Blood Service (For people in England and Wales: www.blood.co.uk)

Alcor (www.alcor.org) Perhaps you'd like to store your body in ice-free cryosuspension at the first sign of terminal illness, just in case technology catches up? There's nowhere better than Alcor in Scottsdale, Arizona, where gems such as Ted Williams's head are allegedly stored.

***Transcend: Nine Steps to Living Well Forever* by Ray Kurzweil (www.fourhourbody.com/transcend)** Kurzweil, called the "rightful heir to Thomas Edison" by *Inc.* magazine, proposes that those interested in "radical life extension" should make it their immediate goal to live through the next 20 or so years, in order to see advances like DNA reprogramming and submicroscopic, cell-repairing robots. This book outlines the nine key areas for extending your life.

***Protein-Cycling Diet* by Dr. Ron Mignery (www.fourhourbody.com/protein-cycle)** According to this book, available for free at this link, a single day per week of restricting protein to no more than 5% of maintenance calories can produce effects similar to extended caloric restriction.

Methuselah Foundation (www.mfoundation.org) The Methuselah Foundation is a non-profit medical charity dedicated to extending healthy human life. The foundation also offers the NewOrgan Network for those in need of replacement organs, making it easier to reach out to friends and family for support.

Immortality Institute (www.imminst.org) The Immortality Institute is an international not-for-profit organization. Its mission is "to conquer the blight of involuntary death". Though I don't love the word *blight,* I do love the forum on this site, where hundreds of self-experimenters (including published scientists who post pseudonymously) report on surprising results and advances from using experimental supplements, drugs and other off-label therapies.

Snowball (www.fourhourbody.com/snowball) If you think about death too much, life seems too goddamn serious. Take a look at this site. It will put things in perspective. Trust me.

CLOSING THOUGHTS

CLOSING THOUGHTS

The Trojan Horse

We either make ourselves miserable or we make ourselves strong. The amount of work is the same.

—Carlos Castaneda

"Running an ultramarathon can't be good for you. I can't imagine how it's possibly good for your body," I said.

I wasn't biting on endurance. Running wasn't my thing and it never had been. Brian MacKenzie laughed: "Good for you physically? No. But you'll recover. And I assure you: if you run 50K (30 miles) or 161km (100 miles), when you finish, you won't be the same person who started."

I thought for a minute, and that's when I bit.

I'd seen a strange ripple effect dozens of times in the world of strength, but for some reason I'd never connected the dots with endurance. Perhaps just as you haven't connected the dots with some subjects in this book. After all, in a knowledge economy, what's the value of deadlifting more or losing 2% body fat? Of hitting a home run?

In a word: transfer.

My father lost 70+lb (32+kg) of fat in 10 months and tripled his strength. During his annual check-up, his doctor declared that he might live forever.

The physical changes were incredible, but the

curious side effects of the programme were the strongest incentives to continue. As my dad explained:

> *It's very odd. I used to feel like the invisible man, but now people more readily ask my opinion and take me more seriously. I went from not being noticed to being noticed. Quite apart from the aesthetic and performance benefit, there's a huge social benefit. I lost my invisibility.*
>
> *Also, after losing 50 or 60 pounds and doing what you once thought impossible, you start to see the other "impossibles"—doubling income in 12 months or whatever—as "possibles".*

This book is a Trojan horse full of unexpected transfers.

It's intended to make you a better all-round human. It's also intended to make you a role model for those around you.

Partial Completeness

Most of us have resigned ourselves to a *partial completeness*, just as Chad Fowler did before losing more than 7.1st (45kg). Partial completeness can take many forms, usually in the form of self-talk like:

"I'm just not [thin, fast, strong, muscular, etc.]. That's the way it is."

"XYZ doesn't matter. It's not that important."

These are said or thought for many reasons. Oftentimes, they're used to excuse something on the outside that people believe they can't change.

The beauty is, almost all of it can be changed.

More important, the reason to change the physical isn't physical at all.

In 2007, I was interviewed for the monthly newsletter of Eben Pagan, who runs a $30 million (£18 million) per year relationship-advice empire. One of his first questions was:

"What's the fastest way for someone to improve their inner game?"

To which I responded:

"Improve your outer game."

If you want to be more confident or effective, rather than relying on easily defeated positive thinking and mental gymnastics, learn to run faster, lift more than your peers, or lose those last 10lb (4.5kg). It's measurable, it's clear, you can't lie to yourself. It therefore works.

Recall Richard Branson's answer to the question, "How do you become more productive?": work out.

The Cartesian separation of mind and body is false. They're reciprocal. Start with the precision of changing physical reality and a domino effect will often take care of the internal.

Becoming Complete

Your body is almost always within your control.

This is rare in life, perhaps unique. Simply focusing on some measurable element of your physical nature can prevent you from becoming a "Dow Joneser", someone whose self-worth is dependent on things largely outside of their control.

Job not going well? Company having issues? Some idiot making life difficult? If you add ten laps to your swimming, or if you cut five seconds off your best mile time, it can still be a great week.

Controlling your body puts you in life's driver's seat.

Fifteen months after giving birth to her first child, Dara Torres took home the U.S. Nationals gold medal in the 100-metre freestyle. . . at age 40. Three days later she broke her own record in the youth-dominated 50-metre freestyle, a record she'd set at age 15.

At age 45, George Foreman knocked out Michael Moorer, age 26, to become heavyweight boxing champion of the world, reclaiming the title he'd lost to Muhammad Ali two decades earlier.

Jack "The Dipsea Demon" Kirk ran the infamous Dipsea trail race for the first time in 1905. He proceeded to run it 67 times, the last at age 94, and broke the record for consecutive foot races held by Boston Marathon legend Johnny Kelley. Jack's oft-repeated saying was, "You don't stop running 'cause you get old. You get old if you stop running!"

Refuse to accept partial completeness.

Take the next step: uncap a pen and take an inventory of all the things in the physical realm that you've resigned yourself to being poor at. Now ask: if I couldn't fail, what would I want to be exceptional at? Circle these alternate realities.

This list, circles staring back at you, gives you a blueprint for not just a new body, but an entirely new life.

It's never too late to reinvent yourself.

Computer scientist Alan Kay once said, "The best way to predict the future is to invent it."

Where will you start?

APPENDICES AND EXTRAS

HELPFUL MEASUREMENTS AND CONVERSIONS

Weight (Food)

GRAMS	OUNCES
28g	1 ounce
1135g	4 ounces
150g	5 ounces
230g	8 ounces
300g	10 ounces
340g	12 ounces
450g	16 ounces or 1 pound

Body Weight

KILOGRAMS (KG)	POUNDS (LB)
45.4	100
54.4	120
63.5	140
72.6	160
81.6	180
90.7	200
99.8	220
108.9	240

Volume (Food)

STARTING COLUMN (BELOW)	GRAM (G) (WATER)	TEA-SPOON (TSP)	TABLE-SPOON (TBSP)	FLUID OUNCE (FL OZ)	PINT	LITRE (L)	GALLON (IMPERIAL)
1 gram (water)	1	0.203	0.068	0.034	0.0021	0.0010	0.0002
1 teaspoon	4.92	1	1/3	1/6	0.010	0.005 (5 mL)	0.0011
1 tablespoon	14.75	3	1	1/2	1/32	0.015 (15 mL)	0.003
1 fluid ounce	29.5	6	2	1	1/16	0.030	0.007
1 pint	472	96	32	16	1	0.473	0.104
1 litre	997.51	202.88	67.63	33.81	2.113	1	0.220
1 gallon (Imperial)	4534.79	922.33	307.44	153.72	9.61	4.546	1

GETTING TESTED–
FROM NUTRIENTS TO MUSCLE FIBRES

There's no need to spend a fortune on testing.

The critical few in this section are ordered from least to most expensive,[1] and I've put asterisks (***) next to the tests that yielded the most actionable results for me and other test subjects in the book.

Of the blood tests, SpectraCell was, across the board, the most immediately impactful for the case studies I supervised. It's on page 475.

Use these tests as a starting point, beginning with the least expensive and adding only when needed or as budget allows. More sophisticated tests can be prescribed by a physician if the basics show abnormalities.

Not sure what *CBC* or *TSH* is? In the beginning, I wasn't either, but you can learn any of them in 60 seconds. For that matter, you could learn *all* of them in 60 minutes. Use www.fourhourbody.com/bloodtests to look up unfamiliar blood test terms, or to get a better understanding of your own results.

Here are a few guidelines to prevent you from going Woody Allen neurotic:

1. **If you can't act on it or enjoy it, don't bother testing it.** No one needs to learn they're predisposed to a disease they can do nothing to fix. Focus on actionable items and ignore the rest.
2. **Take the same tests at the same time.** Timing matters. . . a lot. To compare before and after results for a given test, aim for the same time of day, same day of the week, and (if female) same point in your menstrual cycle. Testosterone levels, as just one example, can easily change more than 10% from 8 A.M. to 12 noon.
3. **If you get an alarming result, repeat the test before making big changes.** One acquaintance removed almost every food from his diet—"I'm

1. If there is a range for cost, I have used the lower range for putting them in order.

allergic to them all!"—without realizing that food allergy testing is notoriously error-prone. If you get an alarming result, repeat the test. If you have the budget, consider using a different lab or, better still, sending two identical samples to the same lab under different names. I did the latter with several tests, including 23andMe, to ensure the results were consistent. 23andMe passed, but many others did not. Get a second opinion before doing anything drastic.

I owe special thanks to Dr. Justin Mager for helping me navigate the world of testing.

THE MENU

Insurance will often cover the first one or two comprehensive tests you have performed, and I encourage you to speak with your doctor about this option.

I prefer to keep my testing activities (and results) out of insurance files and usually pay with a credit card. For this reason, I've listed the cash costs for each test. Skip to "BodPod" if your eyes gloss over with the blood details.

Comprehensive Blood Panel: Free–$600 (£375)

These standard blood draws were performed at the Clear Center of Health near San Francisco and analyzed by Hunter Laboratories (www.hunterlabs.com):

***Chem 6: $210 (£130)

Includes: CMP, lipid panel, ferritin, iron, MG, TSH, FT3, FT4, cortisol, insulin, CBC, UA, Plac, vitamin D

***Male V: $360 (£225)

Includes: estradiol, PSA, DHEA-S, LH, pregnenolone, cortisol, free and total testosterone, IGF-1 (indicative of growth hormone)

Additional Male Tests:

DHT: $22.80 (£14)

FSH: $40 (£25)

Progesterone: $40 (£25)

Female Health Profile[2]
(can overlap with Chem 6): $400–700 (£250–435)

2. Since I am not a woman, this test was found from a non-Hunter source: http://www.anylabtestnow.com/Tests/Female_Tests.aspx

Includes: homocysteine, lipoprotein (a), prealbumin, thyroid panel, DHEA-S, estradiol, progesterone, FSH, LH, C-Reactive Protein (hs-CRP), iron, ferritin, hepatitis, HIV.

Inflammatory markers: Detect bleeding disorders, abnormal blood clotting, and assess your risk of having a heart attack.

Cardio C-Reactive Protein (CRP):	$30 (£19)
Homocysteine:	$30 (£19)
Fibrinogen:	$40 (£25)
Glyco A1C:	$25 (£16)

Liver enzymes: Use these tests to assess whether your liver has a disorder, a disease or has been damaged, whether by diet, supplements or something else.

ALT:	$6 (£4)
AST:	$6 (£4)

*****BodPod (www.fourhourbody.com/bodpod): $25–50 (£16–31) per session** The official body fat measurement device of the NFL Combine. Just sit inside a sealed capsule and alternating air pressure will determine body composition.

*****DEXA (search "DEXA body fat" in Google): $50–100 (£31–62) per session** Dual energy X-ray absorptiometry (DEXA) is my favourite option for measuring body fat percentage, as the results include valuable information besides body composition, including mass imbalances and bone density.

*****ZRT at-home Vitamin D test kits (www.zrtlab.com/vitamindcouncil): $65–220 (£41–137)** Determine your vitamin D levels before supplementing. The ZRT tests are saliva-based and reasonably accurate. Note that vitamin D is often included in the comprehensive bloodwork (in our example, "Chem 6"), and it is always included in the SpectraCell testing I recommend.

Genetic insights (www.23andme.com and www.navigenics.com): $99–1,000 (£62–624) per test If you'd like to determine your genetic indicators for fast-twitch muscle fibre, caffeine metabolism or ethnic make-up, these tests will offer answers.

Berkeley Heart Labs or Advanced Cardio Lipid Panel: $120–260 (£75–162) If you adhere to the Lipid Hypothesis of cardiovascular disease (in essence, that cholesterol and fats cause it) these laboratories offer comprehensive lipid analyses, including tests that measure LDL and HDL particle size as a distribution of seven and five subclasses, respectively.

Food Allergy Testing (Meridian E95 Basic Food Panel): $140 (£87) I've included this as more of a warning than a recommendation. Interviewing doctors who review Meridian tests on a regular basis, it became clear that certain foods (pineapple, kidney beans, egg whites, etc.) often come back as positive for almost 100% of the patients, but there are also periods of lower "allergic response", again across nearly all patients. This seems reflective of bad testing processes, or a bad test in general, and the questionable results seem common across most labs. This is also true for "gut permeability" tests.

There are, however, two main takeaways from my food allergy experiments and polling: most problems are caused by gluten, which you shouldn't be eating much of in the first place; and you can *create* food allergies if you eat the same foods and same protein sources all the time. The fix: Follow the Slow-carb Diet, and change your main protein sources and staple meals every month or so.

*****Doctor's Data Urine Toxic Metals: $160/£100 ($60/£37 kit + $100/£62 for DMPS injection)** In this test, you are injected with a chemical that binds to heavy metals in your blood (i.e. a *chelating* agent like DMPS), which are then excreted in your urine. Using a large plastic jug, you collect urine for a 6-hour period and then bottle a well-shaken sample for analysis. To test the effects of larger fish, I ate swordfish and tuna before injection. The result? I doubled my mercury levels after one meal. Don't do that.

*****Comprehensive Stool Analysis and Parasitology: $245 (£153)** This test, offered by Doctor's Data, Genova, MetaMetrix, and others, looks at the health of your largest interface with the enviroment: your gut. This will help identify digestive issues or parasite-induced problems. If you can't gain weight, this test should be a high priority.

*****SpectraCell Nutrient Testing (www.fourhourbody.com/spectracell): $364 (£227)** This test is used to pinpoint vitamin and micronutrient deficiencies. This test helped me identify a selenium deficiency, which—once corrected—helped me to triple my testosterone levels. One other test subject identified enormous B-12 and vitamin D deficiencies, which—once corrected—made him so energetic that he felt like he was on cocaine. In a good way, that is. Highly, highly recommended.

BioPhysical (www.fourhourbody.com/biophysical): $3,400–8,000 (£2,120–4,990) The Biophysical is an all-in-one test. By surveying the biomarkers in your blood, Biophysical will detect medical conditions and diseases, including: cardiovascular disease, cancer (including breast, colon, liver, ovarian, prostate and pancreatic), metabolic disorders (such as diabetes and metabolic syndrome), autoimmune disease (including rheumatoid arthritis and lupus), viral and bacterial diseases (such as mononucleosis and pneumonia), hormonal imbalance (including menopause, testosterone deficiency, and thyroid deficiency) and nutritional status (such as vitamin and protein deficiencies).

MUSCLES OF THE BODY (PARTIAL)

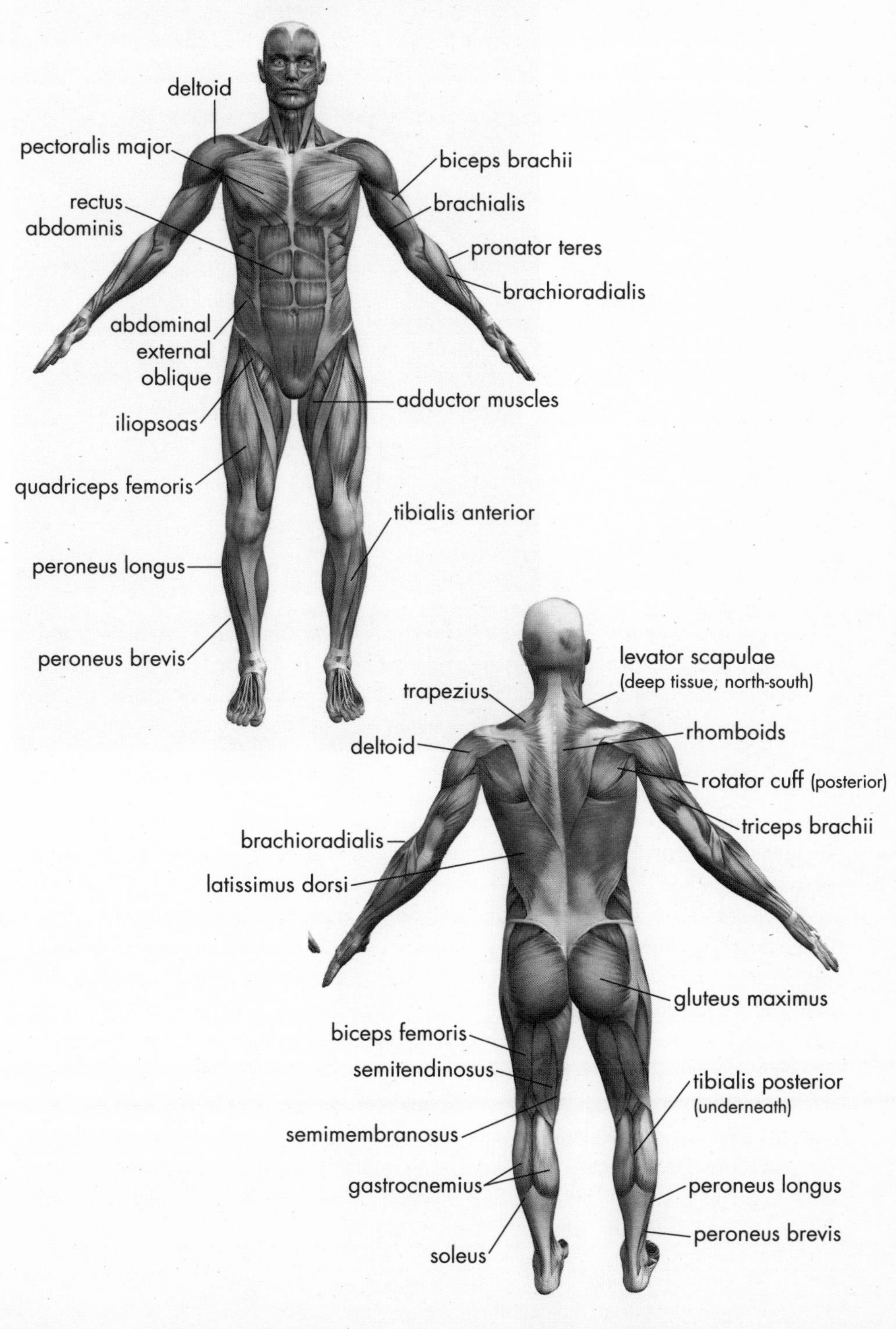

THE VALUE OF SELF-EXPERIMENTATION

All life is an experiment. The more experiments you make the better.
—Ralph Waldo Emerson

It doesn't matter how beautiful your theory is, it doesn't matter how smart you are. If it doesn't agree with experiment, it's wrong.
—Richard Feynman

This chapter was written by Dr. Seth Roberts, professor emeritus of psychology at the University of California–Berkeley and professor of psychology at Tsinghua University. His work has appeared in the New York Times Magazine *and* The Scientist, *and he is on the editorial board of the journal* Nutrition.

I started self-experimentation when I was a grad student. I was studying experimental psychology; self-experimentation was a way to learn how to do experiments.

One of my first self-experiments was about acne. My dermatologist had prescribed tetracycline, an antibiotic. Just for practice, I did an experiment to measure its effect. I varied the dosage of tetracycline—the number of pills per day—and counted the number of pimples on my face each morning. First I compared six pills per day (a high dose) and four pills per day (the prescribed dose). Somewhat to my surprise, they produced the same number of pimples. I tried other dosages. Eventually I tried zero pills per day. To my shock, zero pills per day produced the same number of pimples as four or six pills per day. The conclusion was unavoidable: the drug had no effect. (Many years later, research articles about antibiotic-resistant acne began to appear.) Tetracycline is a prescription drug; it's not completely safe. I'd been taking it for months.

My dermatologist had also prescribed benzoyl peroxide, which comes in a cream. When my self-experimentation started, I believed that tetracycline was powerful and benzoyl peroxide weak, so I rarely used the cream. One day I ran low on tetracycline. Better use the cream, I thought. For the first time, I used the cream regularly. Again I was shocked: it worked well. Two days after I started using it, the number of pimples clearly went down. When I stopped the cream, two days later the number of pimples rose. When I restarted the cream, the number of pimples went down again.

My data left no doubt that (a) tetracycline didn't work and (b) benzoyl peroxide did work—the opposite of my original beliefs. My dermatologist thought both worked. He'd seen hundreds of acne patients and had probably read hundreds of articles about acne. Yet in a few months I'd learnt something important he didn't know.

This wasn't the usual line about self-experimentation. Read any book about it, such as Lawrence Altman's *Who Goes First? The Story of Self-Experimentation in Medicine*, and you will come away thinking that self-experimentation is done by selfless doctors to test new and dangerous treatments. My experience was different. I wasn't a doctor. I wasn't trying to help someone else. I didn't test a dangerous new treatment. Unlike the better-known sort of self-experimentation, which usually confirms what the experimenter believes, my self-experiments had shown I was wrong.

From my acne research I learned that self-experimentation can be used by non-experts to (a) see if the experts are right and (b) learn something they don't know. I hadn't realized such things were possible. The next problem I tried to solve this way was early awakening. For years, starting in my twenties, I woke up early in the morning, such as 4 A.M., still tired but unable to go back to sleep. Only a few dreary hours later would I be able to fall back asleep. This happened about half of all mornings. It showed no sign of going away. I didn't want to take a pill for the rest of my life—not that there are any good pills for this—so I didn't bother seeing a doctor. The only hope for a good solution, as far as I could tell, was self-experimentation.

So I did two things:

1. I recorded a few details about my sleep. The main one was whether I fell back asleep after getting up. How often this happened was my measure of the severity of the problem. In the beginning, I couldn't fall back asleep about half of all mornings.
2. I tested possible solutions.

The first thing I tried was aerobic exercise. It didn't help. Early awakening was just as common after a day with exercise as after a day without exercise. I tried eating cheese in the evening. It didn't help. I tried several more possible remedies.

None helped. After several years, I ran out of things to try. All my ideas about what might help had proved wrong.

Yet I managed to make progress. For unrelated reasons, I changed my breakfast from porridge to fruit. A few days later, I started waking up too early *every* morning instead of half the time. The problem was now much worse. This had never happened before. I recorded the breakfast change on the same piece of paper I used to keep track of my sleep, so the correlation was easy to see. To make sure the correlation reflected causality, I went back and forth between fruit and porridge. The results showed it was cause and effect. Fruit for breakfast caused more early awakening than porridge for breakfast. After ten years when nothing I'd done had made a difference, this was a big step forward. I eventually figured out that any breakfast made early awakening more likely. A long experiment confirmed this. The best breakfast was no breakfast.

I was less surprised than you might think. I knew that in a wide range of animals, including rats, a laboratory result called *anticipatory activity* is well established. If you feed a rat every day at the same time, it will become active about three hours earlier. If you feed it at noon, it will become active about 9 A.M. I had been eating breakfast at about 7 A.M. and waking up about 4 A.M. I had essentially found that humans were like other animals in this regard.

Not eating breakfast reduced early awakening but didn't eliminate it. In the following years, self-experimentation taught me more about what caused it. By accident, I found that standing helped. If I stood more than eight hours in a day, I slept better that night. That wasn't practical—after trying to stand that much for several years, I gave up—but the realization helped me make another accidental discovery 10 years later: standing on one leg to exhaustion helps. If I do this four times (left leg twice, right leg twice) during a day, even in the morning, I sleep much better that night. More recently, I've found that animal fat makes me sleep better.

Both effects are dose-dependent. I can get great sleep if I stand enough and great sleep if I eat enough animal fat.

How much animal fat is "enough"? I've just started trying to figure this out using pig fat, which I consume in a cut called pork belly (the part of the pig used for bacon). I found that 150g (5oz) of pork belly had a little effect; 250g (9oz) of pork belly had a much clearer effect. The effect seems to get larger with more pork belly (e.g., 350g/12oz). Because pork belly may be more than 90% fat by calories (there is great variation from one piece to the next), it's a lot of calories of fat to get the maximum possible effect. I need to burn a lot of calories per day to make that many calories easy to eat, but it's in some respects more convenient than standing on one foot.

Acne and sleep were my first self-experimental topics. Later I studied mood, weight control, and the effects of omega-3 on brain function. I learnt that self-experimentation has three uses:

1. **To test ideas.** I tested the idea that tetracycline helps acne. I tested ideas about how to sleep better. And I've tested ideas derived from surprises. A few years ago, while trying to put on my shoes standing up, I realized my balance was much better than usual. I'd been putting on my shoes standing up for more than a year; that morning it was much easier than usual. The previous evening I'd swallowed six flaxseed-oil capsules. I did self-experiments to test the idea that flaxseed oil improves balance. (It did.)
2. **To generate new ideas.** By its nature, self-experimentation involves making sharp changes in your life: you don't do X for several weeks, then you do X for several weeks. This, plus the fact that we monitor ourselves in a hundred ways, makes it easy for self-experimentation to reveal unexpected side effects. This has happened to me five times. Moreover, daily measurements—of acne, sleep, or anything else—supply a baseline that makes it even easier to see unexpected changes.
3. **To develop ideas.** That is, to determine the best way to use a discovery and to learn about the underlying mechanism. After I found that flaxseed oil improved balance, I used self-experimentation to figure out the best dose (three to four tablespoons per day).

One complaint about self-experimentation is that you're not "blind". Maybe the treatment works because you expect it to work. A placebo effect. I have never seen a case where this appeared to have happened. When treatment 10 helps after treatments 1 through 9 have failed to help (my usual experience), it's unlikely to be a placebo effect. Accidental discoveries cannot be placebo effects.

My experience has shown that improve-your-life self-experimentation is remarkably powerful. I wasn't an expert in anything I studied—I'm not a sleep expert, for example—but I repeatedly found useful cause-and-effect relationships (breakfast causes early awakening, flaxseed oil improves balance, etc.) that the experts had missed. This isn't supposed to happen, of course, but it made a lot of sense. My self-experimentation had three big advantages over conventional research done by experts:

1. **More power.** Self-experiments are far better at determining causality (does X cause Y?) than conventional experiments. Obviously they're much faster and cheaper. If I have an idea about how to sleep better, I can test it on myself in a few weeks for free. Conventional sleep experiments take a year or more (getting funding takes time) and cost thousands of pounds. A less obvious advantage of self-experimentation is that more wisdom is acquired. We learn from our mistakes. *Fast* self-experimentation means you make more mistakes. One lesson I learned stands out: *Always do the minimum*—the simplest, easiest experiment that will make progress. Few professional scientists seem to know

this. Finally, as I mentioned earlier, self-experimentation is much more sensitive to unexpected side effects.

2. **Stone Age-like treatments are easy to test.** I repeatedly found that simple environmental changes, such as avoiding breakfast and standing more, had big and surprising benefits. In each case, the change I'd made resembled a return to Stone Age life, when no one ate breakfast and everyone stood a lot. There are plenty of reasons to think that many common health problems, such as diabetes, high blood pressure and cancer, are caused by differences between modern life and Stone Age life. Modern life and Stone Age life differ in many ways, of course; the fraction of differences that influence our health is probably low. If so, to find aspects of Stone Age life that matter, you have to do many tests. Self-experiments, fast and cheap, can do this; conventional experiments, slow and expensive, cannot. In addition, conventional research is slanted towards treatments that can make money for someone. Because conventional research is expensive, funding is needed. Drug companies will fund research about drugs, so lots of conventional research involves drugs. Elements of Stone Age life (such as no breakfast) are cheap and widely available. No company will fund research about their effectiveness.
3. **Better motivation.** I studied my sleep for 10 years before making clear progress. That sort of persistence never happens in conventional health research. The reason is a difference in motivation. Part of the difference is how much the researcher cares about finding solutions. When you study your own problem (e.g., acne), you care more about finding a solution than others are likely to care. Acne researchers rarely have acne. And part of the motivation difference is the importance of goals other than solving the problem. When I studied my sleep, my only goal was to sleep better. Professional scientists have other goals, which are enormously constraining.

One set of prison bars involves employment and research funding. To keep their jobs (e.g., get tenure, get promoted, get jobs for their students and get grants), professional scientists must publish several research papers per year. Research that can't provide this is undoable. Another set of prison bars involves status. Professional scientists derive most of their status from their job. When they have a choice, they try to enhance or protect their status. Some sorts of research have more status than others. Large grants have more status than small grants, so professional scientists prefer expensive research to cheap research. High-tech has more status than low-tech, so they prefer high-tech. As Thorstein Veblen emphasized in *The Theory of the Leisure Class* (1899), useless research has higher status than useful research. Doing useless work, Veblen said, shows that you are higher-status than those who must do useful work. So researchers prefer useless research, thus the term "ivory tower". Fear of loss of job, grant or status also makes it hard for professional scientists to propose radical new ideas. Self-experimenters, trying to solve their own problem on their own time, are not trapped like this.

Acne illustrates the problem. The dermatological party line is that diet doesn't cause acne. According to a website of the American Academy of Dermatology, "extensive scientific studies" show it's a "myth" that "acne is caused by diet". According to "guidelines for care" for dermatologists published in 2007, "dietary restriction (either specific foods or food classes) has not been demonstrated to be of benefit in the treatment of acne". In fact, there is overwhelming evidence linking diet and acne. Starting in the 1970s, a Connecticut doctor named William Danby collected evidence connecting dairy consumption and acne; it is telling that Danby wasn't a professional scientist. When his patients gave up dairy, it often helped. In 2002, six scientists (none a dermatologist) published a paper with the Weston Price–like conclusion that two isolated groups of people (Kitava Islanders and Ache hunter-gatherers) had no acne at all. They had examined more than 1,000 subjects over the age of 10 and found no acne. When people in these groups left their communities and ate differently, they did get acne. These observations suggest that a lot of acne—maybe all of it—can be cured and prevented by diet.

Why is the official line so wrong? Because the painstaking research needed to show the many ways diet causes acne is the sort of research that professional researchers can't do and don't want to do. They can't do it because the research would be hard to fund (no one makes money when patients avoid dairy) and because the trial and error required would take too long per publication. They don't want to do it because it would be low-tech, low-cost and very useful—and therefore low-status. While research doctors in other specialities study high-tech expensive treatments, they would be doing low-cost studies of what happens when you avoid certain foods. Humiliating. Colleagues in other specialities might make fun of them. To justify their avoidance of embarrassment, the whole profession tells the rest of us, based on "extensive scientific studies", that black is white. Self-experimentation allows acne sufferers to ignore the strange claims of dermatologists, not to mention their dangerous drugs (such as Accutane). Persons with acne can simply change their diets until they figure out what foods cause the problem.

Gregor Mendel was a monk. He was under no pressure to publish; he could say whatever he wanted about horticulture without fear for his job. Charles Darwin was wealthy. He had no job to lose. He could write *On the Origin of Species* very slowly. Alfred Wegener, who proposed continental drift, was a meteorologist. Geology was a hobby of his. Because they had total freedom and plenty of time, and professional biologists and geologists did not (just as now), Mendel, Darwin and Wegener were able to use the accumulated knowledge of their time better than the professionals. The accumulated knowledge of our time is more accessible than ever before. Self-experimenters, with total freedom, plenty of time and easy access to empirical tests, are in a great position to take advantage of it.

TOOLS AND TRICKS

Seth Roberts, "Self-Experimentation as a Source of New Ideas: Ten Examples Involving Sleep, Mood, Health, and Weight", ***Behavioral and Brain Science*** **27 (2004): 227–88 (www.fourhourbody.com/new-ideas)** This 61-page document about self-experimentation provides an overview of some of Seth's findings, including actionable sleep examples.

The Quantified Self (www.quantifiedself.com) Curated by *Wired* co-founding editor Kevin Kelly and Gary Wolf, a managing editor of *Wired*, this is the perfect home for all self-experimenters. The resources section alone is worth a trip to this site, which provides the most comprehensive list of data-tracking tools and services on the web (www.fourhourbody.com/quantified).

Alexandra Carmichael, "How to Run a Successful Self-Experiment" (www.fourhourbody.com/self-experiment) Most people have never systematically done a self-experiment. And yet, it's one of the easiest methods for discovering what variables are affecting your well-being. This article shows you the five principles that will help you get started in running successful self-experiments. Bonus: an 11-minute video from Seth Roberts, discussing experiment design.

CureTogether (www.curetogether.com) CureTogether, which won the Mayo Clinic iSpot Competition for Ideas That Will Transform Healthcare (2009), helps people anonymously track and compare health data to better understand their bodies and make more informed treatment decisions. Think you're alone with a condition? Chances are you'll find dozens of others with the same problem on CureTogether.

Daytum (www.daytum.com) Conceived by Ryan Case and Nicholas Felton, Daytum is an elegant and intuitive service for examining and visualizing your everyday habits and routines.

Data Logger (http://apps.pachube.com/datalogger) Data Logger for iPhone enables you to store and graph any data of your choosing along with a time-stamp and location. It can be used for anything, whether food-related, animal sightings or temperature sensor readings around your neighbourhood. If you can think of it, it can be recorded and tracked.

SPOTTING BAD SCIENCE 101

How Not to Trick Yourself

Nothing is more irredeemably irrelevant than bad science.
—John Polanyi, Nobel Prize winner in chemistry

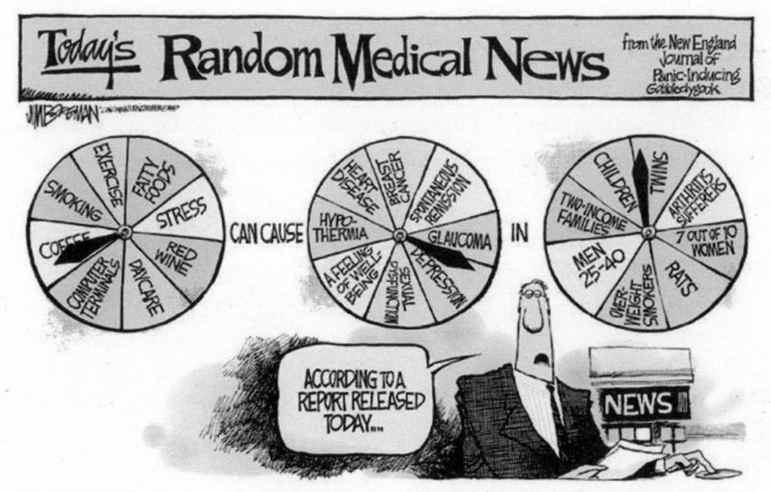

JIM BORGMAN © *Cincinnati Enquirer*. Reprinted with permission of UNIVERSAL UCLICK. All rights reserved.

"Panel Urges Hour of Exercise a Day"
—***New York Times***, September 2002

"Why Exercise Won't Make You Thin"
—***Time***, August 2009

"Low-Carb Fad Fades, and Atkins Is Big Loser"
—***Washington Post***, September 2005

"Low-Carb Diets Combat Metabolic Syndrome"
—***Washington Post***, July 2007

It gets tiring, doesn't it? Scientists seem to change their minds every six months. Eggs and butter will kill you, so you turn to margarine and turkey bacon. Now margarine will kill you and one egg a day is okay?! It almost seems better to opt out completely and live in ignorance.

Fortunately, science isn't arbitrary. In fact, you just need to learn a few simple concepts to separate the truth (or probable truth) from complete fiction.

Most research is presented to the public through media or propagandists with agendas. Since diet is most often hijacked for selling newspapers and ideologies, we'll use *almost*-believable diet nonsense to develop our BS metre. To create the most perfect you, you need to know which science to follow and which "science" to ignore.

After reading the next eight pages, you will know more about research studies than the average MD.

The Big Five

The Big Five are important to understand, as they are the tools most often used to exaggerate and brainwash.

They are also critical to grasp so you don't trick yourself or waste time with false leads as a self-experimenter. I've phrased each concept as a question you should ask yourself when looking at diet advice or the "latest research".

1. IS A RELATIVE CHANGE (LIKE PERCENTAGES) BEING USED TO CONVINCE?

This concept is best illustrated with two potential news headlines.

"Studies Show People Who Avoid Saturated Fat Live Longer"

Should you start avoiding saturated fat?

First, find out exactly what "longer" means. Based on available data, it turns out that reducing your saturated fat intake to 10% of daily calories for your entire adult life would add only 3–30 days to your lifespan. Considering this, is the trouble worth it if a rib-eye steak is one of your pleasures in life? Probably not.

"People Who Drink Coffee Lose 20% More Fat
Than Those Who Don't"

Should you start drinking coffee?

Leaving aside the question of whether or not this is an observational study (discussed next), it's worth looking at that mighty impressive 20%.

Relative increases or decreases, most often expressed as percentages, can be misleading.

Relative isn't enough. It's critical to ask what the *absolute* increase or decrease was—in this case, how many kilograms of fat did both groups actually lose, and over what period of time? In most cases, percentages are used in media and sales brochures to mask the fact that changes were minuscule.

If it were 113g (0.25lb) lost for the control group and 136g (0.30lb) (20% more) for the coffee group over eight weeks at three cups per day, is picking up the coffee habit worth the side effects of high-dose caffeine? Nope.

Distrust percentages in isolation.

2. IS THIS AN OBSERVATIONAL STUDY CLAIMING TO SHOW CAUSE AND EFFECT?

This is the mother lode. If you learn just one concept in this chapter, learn this one. It's the cardinal sin.

Observational studies,[3] also referred to as *uncontrolled* experiments, look at different groups or populations outside the lab and compare the occurrence of specific phenomena, usually diseases. One example is the often misinterpreted "China study".

Here is the most important paragraph in this chapter:

Observational studies cannot control or even document all of the variables involved. Observational studies can only show correlation: A and B both exist at the same time in one group. They cannot show cause and effect.[4]

In contrast, randomized and controlled experiments control variables and can therefore show cause and effect (causation): A causes B to happen.

The satirical religion Pastafarianism purposely confuses correlation and causation:

> *With a decrease in the number of pirates, there has been an increase in global warming over the same period.*
>
> *Therefore, global warming is caused by a lack of pirates.*

Even more compelling:

> *Somalia has the highest number of Pirates AND the lowest carbon emissions of any country. Coincidence?*

Drawing unwarranted cause-and-effect conclusions from observational studies is the bread-and-butter of media and cause- or financially driven scientists blind to their own lack of ethics.

Don't fall for Pastafarianism in science.

3. Also called *population, cohort* or *epidemiological* studies.
4. The one exception is if the effect is so huge that it can't be explained in any other way. For instance, the twentyfold increased risk of lung cancer that is associated with cigarette smoking in multiple studies.

It is critical *not* to take advice based purely on observational studies. In 2004, a commentary published in the *International Journal of Epidemiology* titled "The hormone replacement–coronary heart disease conundrum: is this the death of observational epidemiology?" highlighted the dangers of doing so. Observation of one group of women using hormone replacement therapy (HRT) showed lower heart disease, and media and HRT proponents were fast to promote this sound-bite conclusion: **HRT reduces heart disease!** Sadly, randomized and controlled trials (RCT) later showed no protective effects, and even a slight increase of risk, for heart disease among those using HRT.

How was this possible?

It turns out that the observational studies didn't sufficiently account for different socioeconomic statuses between groups, or for the influence of doctors selecting women for HRT who were less predisposed to heart disease to begin with. The latter is an example of how failing to randomly assign subjects to groups (randomization) leaves observational studies open to bias from experimenters.

The 2004 hindsight commentary stated, rightly:

> *The differing results between observational studies and RCT [randomized and controlled trials] in the association between HRT and CHD throw this idea [that well-conducted observational studies can produce similar estimates of treatment effects as RCT] into question and may signify the death of observational epidemiology.*

Observational studies are valuable for developing hypotheses (educated guesses that can then be tested in controlled settings) but they cannot and should not be used to show cause and effect. To do so is both irresponsible and potentially dangerous.

3. DOES THIS STUDY DEPEND ON SELF-REPORTING OR SURVEYS?

In 1980, scientists at an isolated research station in Antarctica had test subjects weigh and record all of the food they consumed. Once a week, the subjects were asked to recall what they had eaten the day before (food, keep in mind, they had weighed and recorded in their notebooks). Despite all the attention to logging meals, the men still underestimated their intake by 20–30%.

Granted, these might have been blizzard-blind men. Hardly normal circumstances. Let's look at how the real professionals do it.

The Women's Health Initiative (WHI) was a massive $415 million (£259 million) project conducted under the auspices of the National Institutes of Health (NIH) and involving nearly 49,000 women. It was designed to investigate a number of health issues, including the effect of low-fat diets on cancer, over an eight-year period. It was a large-scale intervention study, often viewed by media as the gold standard in nutrition research. Dr. Michael Thun of the American Cancer Association went so far as to call the WHI "the Rolls-Royce of studies".

The *New York Times* announced the results in 2006 with a headline that was crystal clear:

"LOW-FAT DIET DOES NOT CUT HEALTH RISKS, STUDY FINDS"

Though I agree with the conclusion based on other data, the WHI study couldn't possibly conclude this. Let's look to Michael Pollan for a peek under the hood at one of the most common weaknesses of nutritional studies: self-reporting.

> *To try to fill out the food-frequency questionnaire used by the Women's Health Initiative, as I recently did, is to realize just how shaky the data on which such trials rely really are.... It asked me to think back over the past three months to recall whether when I ate okra, squash or yams, were they fried, and if so, were they fried in stick margarine, tub margarine, butter, "shortening" (in which category they inexplicably lump together hydrogenated vegetable oil and lard), olive or canola oil or nonstick spray? I honestly didn't remember, and in the case of any okra eaten in a restaurant, even a hypnotist could not get out of me what sort of fat it was fried in....*
>
> *This is the sort of data on which the largest questions of diet and health are being decided in America today.*

Other WHI questions include:

> *When you ate chicken or turkey, how often did you eat the skin?*
> *Did you usually choose light meat, dark meat or both?*
> *In the last three months, how many times have you eaten a 78g (2¾oz) serving of broccoli?*[5]

How would you do? Think you can pull off recollection within 20% of reality? Let's test the last 24 hours.

Do this: estimate the number of calories you ate and drank yesterday, without using any references, as well as the fat calories you consumed. Then eat the same meals and snacks, but weigh it all in grams on a portable kitchen scale. Measure drinks using a measuring jug. Use www.nutritiondata.com to determine the 100-gram caloric value of each food and do the maths.[6]

Unless you are a professional athlete and can distinguish between a 150g (5oz) serving of steak and a 200g (7oz) serving, the difference between your self-reporting and your weighing analysis will shock you. Combine that misreporting across 49,000 people and you can imagine the rather Picasso-like picture it creates.

Granted, self-reported data can be useful, especially when recording in real time (i.e., recording something as it happens). This has become easier with technology that

5. Michael Pollan, "Unhappy Meals", *New York Times*, 28 January 2007, sec. Magazine.
6. Caloric-value-of-100g/100g = X/number-of-grams-weighed.

takes memory out of the equation, such as DailyBurn's FoodScanner iPhone application and the Withings wifi scale.[7]

To the greatest extent possible, avoid studies that depend on *after-the-fact* self-reporting. Trust your own data. Just record it when things happen.

4. IS THIS DIET STUDY CLAIMING A CONTROL GROUP?

Desirable as it may be, it is almost impossible to change just one macronutrient variable (protein, carbohydrate, fat) in a diet study. It is therefore almost impossible to create a control group.

If a researcher makes such a claim and vilifies a single macronutrient, your sceptical spider sense should tingle.

Let's suppose that someone claims that a study on the effects of a low-fat diet proves it's healthier than a higher-fat diet. There is a control group.

First things first: if you decrease fat or cholesterol in a whole-food diet, you'll be removing fat *and* protein, which means you must add carbohydrate to make the diets equal in calories. If you don't, you have unequal calories as another variable. If you make this caloric correction by adding carbohydrate elsewhere, now you face a conundrum: not only are you comparing a higher-fat and a lower-fat diet, but you're simultaneously comparing a higher-protein and a lower-protein diet, as well as a higher-carb and a lower-carb diet.

How can we know which is responsible for what?

We can't.

Self-experimentation actually offers an unexpected advantage here.

The "control" is everything you've tried up to a certain point that hasn't produced a desired effect. Isolating one variable is often less important than the sum impact of a group of changes. In other words, has *your* body fat per centage gone up or down in the last two weeks of replacing diet A with diet B? If you weren't losing fat on A and now you are, A was your control.

In an ideal (but unattractive) test, you would go back to A and see if body fat then moves in the other direction. Then repeat the switch again. This would minimize the possibility that the first change in body fat just happened to coincide with the change in diet to B.

Alas, this switching would also maximize your likelihood of going insane. If something seems to be working, just stick with it.

5. DO THE FUNDERS OF THE STUDY HAVE A VESTED INTEREST IN A CERTAIN OUTCOME?

Beware of unholy unions between scientists and funding sources.

Fred Stare, founder and chair of the Nutrition Department at Harvard University, obtained a $1,026,000 (£640,000) grant from General Foods in 1960.

7. Even without such tools, if you have large samples and the analysis is good, it is *sometimes* possible to correct for subjective error and reconstruct the information you want.

These manufacturers of the sugar-rich Post cereals, Kool-Aid, and the Tang breakfast drink would be subsidizing the "expansion of the School's Nutrition Research Laboratories". In the decade that followed, Stare became the most public and reputable defender of sugar and modern food additives, all the while receiving funding from Coca-Cola and the National Soft Drinks Association, among others. Does this prove malfeasance? No. Does it show that funding, support that can be discontinued, often comes from those most likely to benefit? Yes. People respond to incentives.

Simple due diligence: Peruse the required "conflicts of interest" section in studies or reviews related to diet and look for "consulting fees". If McCorporation or the XYZ Lobby decides it's too obvious to fund studies directly, hiring researchers as consultants can be an indirect means to the same end. James Hill of the University of Colorado, as one example, is well known for attempting to discredit the relationship between obesity and higher insulin levels caused by sugar consumption. In his stated conflicts of interest, you will see that he has received consulting fees from Coca-Cola, Kraft Foods and Mars Corporation (makers of Snickers, M&Ms and Mars Bars).

Does this make him guilty of skewing data to serve corporate interests? No. But it should make you look closely at the studies themselves before accepting the headlines and making behavioural changes in your life.

The Goal of this Chapter v. the Goal of this Book

Understanding how to act under conditions of incomplete information is the highest and most urgent human pursuit.
—*Nassim Taleb,* The Black Swan

Are the experiments in this book bulletproof? Far from it. All studies are flawed in some respect, often for legitimate cost or ethical considerations.

I use myself as a single subject, and (with a few exceptions) I neither randomize nor create a control. Some scientists will, no doubt, have a field day picking these self-experiments apart.

This doesn't bother me, and it shouldn't bother you.

The goal of this chapter is simple: since we often use published research as a starting point for self-experimentation, we want to ensure that we don't take false leads from tricksters or misinformed journalists with good intentions. Understanding the Big Five questions and the hallmarks of sensationalism puts you in a rare group: those who can depend on themselves, not the media, for nutritional guidance.

This opens doors that we can then crowbar and leverage for incredible effect.

My goal for the book is not, first and foremost, to identify the single variables that produce target changes. That is often the goal of clinical research for publication, but experimentation for self-improvement is a different beast.

It may be that alpha-lipoic acid does nothing in a given fat-loss cocktail; perhaps it's the angle of an exercise and not the load that triggers muscular gain; or it could be that spinach has none of the effects I predict, but other foods in the prescribed meal do. The exact mechanism doesn't much matter if we get the effects we want. . . without side effects.

Dr. Martin Luther King Jr. famously wrote that "justice too long delayed is justice denied". In the world of self-experimentation, where the outcomes are of personal importance, results too long delayed are results denied. This doesn't mean being haphazard. It's more than possible to tinker without hurting yourself. It means, however, that waiting for perfect conditions often means waiting forever.

In the world I live in, people want to lose fat or improve sexual performance now, not in five or ten years.

Let the journals catch up later—you don't have to wait.

GA

P-Value: One Number to Understand

Statistical thinking will one day be as necessary for effective citizenship as the ability to read and write.
—*H. G. Wells, who created national hysteria with his radio adaptation of his science fiction book* The War of the Worlds

British MD and quack buster Ben Goldacre, contributor of the next chapter, is well known for illustrating how people can be fooled by randomness. He uses the following example:

If you go to a cocktail party, what's the likelihood that two people in a group of 23 will share the same birthday? One in 100? One in 50? In fact, it's one in two. Fifty per cent.

To become better at spotting randomness for what it is, it's important to understand the concept of "p-value", which you'll see in all good research studies. It answers the question: how confident are we that this result wasn't due to random chance?

To demonstrate (or imply) cause-and-effect, the gold standard for studies is a p-value of less than 0.05 ($p < 0.05$), which means a less than 5% likelihood that the result can be attributed to chance. A p-value of less than 0.05 is also what most scientists mean when they say something is "statistically significant".

An example makes this easy to understand.

Let's say you are a professional coin flipper, but you're unethical. In hopes of dominating the coin-flipping gambling circuit, you've engineered a penny that should come up heads more often than a normal penny. To test it, you flip it and a normal penny 100 times, and the results seem clear: the "normal" penny came up heads 50 times, and your designer penny came up heads 60 times!

Should you take out a second mortgage and head to Vegas?

		RELATIVE IMPROVEMENT						
		1%	2%	5%	10%	20%	30%	50%
CONFIDENCE LEVEL	80%	44,750	11,225	1,814	461	119	119	21
	85%	87,891	17,030	2,757	699	180	180	31
	90%	103,830	26,045	4,209	1,069	275	275	47
	95%	171,069	42,911	6,934	1,761	453	453	78
	98%	266,691	66,897	10,809	2,745	706	706	121

The above sample size estimation tool, created by the web design and analytics firm WebShare, says: probably not, if you want to keep the house.

If we look at 20% improvement (60 flips v. 50 flips = 10 more flips) at the top and scan down to see how many coin flips you'd need per coin to be 95% confident in your results (p = 0.05), you'd need 453 flips.

In other words, you better make sure that 20% holds up with at least 453 flips with each coin. In this case, 10 extra flips out of 100 doesn't prove cause-and-effect at all.

Three points to remember about p-values and "statistical significance":

- **Just because something seems miraculous doesn't mean it is.** People are fooled by randomness all the time, as in the birthday example.
- **The larger the difference between groups, the smaller the groups can be.** Critics of small trials or self-experimentation often miss this. If something appears to produce a 300% change, you don't need that many people to show significance, assuming you're controlling variables.
- **It is not kosher to combine p-values from multiple experiments to make something more or less believable.** That's another trick of bad scientists and mistake of uninformed journalists.

TOOLS AND TRICKS

***The Black Swan* by Nassim Taleb (www.fourhourbody.com/blackswan)** Taleb, also author of the bestseller *Fooled by Randomness,* is the reigning king when it comes to explaining how we fool ourselves and how we can limit the damage. Our instinct to underestimate the occurrence of some events, while overestimating others, is a principal cause of enormous pain. This book should be required reading.

***The Corporation,* DVD (www.fourhourbody.com/corporation)** This is a disturbing documentary about the American corporation and its relentless pursuit of profit at the expense of our culture. This film gives you a glimpse into how heavily companies can skew health reports when they have a vested interest in the findings. See the next chapter.

"List of Cognitive Biases" (www.fourhourbody.com/biases) We are all susceptible to cognitive biases, including the scientists who produce "bad science". Review the list at this URL and ask yourself whether you're mindlessly accepting as fact things you hear or read.

SPOTTING BAD SCIENCE 102

So You Have a Pill...

This chapter was written by Dr. Ben Goldacre, who has written the weekly "Bad Science" column in the Guardian *since 2003 and is a recipient of the Royal Statistical Society's Award for Statistical Excellence in Journalism. He is a medical doctor who, among other things, specializes in unpacking sketchy scientific claims made by scaremongering journalists, questionable government reports, evil pharmaceutical corporations, PR companies and quacks.*

What I'm about to tell you is what I teach medical students and doctors—here and there—in a lecture I rather childishly call "Drug Company Bullshit". It is, in turn, what I was taught at medical school,[1] and I think the easiest way to understand the issue is to put yourself in the shoes of a big pharma researcher.

You have a pill. It's OK, maybe not that brilliant, but a lot of money is riding on it. You need a positive result, but your audience aren't homeopaths, journalists or the public: they are doctors and academics, so they have been trained in spotting the obvious tricks, like "no blinding" or "inadequate randomization". Your sleights of hand will have to be much more elegant, much more subtle, but every bit as powerful.

What can you do?

Well, firstly, you could study it in winners. Different people respond differently to drugs: old people on lots of medications are often no-hopers, whereas younger people with just one problem are more likely to show an improvement. So only study your drug in the latter group. This will make your research much less applicable to the actual people that doctors are prescribing for, but hopefully they won't notice. This is so commonplace it is hardly worth giving an example.

1. In this subject, like many medics of my generation, I am indebted to the classic textbook *How to Read a Paper* by Professor Greenhalgh at UCL. It should be a best-seller. *Testing Treatments* by Imogen Evans, Hazel Thornton and Iain Chalmers is also a work of great genius, appropriate for a lay audience, and, amazingly, also free to download from www.jameslindlibrary.org. For committed readers I recommend *Methodological Errors in Medical Research* by Bjorn Andersen. It's extremely long. The subtitle is *An Incomplete Catalogue.*

Next up, you could compare your drug against a useless control. Many people would argue, for example, that you should *never* compare your drug against placebo, because it proves nothing of clinical value: in the real world, nobody cares if your drug is better than a sugar pill; they only care if it is better than the best currently available treatment. But you've already spent hundreds of millions of pounds bringing your drug to market, so stuff that: do lots of placebo-controlled trials and make a big fuss about them, because they practically guarantee some positive data. Again, this is universal, because almost all drugs will be compared against placebo at some stage in their lives, and "drug reps"—the people employed by big pharma to bamboozle doctors (many simply refuse to see them)—love the unambiguous positivity of the graphs these studies can produce.

Then things get more interesting. If you do have to compare your drug with one produced by a competitor—to save face, or because a regulator demands it—you could try a sneaky underhand trick: use an inadequate dose of the competing drug, so that patients on it don't do very well; or give a very high dose of the competing drug, so that patients experience lots of side effects; or give the competing drug in the wrong way (perhaps orally when it should be intravenous, and hope most readers don't notice); or you could increase the dose of the competing drug much too quickly, so that the patients taking it get worse side effects. Your drug will shine by comparison. You might think no such thing could ever happen. If you follow the references in the back, you will find studies where patients were given really rather high doses of old-fashioned antipsychotic medication (which made the new-generation drugs look as if they were better in terms of side effects), and studies with doses of SSRI antidepressants which some might consider unusual, to name just a couple of examples. I know. It's slightly incredible.

Of course, another trick you could pull with side effects is simply not to ask about them; or rather—since you have to be sneaky in this field—you could be careful about how you ask. Here is an example. SSRI antidepressant drugs cause sexual side effects fairly commonly, including anorgasmia. We should be clear (and I'm trying to phrase this as neutrally as possible): I *really* enjoy the sensation of orgasm. It's important to me, and everything I experience in the world tells me that this sensation is important to other people, too. Wars have been fought, essentially, for the sensation of orgasm. There are evolutionary psychologists who would try to persuade you that the entirety of human culture and language is driven, in large part, by the pursuit of the sensation of orgasm. Losing it seems like an important side effect to ask about.

And yet, various studies have shown that the reported prevalence of anorgasmia in patients taking SSRI drugs varies between 2 per cent and 73 per cent, depending primarily on how you ask: a casual, open-ended question about side effects, for example, or a careful and detailed enquiry. One 3,000-subject review on SSRIs simply did not list any sexual side effects on its twenty-three-item side effect table. Twenty-three other things were more important, according to the researchers, than losing the sensation of orgasm. I have read them. They are not.

But back to the main outcomes. And here is a good trick: instead of a real-world outcome, like death or pain, you could always use a "surrogate outcome", which is easier to attain. If your drug is supposed to reduce cholesterol and so prevent cardiac deaths, for example, don't measure cardiac deaths; measure reduced cholesterol instead. That's much easier to achieve than a reduction in cardiac deaths, and the trial will be cheaper and quicker to do, so your result will be cheaper *and* more positive. Result!

Now you've done your trial, and despite your best efforts things have come out negative. What can you do? Well, if your trial has been good overall, but has thrown out a few negative results, you could try an old trick: don't draw attention to the disappointing data by putting it on a graph. Mention it briefly in the text, and ignore it when drawing your conclusions. (I'm so good at this I scare myself. Comes from reading too many rubbish trials.)

If your results are completely negative, don't publish them at all, or publish them only after a long delay. This is exactly what the drug companies did with the data on SSRI antidepressants: they hid the data suggesting they might be dangerous, and they buried the data showing them to perform no better than placebo. If you're really clever and have money to burn, then after you get disappointing data you could do some more trials with the same protocol in the hope that they will be positive. Then try to bundle all the data up together, so that your negative data is swallowed up by some mediocre positive results.

Or you could get really serious and start to manipulate the statistics. For two pages only, this will now get quite nerdy. Here are the classic tricks to play in your statistical analysis to make sure your trial has a positive result.

Ignore the protocol entirely

Always assume that any correlation *proves* causation. Throw all your data into a spreadsheet programme and report—as significant—any relationship between anything and everything if it helps your case. If you measure enough, some things are bound to be positive just by sheer luck.

Play with the baseline

Sometimes, when you start a trial, quite by chance the treatment group is already doing better than the placebo group. If so, then leave it like that. If, on the other hand, the placebo group is already doing better than the treatment group at the start, then adjust for the baseline in your analysis.

Ignore drop-outs

People who drop out of trials are statistically much more likely to have done badly, and much more likely to have had side effects. They will only make your drug look bad. So ignore them, make no attempt to chase them up, do not include them in your final analysis.

Clean up the data
Look at your graphs. There will be some anomalous 'outliers', or points which lie a long way from the others. If they are making your drug look bad, just delete them. But if they are helping your drug look good, even if they seem to be spurious results, leave them in.

"The best of five... no... seven... no... nine!"
If the difference between your drug and placebo becomes significant four and a half months into a six-month trial, stop the trial immediately and start writing up the results: things might get less impressive if you carry on. Alternatively, if at six months the results are "nearly significant", extend the trial by another three months.

Torture the data
If your results are bad, ask the computer to go back and see if any particular subgroups behaved differently. You might find that your drug works very well in Chinese women aged 52 to 61. 'Torture the data and it will confess to anything," as they say at Guantanamo Bay.

Try every button on the computer
If you're really desperate, and analysing your data the way you planned does not give you the result you wanted, just run the figures through a wide selection of other statistical tests, even if they are entirely inappropriate, at random.

And when you're finished, the most important thing, of course, is to publish wisely. If you have a good trial, publish it in the biggest journal you can possibly manage. If you have a positive trial, but it was a completely unfair test, which will be obvious to everyone, then put it in an obscure journal (published, written and edited entirely by the industry). Remember, the tricks we have just described hide nothing, and will be obvious to anyone who reads your paper, but only if they read it very attentively, so it's in your interest to make sure it isn't read beyond the abstract. Finally, if your finding is really embarrassing, hide it away somewhere and cite "data on file". Nobody will know the methods, and it will only be noticed if someone comes pestering you for the data to do a systematic review. Hopefully, that won't be for ages.

THE SLOW-CARB DIET—194 PEOPLE

The following Slow-carb Diet data was collected with detailed questionnaires using CureTogether.com. 194 people responded to all questions, and 58% indicated it was the first diet they had ever been able to stick with.

The subjects were recruited via my top-1,000 blog (www.fourhourblog.com), Twitter (www.twitter.com/tferriss), and Facebook (www.facebook.com/timferriss).

	Average Weight Lost (st/kg)	**Number of People**
Everyone	1.5/9.5	194
Vegetarian	1.6/10.4	10
Non-vegetarian	1.5/9.5	178
Age		
15–20	1.1/7.3	19
21–30	1.4/9	86
31–40	0.7/10	56
41–50	1.5/9.5	26
51–60	2.1/13.6	5
61+	0.8/5	2
Men	1.6/10.4	150
Women	0.8/5.4	44
Kids	1.5/9.5	60
No kids	1.4/9	118
First-week loss	0.2/1.5	194
Second-week loss	0.22/1.4	194

	Average Weight Lost (st/kg)	Number of People
Third-week loss	0.23/1.5	194
Fourth-week loss	0.28/1.8	194
Skipped breakfast	1.6/10.4	29
Did not skip breakfast	1.5/9.5	157
Had breakfast within one hour	1.4/9	127
Did not have breakfast within one hour	1.6/10.4	61
Meals per day		
Two	2.8/17.7	8
Three	1.4/8.6	80
Four	1.4/9	64
Five	1.6/10.4	36
Followed the diet strictly	1.3/8.2	84
Modified the diet	1.6/10.4	104
Counted calories	1.9/12.2	35
Did not count calories	1.4/9	152
Exercised while dieting	4.5/10	144
Did not exercise while dieting	1.3/8.2	41
Started exercise after starting diet	1.8/11.3	68
Did not start exercise after starting diet	1.4/8.6	116
Women with children	0.9/5.4	16

DISTRIBUTION OF RESULTS	NUMBER OF PEOPLE
Gained 0–4.5st/0–10kg	4
Lost 0–0.7st/0–4.5kg	39
Lost 0.78–1.4st/5–9kg	68
Lost 1.5–2.14st/9.5–13.6kg	35
Lost 2.2–2.8st/14–18kg	16
Lost 2.9–3.6st/18.6–22.7kg	11
Lost >3.6st/>22.7kg	10

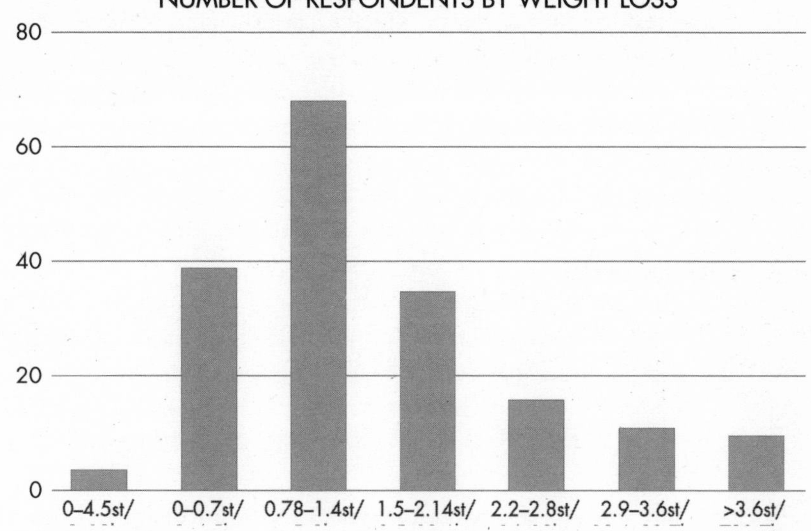

(Potential) Weaknesses of the Data

The data here, while fascinating, are not perfect. Here are two stand-out weaknesses of the methodology, and of polls in general:

PEOPLE COULD BE MAKING THINGS UP.

Though we removed obvious duplicates, omitted rubbish data ("I lost 11.8st/75kg!", "I weighed 2.5st/15.9kg at the beginning", etc.), and flagged questionable entries, no one was checking IDs or making in-person visits. Unless you're conducting a controlled trial, it's hard to avoid this problem.

THIS DATA SET MIGHT NOT ACCOUNT FOR DROP-OUTS—THE PEOPLE WHO TRIED AND GAVE UP.

Given the number of failures in the 3,000 comments reviewed, between 3% and 5%, one would expect more failures reported. Of 194 respondents, only four gained weight or remained the same. Don't forget: these respondents were reached after leaving comments on a blog post or self-selecting by responding to Twitter or Facebook.

The challenge of the missing drop-outs belies a common weakness with questionnaires that are open to the public: those most likely to respond are often those who have had positive results.[8] This is a form of *survivorship bias*, a concept well worth understanding.

8. Unless we're dealing with customer service complaints, in which case there is an incentive: something can be fixed after-the-fact.

Looking at average mutual fund returns from last year to pick a winner? Don't forget that you are asking the survivors. The casualties—what Nassim Taleb refers to as "silent evidence"—aren't around to be polled. The "average" returns are less impressive if you can include the people who bet the farm and lost. Finding those dead bodies is hard, especially in finances, when there is so much incentive to cover them up.

In practical terms, does this mean our diet results are bogus? Not at all. The possibility of survivorship bias isn't proof that the numbers aren't representative. Two things to keep in mind:

1. Based on all available empirical reports on the diet, the failure rate shouldn't exceed 5%. This is incredible by any conventional measure of diet compliance.
2. Nearly all reported failures are due to not following instructions.

If we include only those people who followed directions exactly and provided feedback, the success per centage is as close to 100% as I've seen anywhere.

Discussion of Results

How should you read these data? How should you plan or change your diet based on these results?

Let's look at where you might make common mistakes. This is a practice run of our Spotting Bad Science 101 training.

Taking a first glance at the data, there are a few things we might conclude produce greater fat loss, especially if we're presented with impressive-looking graphs that omit important details:

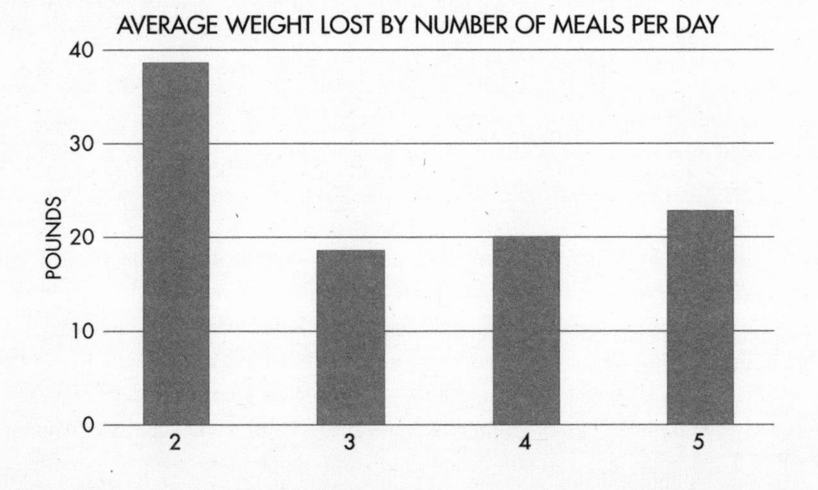

Based on the data, here are some knee-jerk conclusions we could make about variables that result in more weight loss (bolded below):

Eating just two meals per day, v. five meals, the second-most-common number of meals (2.8-v. 1.6st/17.7-v. 10.4-kg average loss)
Eating a vegetarian diet (1.6-v. 1.5st/10.4-v. 9.5-kg average loss)
Counting calories (1.9-v. 1.4st/12.2-v. 9kg average loss)
Skipping breakfast (1.6-v. 1.5st/10.4-v. 9.5-kg average loss)

Those of you who've been paying attention will realize that, for most people, I recommend the opposite of these four conclusions. Did I just get it all wrong? It wouldn't be the first time.

But let's look at those bolded conclusions again.

This time, the numbers in parentheses before 194 (X/194) indicate how many people (X) did what is mentioned out of the total number of subjects (194).

Eating just two meals per day v. five (2.8-v. 1.6st/17.7-v. 10.4-kg average loss) (8/194)
Eating a vegetarian diet (1.6-v. 1.5st/10.4-v. 9.5-kg average loss) (10/194)
Counting calories (1.9-v. 1.4st/12.2-v. 9-kg average loss) (35/194)
Skipping breakfast (1.6-v. 1.5st/10.4-v. 9.5-kg average loss) (29/194)

Remember that it's impossible to determine cause and effect from the above. These are correlations. The next step would be to test them with both control and experimental groups.

But in the meantime, let's look at two of our bolded knee-jerk conclusions:

EATING TWICE A DAY SEEMS LIKE A NO-BRAINER, BUT IT'S NOT.

2.8st (17.7kg) lost v. 1.6st (10.4kg) seems to paint a clear picture. But let's ask ourselves what we don't know: how many people tried two meals and dropped out because it didn't work? Only eight of 194 people ate two meals a day. Also, how big were the people who ate twice a day? Perhaps they were 17.8–21.4st (113–136kg), making it easier to rack up total stone (kilograms) lost, even though the weight lost as a per centage of body mass was more impressive for other smaller people. The vast majority of the total (144), those who averaged 1.3–1.4st (8.6–9kg) lost, ate three or four times per day, as recommended.

COUNTING CALORIES SEEMS LIKE A NO-BRAINER, BUT IT'S NOT.

1.9st (12.2kg) lost v. 1.4st (9kg)—again, the conclusion may seem obvious: calorie counting helps. Alas, it just ain't that simple. First, more than in any other cohort in these data, this is where I suspect survivorship bias applies. 35 of 194 respondents counted calories. How many tried to count calories, which I do not recommend, and quit the diet altogether after finding counting tedious, impossible or inconvenient? Second, do calorie counters really lose more weight because of counting calories? Or is it because they're more attentive to the tracking in general and hold themselves more accountable? I suspect these calorie counters did a better job, on average, in more important areas like tracking protein intake and recording exercise progression.

Does this mean you shouldn't track calories? Not necessarily. Feel free to test it. It's possible you'll be in the minority who benefit. If not, and if you're in the majority who find it boring and awful, just be sure to stop the calorie counting and return to basics before you quit the entire programme.

Conclusion

Though the data can point in interesting directions for further testing, I'll let someone with more budget and interest attempt the controlling. The upshot is: The Slow-carb Diet works.

If you want to replicate the formula that has proven most effective for the most people, follow the rules in "The Slow-carb Diet".

Enjoy cheat day. For that matter, eat a chocolate croissant for me. Those bad boys are delicious.

SEX MACHINE II

Details and Dangers

Too much of a good thing can hurt you. Toxicity is serious business. If the topics of testosterone and libido are important to you, it's better to know too much rather than too little. This chapter will help you avoid problems, provide more background, and amplify results by personalizing the prescription.

If overwhelmed after your first pass-through, just remember the synopsis in Sex Machine I, which wraps up the general programme in concise terms. That said, do not ignore the warnings here.

Here's the nitty-gritty on both protocols.

Protocol #1: Long-term and Sustained

FERMENTED COD LIVER OIL + VITAMIN-RICH BUTTER FAT— TWO CAPSULES UPON WAKING AND TWO CAPSULES BEFORE BED

I began taking fermented cod liver oil and butter fat after conversations with several MDs trained at Harvard and UCSF who cited the findings of Weston A. Price (1870–1948).

Price, nicknamed "the Charles Darwin of Nutrition", was a researcher and dental surgeon who travelled the world throughout the 1930s recording the health and whole-food diets of isolated indigenous populations. Using meticulous notes and hundreds of photographs, he then compared each group with members of the same populations who had moved into cities and adopted industrialized diets. Through hundreds of settlements in 14 countries, from the remote villages of Lötschental, Switzerland, to the Jalou tribes of Kenya, from the American Indians to the Aborigines, he documented a diverse range of traditional diets.

Some contained almost no plants, while others contained a plethora; some ate nearly all food cooked, whereas others preferred all foods, even animal meats, raw. Despite these differences, there were a few commonalities among the diets of the groups with the least incidence of disease. Three types of food are of particular interest in our libido discussion:

1. Lacto-fermented foods such as sauerkraut, kimchi or Japanese natto, which appear a few times in this book, were staples.
2. 10 -fold the U.S. consumption level of vitamin D and vitamin A (animal-based retinol, not plant-based carotene) were consumed from sources such as egg yolks, fish oils, butter, lard and foods with fat-rich cellular membranes (fish eggs, shellfish and offal).
3. The diets included foods rich in what Price called "Activator X", now thought to be vitamin K(2) based on analysis performed by Chris Masterjohn. Common sources included fish eggs, cod liver oil, offal, and the deep yellow butter from cows eating rapidly growing green grass. If "Activator X" is, in fact, vitamin K(2), then Japanese natto is perhaps the best traditional source at 1,103.4 micrograms per 100 grams. It outguns goose liver pâté (yum) (369 micrograms) in second place and the hard cheeses (76.3 micrograms) in third place by almost 3 times and 14 times, respectively.

Why are these three relevant to our discussion?

Vitamin A has a direct positive effect on testosterone production in adult testes, and supplementation along with zinc has been shown to be as effective as anabolic steroid administration (oxandrolone and testosterone depot) in stimulating growth and puberty, the latter defined as an increase in testicular volume of 12 milliliters or more.

Vitamin K(2) activates vitamin A- and D-dependent proteins by conferring upon them the physical ability to bind calcium. Dr. Price had no shortage of real-world examples of how K(2) amplifies the effects of A and D:

Cod liver oil, which is high in both vitamins A and D, partially corrected growth retardation and weak legs in turkeys fed a deficiency diet, but the combination of cod liver oil and high-Activator X butter was twice as effective.

It has also been hypothesized that vitamin D toxicity is often a result of vitamin K deficiency. If you choose to supplement with vitamins A and D, as I do with cod liver oil and liquid vitamin D, it is important to ensure adequate K(2). Suggested sources include butter from grass-fed cows and the aforementioned lacto-fermented foods.

In practice, and as a personal example, this just means I have a few forkfuls of kimchi or sauerkraut in the morning while I wait for my scrambled eggs[9] to cook in—what else?—butter from grass-fed cows. Easy peazy.

VITAMIN D3—6,000–10,000 IU PER DAY FOR FOUR WEEKS

One of the top sports scientists in the United States, who wished to remain anonymous, recounted a single anecdote that led me to a closer re-examination of vitamin D:

9. Don't put the sauerkraut or kimchi in the eggs. I tried it and it's horrific.

One NFL player I ended up treating had experienced debilitating shoulder pain for years and had two surgeries as a result, all to little or no effect. Upon testing his vitamin D levels, it became clear that he was severely deficient. Six weeks after taking vitamin D, his shoulder pain was nonexistent. He had two surgeries for no reason.

Vitamin D, it turns out, does a lot more than most vitamins.

Once vitamin D is activated within the body as calcitriol, it acts as a steroid hormone and regulates more than 1,000 vitamin D-responsive genes, including those that code for specific muscle fibres. It can increase the size and number of type 2 (fast-twitch) fibres, which, as indicated earlier, have the greatest potential for growth. It is one of the most overlooked "sleeper nutrients", according to John Anderson, professor emeritus of nutrition at the University of North Carolina.

The effect can be substantial. Even at just 1,000 IU[10] daily for two years, 48 elderly females deficient in vitamin D (as I was) *tripled* their per centage of fast-twitch muscle fibres and *doubled* fibre diametre in functional limbs. The control group experienced no gains.

Peak athletic performance appears to begin when blood levels approach those obtained through *persistent* full-body exposure to natural summer sun: **50 ng/ml**.

Do you think you get enough sun? It's unlikely. Even in the endless summer of subtropical Miami, a surprisingly high incidence of vitamin D deficiency has been recorded, as most people either use sunblock or avoid prolonged sun exposure. Forty per cent of Louisiana-based runners tested in another study, all of whom trained outdoors, registered insufficient vitamin D levels. Indoor workers and athletes are top candidates for major insufficiencies: Lovell and collaborators found 15 of 18 elite female gymnasts tested to have levels below 30 ng/ml, and 6 to have levels below 20 ng/ml.

Simple at-home tests (see the resources listed in the "Getting Tested" appendix) can tell you where you are, and consistent UV-B or sun exposure (20–30 minutes at least twice per week, depending on latitude), along with sublingual D3, can get you to our minimal target of 50 ng/ml. More than 100 ng/ml is considered excessive, and more than 150 ng/ml is considered toxic.

If you don't get tested and blindly take vitamin D, you run the risk of overdose. One mild overdose symptom can be a metallic taste in the mouth, which Neil from "Occam's Protocol" experienced. In our rush to start the programme, and based on the average deficiencies I'd seen in the blood reports of past subjects, we neglected to get his vitamin D tested. I didn't realize that he surfed for several hours a day.

Establish your baseline first.

My Experience

Baseline from first blood test: **32 ng/ml**

Second test on 8/20/09 (after two months of taking 1,000 IU/day and

10. In this case, ergocalciferol, a form I advise against taking; use the more common cholecalciferol instead.

20 minutes of sun exposure daily): **35 ng**
Third test 5 weeks later on 9/25/09 (after increasing intake to 7,200 IU/day): **59 ng/ml**

I split the 7,200 IU into two doses: 1.5 droppers full of Now® liquid vitamin D3 upon waking and again before bed. It's important to test droppers, rather than trust label claims: even though the bottle claims 5,000 IU per dropperful, the average dropper yield was just 24 drops and 4 drops is 400 IU, so the average full dropper therefore contained 2,400 IU—roughly half of the label claim.

I saw the greatest impact on performance once I crossed the 50 ng/ml barrier and reached 55 ng/ml, after which the effects plateaued. The performance enhancement of vitamin D is well documented, at least as a result of using UV lights:

> *In 1944, German investigators irradiated 32 medical students, twice a week for 6 wk, finding irradiated students showed a 13% improvement in performance on a bike ergometer, whereas performance of the control students was unchanged. In 1945, Allen and Curaton measured cardiovascular fitness and muscular endurance for 10 wk in 11 irradiated male Illinois college students, comparing them with 10 matched unirradiated controls, both groups undergoing similar physical training. The treatment group achieved a 19.2% standard score gain in cardiovascular fitness compared with a 1.5% improvement in the control students.*

Shed some light on yourself or take some drops.

Supplemental vitamin D increases your need for vitamin A, so don't forget the aforementioned cod liver, which includes both.

SHORT ICE BATHS AND/OR COLD SHOWERS—10 MINUTES UPON WAKING AND BEFORE BED

Using ice baths and cold showers to affect sex hormones is largely untested in the literature, but there appear to be plausible mechanisms.

The preoptic area of the anterior hypothalamus is responsible for regulating thermogenesis—the generation of heat in response to cold exposure. The very same preoptic area *also* contains most GnRH-releasing neurons, making it a primary site of GnRH production. Pulses of GnRH, you might recall, then trigger either FSH (low-frequency pulses) or LH release (high-frequency pulses).

Looking at blood test changes after removing and then reincorporating both baths and showers as an isolated variable, I believe intermittent cold exposure has a positive impact on high-frequency pulses of GnRH, resulting in higher levels of LH and testosterone.

Protocol #2: Short-term and Fun

20–24 HOURS PRIOR TO SEX

The evening before your target sex day, consume at least 800 milligrams of cholesterol within two hours of bedtime.

I've duplicated the sex-drive-increasing effect in more than a dozen trials, which began with high-dose grass-fed beef at 450–560g (16–20oz) per sitting. I initially thought that higher meat consumption was accountable. Based on the literature, it seems that overfeeding or carnitine could be responsible, the latter of which has been shown to be important for sperm production (spermatogenesis) and quality (motility).

GA

The problem with this hypothesis is that four ounces of beef steak contain 56–162 milligrams of carnitine. Grass-fed beef is higher in L-carnitine content and (in general) the redder the meat, the higher the carnitine content. But even if we assume the higher per gram (ounce) value of 37.5 milligrams (150 milligrams in 115g/4oz) for medium-rare grass-fed beef, we'd need to consume 1.5kg (53oz) of meat to reach the clinical dosing of two grams per day. Even for an avid meat-eater, this is disgusting. Though I suspect there are non-trivial effects at doses less than two grams per day, I wanted to look for alternative explanations.

The simple solution was found in eggs.

I wanted to isolate cholesterol as a variable because of its potential dose-dependent SHBG-lowering effect, and a single large egg yolk provides more than two-thirds of the USRDA cholesterol limit of 300 milligrams, meaning 200 milligrams per yolk.

The minimum threshold for a *very* noticeable effect appeared to be 800 milligrams of cholesterol, or four whole eggs.

If you want a tasty bonus, add in reduced-fat Swiss cheese, which has the highest levels of CLA (conjugated linolenic acid) of all cheeses, with natural Muenster in second place.

FOUR HOURS PRIOR TO SEX

4 Brazil nuts
20 raw almonds
2 capsules of the aforementioned cod/butter combination

Brazil Nut Explanation: I began consuming Brazil nuts for selenium, as I tested deficient in this trace mineral after sending blood samples to SpectraCell, the same micronutrient testing lab allegedly used by Lance Armstrong.

Brazil nuts have been shown in clinical studies to be more effective than supplementation for increasing selenium, which is important in our context, as selenium has been shown to increase sperm production and sperm quality. Both good things for the twins.

But why was I deficient in selenium in the first place? Was it simply because I didn't eat enough selenium-containing foods like beef?

Or, and this is critical, was something else competing with selenium or removing it from my body? This is the more neglected question. It is also a bigger problem, as you can't fix it by slamming pills or potions.

Based on a review of published studies, I formed three hypotheses related to my selenium deficiency:

1. Even though I consumed large quantities of supposedly selenium-rich animal foods, like beef (200g/7oz satisfies the daily USRDA), the animals grazed on grass from selenium-depleted soil.
2. Going in and out of ketosis had created a selenium deficiency. Unbeknownst to me, long-term ketogenic dieting has been associated with selenium deficiency. This was a real lightbulb moment.
3. Selenium protects against mercury by binding to it. Elevated blood mercury levels, which I tested positive for, could therefore also contribute to selenium deficiency.

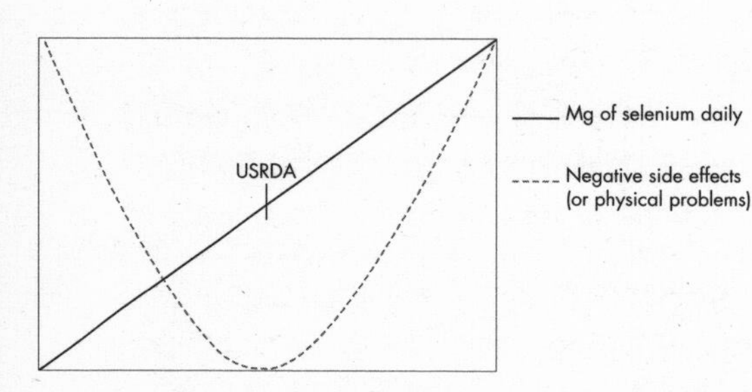

Once I had a few plausible explanations, it was time to test corrective actions:

Corrective action #1: I began to consume three Brazil nuts at breakfast and three Brazil nuts at bedtime. Too much selenium hurts swimmies, so I kept well within the tolerable upper limit for adults, which is 400 micrograms per day. 30g (1oz) of Brazil nuts (approximately 11 nuts) provides 544 micrograms, so 400 micrograms is approximately eight nuts per day (49 micrograms each). I am consuming six to play well within non-toxic ranges. I experimented twice with higher ranges of 8–10 nuts per day; in both cases, I immediately broke out in the worst acne of my life. Though selenium deficiencies can cause skin problems, it appears that excessive selenium, or at least Brazil nuts, can do the same.

Corrective action #2: Second, I am ensuring that I exit ketosis at least once per week by consuming carbohydrates à la the Saturday cheat day on the Slow-carb Diet. Since I have tested deficient, I am also consuming one cheat meal every other week for Wednesday lunch, which generally includes a single bowl of brown rice with a Thai meal.

Corrective action #3: I began to attempt to remove mercury from my body without killing myself. Despite multiple DMPS IV chelation sessions, urine tests showed almost no noticeable changes in mercury levels. To date, chelation has not shown benefits, but I plan to experiment with a more extended protocol of 3 days on, 11 days off using EDTA suppositories (fun, fun!) to avoid the often severe side effects of oral chelation.

Almonds Explanation for Testosterone Boost: Almonds were an accidental discovery.

Late one evening, after realizing my bachelor refrigerator contained nothing but alcohol and various disgusting protein powders, I descended on a single large bag of almonds out of desperation. I was starving and ate about 30 almonds (30g/1oz).

The following day, I had a much higher than normal sex drive and was puzzled. I was able to correlate it with the almond intake only after looking at a detailed food log. But what in almonds could have this effect? The only potential mechanism seemed to be high vitamin E content.

Lo and behold, after this first experience, I tested deficient for vitamin E on the same SpectraCell test that uncovered the selenium issue.

Looking more closely at the research studies on PubMed, I realized vitamin E not only had the potential to counter the oxidative stress that lowers testosterone and sperm production, but it had also been used successfully in combination with selenium and vitamin A (amazing coincidence, right?) for treating partial androgen deficiency in males.

Most interesting to me, vitamin E stimulates the release of luteinizing hormone-releasing hormone (LHRH) from the hypothalamus.

Bingo.

30g/1oz (30 almonds) gives you approximately 40% of your daily value (DV). I consume both raw almonds and organic almond butter to reach no more than 150% DV, often having two heaped tablespoons of the latter on celery sticks with breakfast.

Like most things, too much vitamin E is as bad as too little. Rock it like Goldilocks: get it just right and get levels tested every two to three months. The results appear to be worth it.

• • •

I do not have explanations for the apparent additive impact of several of the ingredients in the protocol cocktail, but removing any one piece seems to decrease the libido effect.

To confirm this, I've systematically removed each item. For example, I stopped vitamin D intake for six weeks while increasing Brazil nuts to eight per day. My testosterone jumped to 835 (normal is 280–800), but my libido and vitamin D decreased, the latter to 31.3 (normal is 32–100).

Be smart and test regularly.

FIXING ONE PROBLEM, CAUSING ANOTHER: DEFICIENCIES CREATED BY COMMON DRUGS AND TRAINING

Even with the perfect diet, it is possible to develop nutrient deficiencies. How? By using drugs that prevent specific nutrient absorption, or by over-engaging in training that taxes a particular biochemical system.

Here is a small sample of drugs and training regimens matched to some of their associated deficiencies.

Have you used any of them?

Oral contraceptives
Used for: birth control
Associated deficiencies: folic acid, vitamins B-2, B-6, B-12 and C, zinc, magnesium

Stimulants (e.g., the "greenies" used by baseball players, the "go pills" used by air force pilots or high-dose run-of-the-mill caffeine)
Associated deficiencies: molybdenum, B-5, potassium, magnesium, vitamin C

Antibiotics
Used for: bacterial infections
Associated deficiencies: B vitamins, folic acid, vitamins D and K[11]

Antidepressants
Used for: depression
Associated deficiencies: vitamin B-2

Alcohol
Used for: recreation
Associated deficiencies: folic acid, thiamine, vitamin B-6

Anti-ulcer and heartburn medications
Associated deficiencies: vitamins B-12 and D, folic acid, and the minerals calcium, iron and zinc

Anticonvulsants
Used for: epilepsy, bipolar disorder
Associated deficiencies: biotin, folic acid, vitamins B-6, D and K

Cholestyramine
Used for: high cholesterol
Associated deficiencies: vitamins A, D, E and K

11. Important note: There is also some evidence that select antibiotics may also make contraceptive pills less effective because of their negative impact on gut flora and absorption of oestrogens. To prevent unplanned pregnancy, consult with your doctor if taking antibiotics while on birth control.

Nitrous oxide
Used for: dental anaesthesia, recreation
Associated deficiencies: vitamin B-12

Chemotherapy drugs
Used for: cancer treatment
Associated deficiencies: folic acid

Antipsychotics
Used for: schizophrenia, bipolar disorder
Associated deficiencies: vitamins B-2 (riboflavin) and D

Anticoagulants (e.g., warfarin)
Used for: atrial fibrillation, preventing blood clots
Associated deficiencies: vitamins E and K

Anti-inflammatories (corticosteroids)
Used for: arthritis, rashes, asthma, hepatitis, lupus, Crohn's disease, eye inflammation, adrenal insufficiency
Associated deficiencies: calcium, DHEA, magnesium, melatonin, potassium, protein, selenium, vitamins B-6, B-9, B-12, C and D, zinc

Metformin
Used for: type 2 diabetes
Associated deficiencies: folic acid, vitamin B-12

Anabolic-androgenic steroids
Used for: muscular growth, athletic performance, wasting/immune disease
Associated deficiencies: vitamins B-6, B-9, B-12, C and D

Clenbuterol
Used for: asthma, fat loss among bodybuilders
Associated deficiencies: taurine and cardiac magnesium (potentially fatal)

Training-specific deficiencies per Charles Poliquin:

Among throwing specialists (pitchers, shot-putters, etc.)
Characteristic: taxed GABA and nervous system
Associated deficiencies: taurine

NFL and NHL players and bodybuilders
Taxed system: muscular damage
Associated deficiencies: lysine

THE MEATLESS MACHINE I

Reasons to Try a Plant-Based Diet for Two Weeks

Bacon: the gateway meat.
—Pin on messenger bag in San Francisco

The Power of Positive Constraints

Limiting options is usually thought of as a bad thing.

But how would your speaking improve if you couldn't use the adjective "interesting" and had to be more precise?

How would your planning skills improve if you had to go without a mobile phone for two weeks?

In reality, there are both negative and *positive* constraints. The latter are often used in business to improve innovation and results in a specific area. The famous "lean manufacturing" at Toyota was a result of applying positive constraints to wasteful processes.

How do you apply this to diet? Simple: by eliminating certain foods for a limited period of time. For most omnivores, removing meat is the hardest, and—therefore—the most valuable. To quote Dr. John Berardi (a meat-eater, like me), whom we'll meet later: "In our quest for filling one-third of our plate with animal flesh, sometimes we forget to think about what the other two-thirds should be filled with."

The constraints of testing a primarily plant-based diet (what I'll refer to as "PPBD"), whether pescatarian, vegan, or elsewhere on the spectrum, demands a knowledge of food that transcends whatever you're eliminating. Even a two-week experiment produces huge permanent benefits.

For example: if you know you might become deficient in B-12 on a PPBD, you learn about B-12, you learn about B vitamins, and you learn about vitamins in general, which might then branch your interest out to desiccated liver (a good source), which leads you to eat grass-fed local beef once a week on Saturdays instead of choosing to be vegan.

It's about finding what's best for you.

I suggest a two-week PPBD test after 3–4 months on the Slow-carb Diet. No matter where you end up afterwards, the awareness will lead to better decisions that benefit appearance, performance and the planet as a whole.

Moving From Ideal to Practical: Five Steps

A few definitions are in order before we get started:

1. The term "vegetarian" is so overused as to be meaningless. I define it here as someone whose food volume is at least 70% plant-based by volume. This is the aforementioned primarily plant-based diet (PPBD), and this is the term I'll use in place of "vegetarian". On the Slow-carb Diet, I consume a 60% minimum PPBD, meaning that most meals are 60%+ plant-based; 6/10ths of each plate is covered in veggies of some sort.

2. I define "vegan" here as someone who consumes no animal products except insect-produced goods such as honey. The latter is controversial for some vegans, but that is an argument for another book.

If you are considering test-driving a PPBD, which I hope you will, I suggest that you make the transition from an animal-based diet gradual.

It's better for the environment if you locally source a 70% PPBD[12] indefinitely, rather than eat 100% vegan for two months and quit because you find it unsustainable. Some vegans, lost in ideological warfare, also lose sight of cumulative effects: getting 20% of the population to take a few steps in the right direction will have an infinitely greater positive impact on the world than having 2% of the population following a 100% plant-based diet. To both uninformed meat-eaters and vegetarians—stop ad hominem attacks and focus on the big picture.

Of course, there are many vegetarians and vegans who object to any consumption of animal products as immoral, even if the animals are raised in humane and sustainable conditions. I won't address that here, as too many subjective definitions are involved. Instead, I will focus on the nutritional and logistical implications of following a PPBD.

The following five-step sequence is simple to implement. Each step will make you a more conscious eater and serve to lessen your environmental impact:

12. This assumes the plants are not coming primarily from monocrops like soya, wheat and corn. I believe that industrial production of annual grains has done as much damage to the environment as factory farms, based on habitat destruction (and therefore species eradication) and carbon footprint data.

Step 1. Remove starches (rice, bread, grains) and add legumes. Dense products, like black bean burgers without buns, are encouraged. Binge on cheat foods once per week. Read the chapters on the Slow-carb Diet as a refresher, if needed.

Step 2. Ensure that all of your meat is pasture-raised, grass-fed, or sourced within 80km (50 miles) of your home.

Step 3. Eat meat only after 6:00 P.M. (what Mark Bittman and others refer to as the "vegan till 6" plan) *or* eat meat only on the weekends or on cheat days.

Step 4. Remove all meat except fish (pescatarian) and/or eggs and dairy (lacto-ovo vegetarian). Bill Pearl won Mr. Universe in 1967 and 1971 as a lacto-ovo vegetarian, and he built 52.5-cm (20 3/8-in) upper arms at 15.6st (99kg). Red meat is not a requirement for growth.

Step 5. Eat a 100% plant-based vegan diet.

Removing too much, too quickly leads to abandoning positive changes. Skipping steps in this process usually creates a caloric void that makes you (1) feel terrible and revert to old habits or (2) fill the void with vegetarian junk food like processed fake meat, chips, agave nectar and sugar milk labelled as soya or almond milk.

Take it one step at a time, and stop when you've reached your sustainable threshold. I have experimented up to #5, but most consistently operate at #2.

Getting Organized

Make no mistake: In a world of ubiquitous meat and cheap animal protein, you will need to be more organized than your carnivorous cousins.

How organized depends on your ambition. Becoming a fit "vegetarian" requires much less diligence than becoming a record-breaking vegan athlete.

We'll look at the entire spectrum with real-world examples, including a slow-carb dieter, one of the most famous ultraendurance athletes of all time, and an omnivore scientist who tested veganism on himself for 28 days.

My goal is to help you follow your own ethical or environmental guidelines without causing undue damage to yourself or your wallet. This chapter will also answer the most popular questions submitted by vegans among my 100,000+ Twitter followers:

How do I get enough protein on a vegan diet?
How can I do it without soya?
What can I eat as a vegan while travelling?
Which supplements should I use to prevent deficiencies?

Since these are the greatest concerns, let's address them before jumping into the case studies:

HOW DO I GET ENOUGH PROTEIN ON A VEGAN DIET. . . WITHOUT SOYA?

Answer: first, we must define "enough".

By most carnivorous standards, the endurance athletes profiled in this chapter consume insufficient protein, yet they are able to compete at the highest levels in their sports. It's not limited to running, either. Mike Mahler, one well-known vegan strength athlete, consumes 100–130g (3½–4½oz) per day on training days and approximately 90g (3¼oz) per day on non-training days. Given his bodyweight of 14st (89kg) and assumed lean body mass of 80kg (177.3lb) (10% body fat), this computes as a high end of 0.73 grams per kilogram of lean bodyweight on training days and 0.51 grams per kilogram of lean bodyweight on non-training days. Dr. John Berardi, whom we'll meet later, consumes a great deal more, but let's adopt Mahler's range as a target.

How do you consume enough if you're aiming for a minimum of 0.5 grams per kilogram of lean bodyweight? To estimate this and err on the high side, just divide your bodyweight in half, (e.g., 10.7st/68kg ⟶ 75 grams of protein).

A high per centage of vegans use soy as their primary source of protein. This is a bad idea.

Based on all of the literature I've reviewed, the phytoestrogens in soya are dangerous for adults and, to a greater extent, children, even when used in moderation. Studies have demonstrated that just 30 grams of soya per day (about two tablespoons) for 90 days can disrupt thyroid function, and that's in Japanese subjects. The Swiss Federal Health Service equated **100 milligrams** of isoflavones (phytoestrogens) to a single birth control pill in terms of oestrogenic impact. How many birth control pills are you inadvertently eating each day?

FOOD	TOTAL ISOFLAVONES (IN 100G/3 ½OZ SERVING)
Instant soya beverage	109.51 mg
Raw soya beans (Japanese)	118.51 mg (in less than 76g/2 ½oz)
Fried tofu	48.35 mg (7–8 small pieces)
Tempeh	43.52 mg (in less than 167g/6oz)
Common infant soya formula	25 mg

Oestrogen overdosing isn't good for either gender, unless you're aiming for sterility.

So, how can you do it without soya?

Answer: Either extensive whole foods, which requires prep time, or powdered protein, which requires budget.

The whole-food options will be covered in the case studies, though you'll see some soya products creep in. For supplementation, the most consistently recommended protein powders among vegan athletes are:

Sun Warrior Chocolate Brown Rice Protein (rice protein)
Pure Advantage Pea Protein Isolate (pea protein)
Nitro Fusion Plant Fusion (rice, pea and artichoke protein)

I have also confirmed each of these as non-vomit-inducing when blended with 1–2 tablespoons of almond butter and either ice water, almond milk or coconut milk.

WHAT CAN I EAT AS A VEGAN WHILE TRAVELLING?

Answer: If we mean whole meals, the easiest is Mexican or Thai food, just as on the Slow-carb Diet.

Vegans opting for Mexican would order a number of side dishes like black beans (no lard), steamed veggies and extra guacamole (this is fat- and calorie-rich and not to be neglected), either eaten alone or with corn tortillas. I suggest avoiding wheat, as do the world-class vegan athletes I interviewed.

If caught in a bind with nothing but McDonald's and Pizza Hut in sight, a bag of 50+ raw almonds can sustain you for 10 or so hours until you find something more substantial. These can be found at almost all petrol stations and airport magazine shops.

Worst-case scenario, choose mild hunger over breaking your rules.

WHAT SUPPLEMENTS SHOULD I USE?

Answer: For essential insurance against serious health issues, ensure the following:

NUTRIENT	RECOMMENDED DAILY AMOUNT (USRDA)
Iodine	150 mcg
Lysine	12 mg/kg body weight
Biotin	30 mcg (no USRDA)
Vitamin K (kimchee, sauerkraut, etc.)	90 mcg women, 120 mcg men
Creatine[13]	5 grams per day (no USRDA)
Coconut milk (for saturated fats)	1/2 cup minimum (no USRDA)
Avocado (fat and potassium)	1–2 avocados (150 g/5 oz) (no USRDA)

13. How do you make vegetarians smarter? Have them take creatine. In one double-blind placebo-controlled study (http://www.ncbi.nlm.nih.gov/pmc/articles/PMC1691485/?tool=pmcenrez), 45 young-adult vegetarians were given 5 grams of creatine daily for 6 weeks, and the researchers concluded that "Creatine supplementation had a significant positive effect (p<0.0001) on both working memory (backward digit span) and intelligence (Raven's Advanced Progressive Matrices)". 2 grams per day did not replicate these results in separate studies.

My additional recommendations:

NUTRIENT	RECOMMENDED DAILY AMOUNT (USRDA)
Vitamin B-12	2.5 mcg
Essential fatty acids (Udo's Oil)	500 mg–4 g
Protein	55 g women, 65 g men
Calcium	1,000 mg
Iron	18 mg women, 8 mg men
Vitamin D	5 mcg minimum (see "Sex Machine")
Zinc	8 mg women, 11 mg men
Folic acid	400 mcg
Selenium	55 mcg
Riboflavin	1.1 mg women, 1.3 mg men
Vitamin E	15 mg

The most important caveat of all: we can only identify deficiencies, and therefore supplementation, for things that scientists have isolated.

See the conclusion of the next chapter for important warnings related to this.

The Case Studies

For each case study, I'll extract the most salient lessons and include both weekly grocery lists and, in athletic examples, go-to staple meals.

Marque Boseman (male)—Vegetarian
Athletics: Non-competitive athlete
Objective: Fat loss using the Slow-carb Diet
Weight: 13.5st (86kg) (15.7st/100kg prior to diet)
Height: 170cm (5ft 7in)
Weekly food cost: $60 (£37)
Weekly food complexity: Low

Scott Jurek (male)—Vegan
Athletics: World-class ultraendurance runner
Objective: Endurance
Weight: 11.8st (75kg)
Height: 188cm (6ft 2in)
Weekly food and supplement cost: $400–500 (£250–312)
Weekly food complexity: High

Dr. John Berardi (male)—Omnivore (tested veganism for 28 days)
Athletics: Pro- and Olympic-level athletic coach, PhD in physiology
Objective: Strength
Weight: 13.3st (85kg)
Height: 175cm (5ft 9in)
Weekly food cost: $80 (£50)
Weekly supplement cost: $60 (£37)
Weekly food complexity: Moderate

The following case studies are not included in this chapter, sadly, due to space restraints, but they can be found at www.fourhourbody.com/vegan-athletes.

Steph Davis (female)—Vegan
Athletics: World-class rock-climber
Objective: Endurance
Height: 166cm (5ft 5½in)
Weight: 8.4st (53kg)
Weekly food cost: $60–80 (£37–50)

Mike Mahler (male)—Vegan
Athletics: Strength athlete
Objective: Strength and metabolic conditioning
Height: 183cm (6ft 0in)
Weight: 14st (89.3kg)
Weekly food cost: $100–125/£62–78 (plus $60/£37 in supplements)

Marque Boseman

Marque Boseman lost 2.2st (14kg) on the Slow-carb Diet (13+ in the first month) while consuming no meat, and he has since moved to veganism.

Here is his basic profile:
35-year-old software engineer
Married, one daughter, one son on the way
Started at 15.7st (98kg) and 33% bodyfat
Ended at 13.5st (85.7kg) and 25% bodyfat

In just under three months, he lost 2.2st (14kg), 1.9st (12kg) of which was fat.
He ran 4.8km (3 miles), four days a week.
His cholesterol dropped from 220 to 160.

MARQUE'S GROCERY LIST

Marque spent just $60 (£37) per week on groceries, and his list requires 10–15 minutes of shopping:

Large cartons of egg whites and/or tofu/milk/veggie protein powder. I tried to get around 19 grams of protein per meal.
About 2 bags of black beans and/or chick peas and/or lentils. (Cheaper than canned.)
3–4 large bags frozen veggies
A jar of natural peanut butter no sugar added, or bulk nuts (easy way to supplement fats)
Flaxseed oil and/or olive oil and/or guacamole
Tahini (combine with chick peas and make hummus, good with the veggies)
Salsa (All natural and no sugar. Make it if you have the time. I put this on my eggs when I got bored.)

Exact portions aren't important, as adjustments will get you to your exact quantities by week three:

People may buy too little or too much the first week or two, but by week three they will know how much they need.

Marque explains his approach to tweaking the boilerplate Slow-carb Diet:

The insight that helped me adapt the slow-carb diet to vegetarianism came from using DailyBurn (www.dailyburn.com) to track my food.

After a few days of entering my food, I noticed that my nutrient ratios, calculated on DailyBurn, were 40:30:30 (carbs:protein:fats). My wife has always been big on the Zone Diet, so I recognized the ratio right away as identical. I was hitting this ratio daily just by following your instructions, but eating only egg whites for my protein. As long as I reduced my carb intake from beans and vegetables, to account for the additional carbs I took in with soy products and dairy, my ratios were the same and I continued to lose weight.

In other words: all of the protein sources in your original version are what I would refer to as "isolated" protein sources (chicken breast, fish, etc.) that contain almost no carbs. It's hard to find whole foods "isolated" protein sources as a vegetarian, so when I adapted this diet for vegetarianism, I thought of all the carbs in the protein-containing dairy or soy products as counting towards a total carb limit. I then subtracted veggies and legumes accordingly. For every 9 grams of carbs I got from a protein or fat source, I ate 9 grams of carb less from vegetable and legume sources. This helped me keep my ratios on track without much effort. The simplest solution to this problem is to avoid dairy and soy altogether, which I did for the most part.

One might ask: why didn't I just switch to the Zone Diet? I didn't switch because the slow-carb diet as described by you is simpler and doesn't allow for "less favorable" foods which give less favorable results. It keeps things simple and is easier to follow. If I had just one last tip for following the slow-carb diet as a vegetarian, it would be simple: eat extra good fats. Since you are missing fats from animal-based protein sources, you need to supplement with flaxseed oil,

(continues on next page)

MIKE MAHLER'S VANILLA WALNUT PROTEIN COOKIES

Mike Mahler does not fit the vegan stereotype.

He's trained athletes like former UFC champion Frank Shamrock, he can one-arm military press a 44-kg (97-lb) kettlebell 10 times, and can one-arm kettlebell snatch a 48-kg (105-lb) kettlebell 17 times with each arm. This is at a lean bodyweight of 14st (89.3kg).

He makes his own protein bars, and the following is his favourite recipe:

4 scoops of vanilla Sun warrior Protein Powder (60 grams of high-quality protein and iron)
2 tbsp almond butter (good protein, fat and magnesium)
1 tbsp cashew nut butter
3 tbsp flaxseed powder (contains omega-3 and fibre; increases ratio of good oestrogens to bad)
1 tbsp Maca (plant sterols, hormone support)
25g (1oz) walnuts
37g (1⅓ oz) Goji berries (high in vitamin A, vitamin C and iron)
2 tbsp mixed spice (loaded with healthy spices)
1 tsp agave nectar
350ml (12fl oz) water

Preheat oven to 220°C (425°F), Gas mark 7. Mix everything in a bowl with a spoon until a thick paste forms. Divide into eight parts, then shape into cookies. Place on baking sheets and bake for 15 minutes.

Total Nutrition Profile (all eight cookies)
Protein: 79 g
Carbohydrates: 63 g
Fat: 30 g

olive oil, and nuts. 0.5–1 tablespoon twice a day did it for me. If I didn't supplement fats, I felt tired and mentally off.

I have since become a vegan and removed soy from my diet completely. Currently my main source of isolated protein is pea and rice protein powders, my favorite being Plant Fusion by Nitro Fusion.

MARQUE'S FAVOURITE MEALS AND STAPLE MEALS

There is no need to complicate things:

> *One thing that has helped me a lot was to let go of the distinction between breakfast foods and "other meal" foods.*
>
> *My most frequent meal was eggs with salsa, some beans, probably some hummus, and some nuts. Often eggs were replaced by protein powder, salsa replaced by mixed veggies, and nuts replaced by flaxseed oil. I tried to keep it really simple.*

Choose a few meals and repeat. Simple wins.

Scott Jurek

Scott Jurek is a veritable demi-god in the sport of ultramarathoning, which involves races of more than marathon length. He has won the 161km (100-mile) Western States Endurance Run an incredible seven consecutive times, twice won the Badwater Ultramarathon, described as "the world's toughest race", and also holds the American record for 24-hour running, in which he logged 266.67km (165.705 miles) to beat Rae Clark's 20-year-old record.

SCOTT'S GROCERY LIST

Get ready to enter the mother lode. Scott's leave-no-stone-unturned approach is a sharp contrast to Marque's minimalism.

I had one of my unsuspecting researchers, Charlie Hoehn, head off to Whole Foods to gather the list and time himself, from entering the store to leaving the shop.

He arrived at Whole Foods at 3:38 P.M. and left at 6:20 P.M. for a total time of: **2 hours, 42 minutes.** This was, of course, a first-time expedition, and Charlie had to search for everything. To account for this, I had him review locations within the store the following day and then repeat the drill the day thereafter.

For the second round of timing, Charlie rearranged all of the items on the list into groups based on areas of the store (to cut down on walking back and forth), and he had a friend tag along to read the list and check off items. Charlie's job was pure speed.

Sprinting around the store behind the cart like a kid on a Nickelodeon shopping spree, he cut the total time in the store down to **1 hour.**

The total cost, regardless of time, was **$541.09 (£338)**.

Some of the items (supplements, protein powder) would be used over several weeks, so I also had Charlie determine the weekly cost for these items based on number of servings. This shaves off $121.83 (£76), giving you a new weekly total of **$419.26 (£262)**.

Scott's weekly shopping list is below, along with the substitute items Charlie bought (bolded) when he couldn't find them at Whole Foods. Keep in mind that this list is for a peak training period, when Scott would be consuming 5,000–6,000 calories/day at approximately 60–70% carbohydrate, 20–30% fat and 15–20% protein. Feel free to skim, as the list is three pages long:

79g (2.8oz) Green Magma by Green Foods
60 veg cap Udo's Choice Adult Probiotics by Flora Health
30 veg cap Udo's Choice Super Bifido Plus by Flora Health **(90 caps Nature's Way Primadophilus Bifidus)**

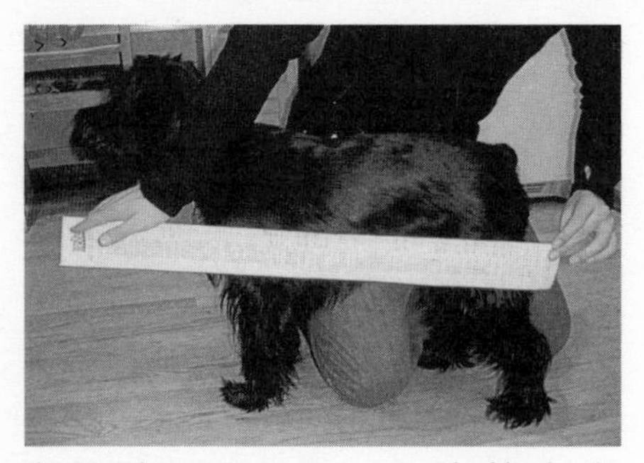

This 30-inch receipt represents one week of food in the life of ultra-runner Scott Jurek. It is compared here to Charlie's free-range black schnauzer, which was also bought at Whole Foods for a BBQ later that evening.

300g (10oz) raw organic almonds
525g (18½oz) raw organic dates from The Date People **(350g/12oz Whole Foods raw organic dates)**
850ml (30fl oz) Organic Hemp Protein + Fibre by Nutiva **(2 × 450ml (16fl oz) Bob's Red Mill organic hemp protein)**
14 organic bananas
2 bags frozen organic wild blueberries from Trader Joe's
1 bag frozen organic strawberries from Trader Joe's
1 bag frozen mango chunks from Trader Joe's
1 bag frozen pineapple chunks from Trader Joe's
1 bag frozen papaya chunks from Trader Joe's **(They didn't have papaya, so I got one more bag of frozen mango chunks; all fruit bags are Whole Foods brand)**
450g (1lb) raw organic carob powder from Earth Circle
225g (8oz) raw organic shredded coconut bulk from Earth Circle **(225g/8oz Let's Do . . . Organic! desiccated coconut)**
400g (14oz) Jarrow Fermented Soy Essence protein powder
115g (4oz) celtic sea salt bulk
60g (2oz) raw organic vanilla powder
225g (8oz) raw organic maca powder from Earth Circle
480ml (17fl oz) Udo's Oil DHA 3-6-9 Blend by Flora Health
480ml (17fl oz) Floradix Iron + Herbs by Flora Health
5 So Delicious Coconut Milk Yogurt Plain by Turtle Mountain

7 organic pink lady apples
8 organic valencia oranges **(Came in a bag of 12)**
6 organic grapefruit
7 organic pears
450g (1lb) raw agave nectar
450g (1lb) raw organic almond butter homemade with a Champion juicer **(Just bought Whole Foods raw organic almond butter instead of making it with a juicer)**
1 loaf Ezekiel 4:9 cinnamon raisin bread by Food 4 Life
450g (1lb) raw organic walnuts **(Got 350g/12oz)**
900g (2lb) dried organic polenta bulk
115g (4oz) raw organic yerba mate bulk **(Bought pre-packaged tea bags)**
60g (2oz) organic green tea bulk
7 Clif C Bars
450g (1lb) organic quinoa bulk
450g (1lb) organic brown rice bulk
225g (8oz) organic dried pinto beans bulk **(Bought 500g/1lb)**
225g (8oz) organic dried red lentils
115g (4oz) organic dried puy lentils
3 pkgs tempeh
850g (30oz) raw nigari tofu by Wildwood **(2 × 540g/9oz Denver Tofu)**
450g (1lb) organic Yukon or baby red potatoes
2 bunches organic lacinato kale
2 bunches organic rocket
1 head organic cos lettuce
4 organic carrots
2 organic yellow onions
2 heads organic garlic
2 organic red peppers
1 head organic broccoli
2 bunches organic collard greens
2 organic avocados
2 organic jalapeños
6 organic Roma tomatoes
225g (8oz) organic buckwheat soba noodles by Eden Foods
450g (1lb) whole wheat noodles by BioNature
1 cup nutritional yeast bulk
225g (8oz) organic Nama Shoyu
175g (9oz) organic miso paste by South Mountain **(8oz Miso Master organic)**
450ml (16fl oz) extra-virgin cold-pressed organic olive oil by Bariani **(480g/17oz Bella extra-virgin cold-pressed organic olive oil)**
425ml (15fl oz) extra-virgin coconut oil by Nutiva

225ml (8fl oz) organic unrefined sesame oil by Eden Foods **(Whole Foods brand)**
4 bars organic dark chocolate in various flavours by Dagoba
4 organic medium sweet potatoes
225g (8oz) raw organic pumpkin seeds bulk
225g (8oz) raw organic sunflower seeds bulk
115g (4oz) raw organic hemp seeds bulk
450g (1lb) ice cream
½ head organic cabbage
900g (2lb) container Clif Electrolyte Drink in Crisp Apple **(2 × 450g (16oz) Clif Quench Limeade)**
10 Clif Shot gels
5 pkgs Clif Shot Blocks

SCOTT'S FAVOURITE MEALS AND STAPLE MEALS

Breakfast or Post-workout Recovery

Blueberry Protein Power Shake

1 banana fresh or frozen (peel, break into 5cm/2in pieces, and freeze overnight in freezer-proof container or bag)
75g (3oz) presoaked almonds (soak the almonds in water 3–4 hours or overnight)
144g (5oz) frozen or fresh blueberries
600ml (20fl oz) water
3 tbsp hemp protein powder
3 tbsp Green Foods vegan protein powder
4 to 6 dates or natural sweetener
3 tbsp Udo's Oil DHA 3-6-9 Blend
½ tsp sea salt
½ tsp vanilla extract or raw vanilla powder

Blend all ingredients in a blender until smooth. Serves 4.

Go Raw Carob Cashew Smoothie

2 bananas fresh or frozen (peel, break into 5cm/2in pieces, and freeze overnight in freezer-proof container or bag)
75g (3oz) pre-soaked raw cashews (soak cashews in water 3–4 hours or overnight)
600ml (20fl oz) cups water
3 tbsp hemp protein powder
20g (¾oz) raw carob powder
3 tbsp Udo's Oil DHA 3-6-9 Blend

½ tsp sea salt
½ tsp vanilla extract or raw vanilla powder

Blend all ingredients in a blender until smooth. Serves 4.

Green Machine Pudding
1 banana
1 avocado
2 apples
2 pears
3 tbsp spirulina

Core apples and pears (leave skin on). Stone and scoop out avocado. Blend all ingredients in high-powered blender like a Vitamix 1–2 minutes or until very smooth. Should have a pudding consistency. Serves 4.

Lunch

Raw Dino Kale Salad
1 large or 2 small bunches black kale
1 small or ½ large ripe avocado
½–1 tsp sea salt
juice from 1–2 lemons or oranges
69g (2 ½oz) raw pumpkin seeds (soaked in 225ml/8fl oz of water, 4–6 hours)
2 tomatoes, chopped
*(for a bit of spice, but optional) Small pinch cayenne powder

Wash and chop off ends of kale (2.5cm/1in) and discard. Chop the rest of kale into 2.5–4cm (1–1½-in) pieces and place in mixing bowl. Deseed, scoop out and chop avocado. Add to kale along with sea salt and juice. Using a mixing spoon, massage the ingredients for 5 minutes until the avocado, salt and juice form a dressing and kale is fully covered. Add remaining ingredients and lightly mix. Salad can be served immediately or marinate for 1–2 hours at room temperature, allowing kale to absorb flavours. Serves 4–6.

On the Go Hummus
720g (1.5lb) beans
3 tbsp tahini
3 tbsp tamari
3 cloves garlic
60ml (2fl oz) lemon, lime or orange juice

½ tsp cumin
60–120ml (2–4fl oz) water

Process all ingredients except water in blender or food processor. Add a small amount of water at a time to keep ingredients moving in blender or processor, as needed. Great with tortillas or pitta and laced with Kalamata olives for trailside lunch on those long runs. For a great sandwich, add slices of red pepper, tomatoes and choice of salad. Serves 6–8.

Dinner

Dinner #1: Scott's Sweet Potatoes, Garlicky Greens, and Tempeh

Sweet Potatoes

4 sweet potatoes, sliced in wedges
1 tbsp olive or sunflower oil
1½ tsp sea salt
1 tsp paprika
1 tsp rosemary

Preheat oven to 190°C (375°F) Gas mark 5. Toss potatoes with oil and seasonings. Arrange on a preseasoned baking sheet. Bake for 20–30 minutes until potatoes are cooked through and lightly browned.

Garlicky Greens

1 tbsp olive oil
2 cloves garlic, finely chopped
1 jalapeño pepper, deseeded and finely chopped (optional)
1 bunch kale, collards or chard, deveined and coarsely chopped
½ tsp sea salt or tamari

Preheat frying pan and olive oil. Sauté garlic and pepper for 1–2 minutes. Add greens and salt. Sauté for 5–8 minutes. Serves 4.
Calories per serving: 230, carbs: 38 g, protein: 4 g, fat: 7 g

Lime Tamari Tempeh

1 225–350g (8–12oz) pkg tempeh
½ tsp olive oil
juice of one lime or lemon
1–2 tbsp shoyu or 2 tbsp miso mixed with 60ml (2fl oz) water

Pre-heat large frying pan with oil over a medium low-medium heat. Slice tempeh into 5–2.5mm (¼–⅛in) strips. Add tempeh to frying pan. Sauté for 5–8 minutes on each side or until lightly browned. Turn heat to very low or off, squeeze lime over tempeh and sprinkle tamari or shoyu and allow flavours to blend for 2–5 minutes.

Dinner #2: Tempeh Tacos

½ medium-sized onion, chopped
3 cloves garlic, finely chopped
1 jalapeño pepper, finely chopped
2 tbsp olive oil
2 300g (10-oz) pkgs tempeh, diced into 2.5mm (⅛in) cubes
4 tbsp Mexican seasoning
1 tsp salt
225ml (8fl oz) water
3 heaped tbsp chopped coriander
12 whole grain or corn tortillas
any combination tomatoes, avocados, cos lettuce, corrinder, peppers and jalapeños to garnish.

Sauté onion, garlic and jalapeño in olive oil until soft. Add diced tempeh and continue to sauté for 2 minutes. Add seasoning, salt and water. Cook the mixture 10–25 minutes, until enough liquid evaporates that you're left with a thickened sauce. Just before serving, add coriander and stir.

Heat tortillas over a griddle or a stove top grill pan or wrapped in foil in the oven. Fill each tortilla with 2–3 tbsp tempeh mixture and your choice of garnishes. Serves 4–6.

So how does an omnivore adapt when they try to move to a PPBD? That's where the next chapter and Dr. John Berardi come in. It's also where we'll look at the dangers of PPBDs and my conclusions.

TOOLS AND TRICKS

None! You'll need to read the next chapter to get those.

THE MEATLESS MACHINE II

A 28-day Experiment

John Berardi PhD specializes in exercise and nutrient biochemistry. He has published studies on subjects ranging from plant-based supplementation and probiotics to the effects of exercise on protein requirements.

Through his company, Precision Nutrition, he has coached more than 50,000 clients in 100+ countries. In the last two winter Olympic games alone, Dr. Berardi's athletes collected more than 20 medals, and he's consulted for teams including the Cleveland Browns, Toronto Maple Leafs, Texas Longhorns and the Canadian Olympic ski teams.

Individual athletes he's advised include:

UFC welterweight champion Georges St. Pierre
2006 Olympic cross-country skiing gold medalist Chandra Crawford
2010 Olympic skeleton gold medalist Jon Montgomery
2006 world rowing champion Jane Rumball
2010 Olympic bobsled gold medalists Steve Holcomb and Steve Messler
2009 Ironman Brazil winner Dede Griesbauer

Berardi is also a meat-eater who decided to follow an almost 100% vegan diet for 28 days (12 January 2009, to 8 February 2009) and attempt to gain muscular weight during it all.

It was an experiment many felt was destined to fail, and . . .

It succeeded.

He gained 0.5st (3.1kg): 4.9lb (2.2kg) of lean body mass and 2.1lb (953g) of fat.

Elegant Is Effective

John consumed the same meals every day for 30 days:

BEFORE BREAKFAST

5 tablets BCAA (Biotest—5 g total)
2 capsules resveratrol (Biotest)
1 multivitamin (Genuine Health)
1 tablet vitamin D (Webber Naturals—1,000 IU total)
1 serving sublingual B-12 (Webber Naturals—1,000 mcg total)
500ml (17fl oz) water

BREAKFAST

3 whole eggs with 1 slice cheese (this was the exception; discussed later)
2 slices sprouted grain bread
130g (4½oz) vegetables
500ml (17fl oz) water
225ml (8fl oz) green tea
1 tsp Lorna Vanderhaeghe's Omega Vega (provides about 150 mg DHA)

SNACK #1

244g (8½oz) homemade granola (mix includes pumpkin seeds, unsweetened coconut, whole oats, almonds, pecans, cashews, pistachios and dried fruit)
1 tbsp honey
225ml (8fl oz) unsweetened soya milk (So Nice® brand)[14]

LUNCH

123g (4½oz)) homemade hummus
2 whole wheat tortillas
130g (4½oz) veggies
88g (3oz) mixed beans (not canned)
1 sweet potato with cinnamon on top

SNACK #2

244g (8½oz) homemade granola (mix includes pumpkin seeds, unsweetened coconut, whole oats, almonds, pecans, cashews, pistachios and dried fruit)
1 tbsp honey
225ml (8fl oz) unsweetened soya milk

14. Berardi emphasized that he would use unsweetened almond milk in place of soya milk if he repeated the experiment.

WORKOUT DRINK

2 tsp BCAA (Xtreme Formulations—14 g total)
2 servings carbohydrate (Avant Labs—22 g total)
1,000ml water

AFTER WORKOUT

176g (6oz) mixed beans
200g (7oz) quinoa (measured uncooked)
260g (9¼oz) green veggies
2 cloves garlic
1 tbsp olive oil
1 tbsp garlic-chilli flaxseed oil from Jarrow Formulas (Omega Nutrition)
1 tbsp curry powder
1 multivitamin (Genuine Health)
1 tablet vitamin D (Webber Naturals—1,000 IU total)

BEDTIME SNACK

2 scoops protein (Genuine Health Vegan)
1 scoop greens (Genuine Health Perfect Skin)
Handful raw nuts
1 natural peanut butter and honey sandwich on 1 slice sprouted grain bread

When Scientists Become Guinea Pigs

As a trained scientist, John was able to pinpoint and explain the non-obvious, both physiologically and logistically.

First, an example of the former, fibre and lectin side effects:

> *High-calorie vegetarian meal plans are hard to digest. Diets high in plant foods contain a ton of fibre and lectins. Fibre is good for us in the right amount, but when fibre is consumed in excess, it prevents the digestion and absorption of other nutrients. It also upsets the stomach, leading to diarrhea, gas, and bloating.*
>
> *Furthermore, lectins can be problematic in and of themselves. Many people are lectin intolerant, and consumption leads to symptoms similar to lactose intolerance: massive bloating, flatulence, and diarrhea. In fact, when I followed my plant-based diet, by the end of the day, my waist circumference, which is 81cm (32in) upon rising, ballooned up to a full 107cm (42in). Not attractive, and very uncomfortable.*

Second, a logistical example: the importance of "batching" food prep and preparing certain foods in bulk a few days or a week in advance. This helps prevent defaulting to vegetarian junk foods:

With all my groceries at home, I did two things right off the bat.

First, I mixed up my granola and ate a big bowl.

Second, I started soaking the dry beans. By soaking beans for about 12 hours with a little baking soda mixed in, you can actually reduce the, ahem, gaseous effects of those little buggers. Also, this strategy helps to remove some of the anti-nutrients present in beans.[15]

About 12 hours later, I boiled two large pots of the pre-soaked legumes. One pot contained a mixture of navy beans, kidney beans, and garbanzo beans, along with red and green lentils. The other contained garbanzo beans only. When prepping the beans, I also pre-chopped some green peppers, red peppers, broccoli, cauliflower, mangetout, and sugar snap peas for the week. This way I couldn't use chopping as an excuse for missing a meal.

The mixed beans were stored in the fridge and the chick peas were then turned into homemade hummus and placed, with my pre-chopped veggies, on the wraps.

Questions with Dr. Berardi

WHAT WAS YOUR DAILY MACRONUTRIENT BREAKDOWN ON THIS DIET?

"The macronutrient breakdown, including supplements, was:

5,589 kcal [about the same as Scott Jurek during training]
247 g fat (38% of total caloric intake)
  68 g saturated
  64.5 g polyunsaturated
  92 g monounsaturated
653.7 g carbohydrate (46% of total caloric intake)
112 g fibre
246 g protein (16% of total caloric intake)

"Even with the high caloric load, without B-12 supplementation and vitamin D supplementation, I would have fallen short of the RDA [recommended daily allowance] for both nutrients. With the supplements, I was more than adequately covered."

15. This is another problem with eating a large volume of raw vegetables: "anti-nutrients". Anti-nutrients are so named because they prevent absorption of other nutrients, often essential minerals. Examples are phytic acid (interferes with calcium, zinc and copper), trypsin inhibitors and our bloat-causing friends, lectins, which act as enzyme inhibitors and prevent proper digestion. This is one of the reasons vegans can eat plenty of everything and still end up nutritionally deficient.

WHAT WAS YOUR FOOD COST FOR THE WEEK?

"During the plant-based experiment, I was spending about $80 (£50) per week for food. That's around $20–30 (£12.50–19) less than normal (i.e., when I'm eating a more varied diet that includes animal foods)."

WHAT IS YOUR BEST ESTIMATE OF YOUR SUPPLEMENT COST PER WEEK (UNDERSTANDING YOU MIGHT NEED TO DIVIDE SOME COSTS, AS A BOTTLE MIGHT LAST A WHILE)?

"During the experiment, I was using about $60 (£37) per week in supplements (BCAA, resveratrol, multi-vitamin, D, B-12, protein, greens, DHA, carb drink). That's about $20–30 (£12.50–19) more than I might normally spend for supplements.

"This means that, combining food and supplement costs, I spent the same amount total as when including animal products."

IF YOU HADN'T EATEN EGGS, WHAT DO YOU THINK WOULD HAVE HAPPENED?

"Same exact results, I think."

IF YOU'D CONTINUED THE PLANT-BASED DIET FOR SIX MONTHS, WHAT DO YOU THINK WOULD HAVE HAPPENED?

"I would have continued to gain weight, for sure.

"However, I think I might have created serious digestive problems. Many experts believe that continually eating foods that cause GI distress can lead to chronic gut inflammation, 'leaky gut syndrome', and a host of autoimmune problems."

VEGANS TALK ABOUT COMBINING FOODS FOR COMPLETE PROTEINS—RICE AND BEANS, FOR EXAMPLE, OR LEGUMES AND SEEDS OR NUTS. WHAT ARE YOUR THOUGHTS?

"The research is showing that, to prevent protein malnutrition, food combining isn't necessary. Rather, if all the essential amino acids are eaten in a single day, people are fine.

"However, from an optimization and sports performance perspective, I think that a complete complement of amino acids should be eaten each meal. There are some data to support that there's an 'amino-stat' in the brain that senses blood amino acids. And if we eat incomplete proteins, the body releases the 'missing' amino acids from muscle to balance out the blood amino acids. . . It's hard to build muscle or recover from training adequately if your diet is kicking off a muscle catabolic sequence."

IS IT POSSIBLE TO BE VEGAN LONG-TERM USING ONLY WHOLE FOODS AND WITHOUT PROTEIN SUPPLEMENTATION?

"Yes, without protein supplementation, it's totally possible, but it's much more difficult. And without some guidance, it's unlikely that people will do it properly if muscle building or high-level sport performance is the goal.

"But it is possible."

WHAT ARE THE MOST COMMON MISTAKES SELF-DESCRIBED "VEGETARIANS" MAKE?

"**Just dropping animal foods.** The worst mistake any would-be vegan could make is to simply stop eating meat. Then their lifestyle choice isn't a positive one, it's about negation.[16] Instead, people should focus on what they'll be eating more of. In other words, a proper vegetarian meal plan is based on eating mostly or only foods that come from plants: fruits, veggies, unprocessed grains, legumes, etc. It's not simply avoiding meat and filling up on processed junk foods. And this is something many vegetarians do. By focusing only on what they're dropping, there's no plan for getting enough calories, enough protein and enough micronutrition to ensure an easy transition to vegetarianism.

"**Using dairy for all their protein.** Many lacto-ovo vegetarians will turn to dairy for all their protein needs when dropping meat. This can be a big mistake for a few reasons. First of all, lactose-intolerance and milk protein allergy are quite common—more common than most people think. Second of all, most shop-bought milk and dairy offerings contain hormone and antibiotic residues, which are now being shown to negatively impact human health. Of course, in small doses (i.e., 225ml (8fl oz) of dairy per day), this isn't much of a problem unless you're highly sensitive, but using dairy multiple times per day can create big problems.

"**Not using supplements.** As discussed above, by dropping entire food groups from your menu, you're bound to create some dietary deficiencies if you're not careful. So you have to supplement, and very few vegetarian athletes know what to do in this regard.

"Use the supplements in my daily menu as a basic guide. It might seem like a pretty long list of nutrients to be mindful of, and it is. If you're going to make the lifestyle choice to become a vegan or vegetarian, you have to accept the responsibilities that such a choice foists upon you. If not, you're just being negligent, and you can expect health problems to follow."

WHAT DID YOU CONCLUDE AFTER THIS EXPERIENCE?

"I've come to conclude that vegetarianism can work, but this usually requires the help of a trained nutrition coach. Done right, vegetarianism can be satisfying, healthy, and performance-boosting.

16. Scott Jurek agrees: "I try to get people to think about what I eat, rather than what I do not eat, as that is how I look at it."

"That said, I've also concluded that vegetarianism is a real challenge for the average person. Without meticulous planning and some nutritional guidance, most are doomed to muscle loss, poor performance and a host of nutritional deficiencies, ranging from mild to severe.

"It's not a change to take lightly, and most people don't have the discipline to prevent digressions and corner-cutting that will have serious consequences over time."

Meat v. Plant—Bridging the Divide

Some of John's meat-eating supporters became enraged by his 28-day experiment, one going so far as to FedEx him grass-fed sirloin packed in dry ice. Carnivores can take vegetarianism very personally.

On the other side of the fence, die-hard vegans tore into him for compromising in a few areas and not going pure 100% vegan. Hate mail abounded.

As usual, the extremists on both sides were missing the point.

It was an experiment, not a moral statement, and there were valuable lessons to be learnt by purists from both sides.

For the militant vegans, the primary lesson is that omnivores can quickly transition to a near-vegan PPBD if they make some allowances for protein (such as two to three eggs per day). If this compromise isn't allowed, crossing the chasm can take months and, more often than not, never happens.

For the omnivores and carnivores, the benefits of considering a vegan diet are multifold, even if it's just a thought experiment: *If I couldn't eat any animal products for 28 days, what would I eat?*

John summarizes a few areas where *proper* vegans (the organized and informed minority) trump 99% of meat-eaters:

"Proper vegans tend to eat more whole, natural, locally produced and unprocessed foods than most omnivores. This means things like raw nuts and seeds, whole grains like quinoa and amaranth, and a locally grown bounty of fruits and veggies. That's all they eat, so they make sure to do it right.

"Speaking as an omnivore, in our quest for filling one-third of our plate with animal flesh, sometimes we forget to think about what the other two-thirds should be filled with. And that can be a big, gut-expanding, health-degrading mistake.

"Proper vegans also tend to spend more time learning about where their food comes from. In other words, they make it a point to understand which foods come from which regions of the world, which foods are in season during certain times of the year, and which methods are best for raising the healthiest food.

"Not only is this environmentally friendly and quite healthy, it's also pretty cool stuff to know."

RAW FOOD AND POTTENGER'S CATS: PANACEA OR MISINTERPRETED SCIENCE?

When Francis M. Pottenger Jr. was a newly graduated California doctor in 1932, he spent 10 years studying cats. Nine hundred cats over three generations, to be precise. Pottenger's experiments are often cited by raw-food enthusiasts as evidence of the superiority of raw food.

Experiment #1: Raw Meat v. Cooked Meat. Pottenger fed one group of cats a diet of two-thirds raw meat, one-third raw milk and cod liver oil. He fed the second group two-thirds cooked meat, one-third raw milk and cod liver oil. The cats fed raw meat were, by all measures, normal and healthy. The cats fed cooked meat produced kittens that had skeletal deformities, heart problems, vision problems, multiple infections, irritability, allergies, difficult births and even paralysis. Rut-roh!

Experiment #2: Raw Milk v. Cooked Milk. This time Pottenger had four groups of cats. The first group got two-thirds raw milk, one-third raw meat and cod liver oil. The other three groups got either two-thirds pasteurized milk, two-thirds evaporated milk or two-thirds sweetened condensed milk in place of the raw milk. He saw the same pattern of happy, healthy cats on raw milk, and all manner of abnormal development in the other groups, getting worse as the milk was more processed.

Based on these experiments, Pottenger concluded that "the elements in raw food which activate and support growth and development in the young appear easily altered and destroyed by heat processing". He went on to extrapolate that humans suffer from the same nutritional deficiencies that are causing more developmental problems with each generation: "canning, packaging, pasteurizing and homogenizing—all contribute to hereditary breakdown".

Hmmm. This sounds like a compelling, fear-inducing argument. But here's what Pottenger didn't know when he said this: cats need taurine.

Taurine is a component of bile acid that cats can't synthesize on their own, but humans can. It helps with digestion and is a supplement in commercial cat food. If cats are taurine-deficient, they show vision problems, heart problems and developmental problems. Sound familiar? Guess what else? Taurine is deactivated by heat. So Pottenger's cooked meat/milk diets would have been taurine-deficient.

Another factor to consider: cats are carnivores, humans are omnivores. It's like comparing apples to oranges, as we have different nutritional requirements. A better animal model for humans would be mice, or rats, or primates. Without even calling into question how well controlled Pottenger's study was, it doesn't make good scientific sense to transfer what he learnt about cats directly to humans.

But back to the crux of the debate: Should humans eat raw food or cooked food? It all depends. Here are some examples, each supported in the scientific literature:

FOOD	RAW OR COOKED?	GUIDELINES
Kidney beans	Cooked	Soak or cook your own, or use canned
Broccoli	Raw	Crunch away
Carrots	Cooked	Steam and purée
Tuna	Raw	Make sure it's sushi-grade tuna
Amaranth (grain)	Cooked	Mix with water, cook ten minutes or more
Beef	Cooked	Fry in pan instead of microwaving
Vegetables	Juiced	Juiced veggies show higher bioavailability nutrients compared to raw or cooked vegetables for breast cancer patients
Mussels	Raw	Slurp directly from shell
Tomatoes	Cooked	Cook with olive oil
Mung bean	Cooked	Germinate first, then cook
Cauliflower, cabbage, brussels sprouts, kale	Cooked	Steam until tender
Bread	Cooked (Duh)	Cut off the crust to avoid acrylamide exposure

By all means, go ahead and eat raw food if you like, or be vegan, or go gluten-free, or eat a few cats (I suggest fajitas). Just make sure you do your homework. Don't confuse ideology with good science. Take an honest look at the available research (applicable to humans) so that you can make a well-informed decision.

It's your body, after all.

Darwin's Rule—Eat for Fertility

So if vegetarianism can be done, why am I not a vegetarian in the usual sense?

To paint a one-sided picture of the benefits would be irresponsible, so allow me to explain the reasons:

1. I have been unable to find a single indigenous population that has thrived on a 100% PPBD, even after asking my 100,000+ Twitter followers to help me find one. Low animal product consumption is simple to find, but even the famous Jains of India are, with rare exception, lacto-ovo vegetarians. Dr. Weston Price (see "Sex Machine II") and others have been similarly unable to find a vegan indigenous culture in anthropological expeditions.

2. Our closest relatives, chimpanzees, are occasional meat-eaters, and humans produce the enzyme elastase, which serves to break down connective tissue for digestion.

There are, on both sides of the fence, avid debates of evolutionary biology and conflicting data points, but the argument-settling experience for me was empirical:

3. In the course of researching and interviewing for this book, I encountered dozens of former vegan women and would-be mothers who had miscarriage after miscarriage until they reintroduced animal products into their diets, after which they were able to become pregnant in a matter of weeks.

Based on the above and my own experiments, I've concluded that some form of animal product is necessary for proper hormone production. This could be due to the longer-chain fatty acids, saturated fat, cholesterol, fat-soluble vitamins, or (more likely) a combination of interdependent elements, some of which we haven't even identified. It's also possible that common vegetarian staples cause the problems, whether soya or gluten. Either way, it's significant that boys born with hypospadias, the opening of the urethra on the underside of the penis rather than at the tip, are five times more likely to have vegetarian v. omnivore mothers. Dr. Richard Sharpe, director of the Medical Research Centre for Reproductive Biology in Edinburgh, Scotland, echoes my conclusion about soya:

> *"I've seen numerous studies showing what soy does to female animals. Until I have reassurance that it doesn't have this effect on humans, I will not give soy to my children."*

Food is complex and humans are overconfident.

Consider the antioxidants we've identified thus far in garden-variety thyme, as listed by Michael Pollan in a *New York Times Magazine* article:

> *4-Terpineol, alanine, anethole, apigenin, ascorbic acid, beta carotene, caffeic acid, camphene, carvacrol, chlorogenic acid, chrysoeriol, eriodictyol, eugenol, ferulic acid, gallic acid, gamma-terpinene isochlorogenic acid, isoeugenol, isothymonin, kaempferol, labiatic acid, lauric acid, linalyl acetate, luteolin, methionine, myrcene, myristic acid, naringenin, oleanolic acid, p-coumoric acid, p-hydroxy-benzoic acid, palmitic acid, rosmarinic acid, selenium, tannin, thymol, tryptophan, ursolic acid, vanillic acid.*

And that's just thyme.

So we must have it all figured out, right? My vote: not a chance. Pollan offered the list to make the same point:

It's also important to remind ourselves that what reductive science can manage to perceive well enough to isolate and study is subject to change, and that we have a tendency to assume that what we can see is all there is to see. When William Prout isolated the big three macronutrients, scientists figured they now understood food and what the body needs from it; when the vitamins were isolated a few decades later, scientists thought, O.K., now we really understand food and what the body needs to be healthy; today it's the polyphenols and carotenoids that seem all-important. But who knows what the hell else is going on deep in the soul of a carrot?

Never forget:

1. We can only determine deficiencies for things we've isolated.
2. Taking those isolated nutrients outside of whole foods can produce side effects we cannot predict.

Scurvy was a mysterious problem for thousands of years. Only in 1932 did scientists isolate vitamin C and determine that the two were related.

Much later, when beta-carotene became popular in the media as a miracle molecule, we took a more proactive approach and began to supplement. Better safe than sorry, right? Unfortunately, as we found out, taking supplemental beta-carotene by itself can cause problems. It can block the absorption of other beneficial carotenoids and increase the risk of prostate cancer and intracerebral haemorrhage, among other things. It's best absorbed in combination with its close cousins in whole foods, in naturally accuring ratios.

There will be similar mistakes and discoveries in years to come.

In cases where I can find an indigenous population that has lived without a food group for hundreds of years (fruit, for example, which is easy), I don't worry much about excluding it. If I can't find such a group, I'd suggest that our science hasn't caught up with Darwinism.

Eater beware.

My general guideline, what I refer to as "Darwin's Rule", is simple: eat for optimal fertility and everything else falls into place.

Moreover, if you eat for optimal fertility, you will have high-level athletic performance and what most define as optimal health. No matter which diet you choose, I encourage you to have the following tests, as a minimum, every six months. If you are eliminating animal products entirely, I suggest every three months.

All of these tests are common enough that your general practitioner or primary care doctor should, in theory, be able to order them. In many cases, insurance will cover them, but be willing to ante up in cash if needed. If you chose to be vegan, this is not the place to cut costs. Some primary care doctors will not feel comfortable administering the fancier gynaecological tests and will refer you to an ob/gyn specialist. That's fine: just get them done.

You don't need to know what all of these mean; you just need to photocopy them and have a conversation with your doctor.[17]

If male, have these tests:

Semen analysis (includes volume, which should be >1.5 ml; concentration/count > 20 million/ml; motility > 40%; morphology > 30% normal by WHO criteria)

Testosterone (both total and free)

Estradiol

Luteinizing hormone (LH)

Follicle-stimulating hormone (FSH) (tests hypothalamus functioning)

Prolactin (pituitary level)

Total cholesterol (160–200)

AST (20–30)

ALT (20–30)

If female, have these tests:

Estradiol

Luteinizing hormone (LH)

Follicle-stimulating hormone (FSH) (tests hypothalamus functioning)

Prolactin (pituitary level)

Total cholesterol (160–200)

AST (20–30)

ALT (20–30)

Day 3 FSH and E2 (estradiol) blood tests (looks at ovarian reserve; the doctor can also do an antral follicular count by ultrasound and/or check anti-muellerian hormone by blood)

Those are the basics. For women, it can pay to take a slightly more detailed look at things:

1) It may seem obvious, but a woman first needs to have periods to see if she is ovulating. It is important to be off of oral contraceptives to determine this. Unfortunately, some doctors prescribe "the pill" to vegetarians to initiate menstruation, which simply masks symptoms instead of addressing root causes. Do an **over-the-counter urine LH test**, starting at approximately day 9 (most women have LH peak and subsequent ovulation 24–36 hours

17. Special thanks to Dr. Nassim Assefi, TED Fellow and internist specializing in women's health and global medicine, for help with this testing section. I added several tests not common to fertility testing, such as total cholesterol and liver enzymes.

later during days 12–15). Using urine LH test strips is much easier than doing basal body temperatures and looking for a rise in temperature after ovulation.

2) To check the uterus and fallopian tubes: do a **hysterosalpingogram (HSG)** (dye shot into cervix and imaging) and/or saline sonohystogram (the former is a better test)

3) To check the luteal phase, do a **"pooled" progesterone test** in the luteal phase—five to nine days after the LH surge, on three days in the second half of the cycle. Determine average progesterone.

The upshot of all this:

There is no sin in considering consuming animal products once per week if you are currently a vegan, if it means you will be healthier and better able to convert others to a similar mode of eating. The ideal is, of course, to find a mode that is farsighted on both a personal and a global level. The mistake is to pursue the latter and ignore the former.

Even Dave "The Man" Scott, six-time winner of the Hawaii Ironman Triathlon and famed vegetarian athlete, returned to eating meat after competing for years on a 99% PPBD. Though he hasn't eaten red meat in 33 years, he now consumes fish, chicken and turkey.

> *The irony of the whole situation is that when I switched back to chicken and fish, I was far leaner and felt more powerful. I mean, I was in better shape in my 40s as a meat eater than I ever was on a strictly plant-based diet.... When I did Ironman in '94, I felt like my strength, recovery, and muscle endurance was better than ever.*

Just because you don't want kids now, there is no reason to create hormonal issues that affect everything from cognition to sexual function. I've seen too many lives disrupted by diet-induced hormonal problems. Think ahead.

For my personal story, see "Sex Machine I: Adventures in Tripling Testosterone".

Good luck and do your homework. It can be a confusing jungle out there, but there are ways to simplify. It's my hope that the five-step progression in the last chapter helps you improve yourself and the world around you, one conscious meal at a time.

Small changes matter.

TOOLS AND TRICKS

The Good Guide (http://www.goodguide.com/) Founded by Professor Dara O'Rourke of the University of California–Berkeley, this "for-benefit" start-up provides a consumer guide to common products, ranking each by health, impact on the environment and impact on society. What chemicals are in your baby shampoo? Was sweatshop labour used to make your T-shirt? Is that whole-grain cereal really good for you? Good Guide can tell you, and help direct your buying behaviour.

Additional Interviews (www.fourhourbody.com/vegan-athletes) Nate Green, who helped research this chapter, was able to interview the following vegans and former vegetarians, among others: Brendan Frazier, Bill Pearl (multiple-time Mr. America and Mr. Universe winner), Mike Mahler, and Dave Scott. I also interviewed Scott Jurek and rock-climbing phenom Steph Davis. All of them are available online.

Howard Lyman, *Mad Cowboy: Plain Truth from the Cattle Rancher Who Won't Eat Meat* (Scribner, 2001) (www.fourhourbody.com/cowboy) This is one of three books (the others were Andrew Weil's *Spontaneous Healing* and *8 Weeks to Optimal Health*) that convinced Scott Jurek to become a vegan. Howard Lyman, a third-generation cattle rancher, appeared on *Oprah* and was a party in her legal battle with Texas cattle ranchers.

Lierre Keith, *The Vegetarian Myth* (www.fourhourbody.com/myth) This is a look at the flip side. Lierre Keith was a vegan for 20 years. She no longer is, and this book explores the moral, eco-political, and nutritional realities of veganism that led her to re-incorporate limited animal products into her diet. Reference-rich and well-written, it is easily the most engrossing book on these topics that I have ever read.

Beyond Vegetarianism (www.beyondveg.com) BeyondVeg, curated by vegetarian Thomas E. Billings, features reports from veterans of raw-food and vegetarian diets (including veganism and fruitarianism), plus new scientific discoveries from clinical nutrition. The intent of the site is to discuss the serious problems that can occur on alternative diets but often go unreported. How have dieters solved their problems, whether by modifying the diet in some "unapproved" way while remaining vegetarian, or by adopting non-vegetarian options? BeyondVeg is one of the best compendiums of answers I've found.

Bonus Material

This book isn't just what you hold in your hands. Using passwords hidden in this book, you can access some of the most entertaining material that didn't make it in. Here are just a few samples:

Spot Reduction Revisited: Removing Stubborn Thigh Fat
Becoming Brad Pitt: Uses and Abuses of DNA
The China Study: A Well-intentioned Critique
Heavy Metal: Your Personal Toxin Map
The Top 10 Reasons Why BMI Is Bogus
Hyperclocking and Related Mischief: How to Increase Strength 10% in One Workout
Creativity on Demand: The Promises and Dangers of Smart Drugs
An Alternative to Dieting: The Body Fat Set Point and Tricking the Hypothalamus

For this and much more, visit the free message boards (where I also post answers and suggestions) at www.fourhourbody.com.

Join us and see how simple big changes can really be.

ACKNOWLEDGEMENTS

First, I must thank the self-experimenters, scientists and athletes whose incredible methods are the lifeblood of this book, including those who preferred to remain anonymous. Even if your name doesn't appear in these pages, your contributions are no less spectacular. If I've omitted anyone by accident, I can only offer my sincerest apologies. Please reach out to me if I somehow lapsed, and I'll make amends.

To Stephen Hanselman, the best agent in the world, I thank you for "getting" the book at first glance and helping to midwife it into existence. From negotiation to non-stop jazz, you amaze me.

Heather Jackson, your insightful editing and incredible cheerleading has made this book a pleasure to write. Thank you for believing in me! To the entire Crown Publishing team, especially those whom I bother (because I love them) more than four hours a week, you are the backbone of this book: Tina Constable, Maya Mavjee, Michael Palgon, Linda Kaplan, Karin Schulze, Jacqueline Lebow, Jill Flaxman, Meredith McGinnis, Jill Browning, Mary Choteborsky, Robert Siek, Elizabeth Rendfleisch, Tara Agroskin and Jennifer Reyes. This book was also first drafted using Scrivener, a gorgeous application, and Keith Blount kept me sane as I tested the limits of the software.

I owe particular gratitude to Charlie Hoehn and Alexandra Carmichael. Where to begin?

Charlie, you were a co-creator and co-conspirator from the very earliest stages. I can only hope that the end product makes you proud. God knows we pulled enough all-nighters over Casino Royale to kill a giraffe, and they only need 1.5 hours of sleep per night. The Photoshop was priceless, and I only regret I didn't have more shiny, full-colour chapters to give you migraines. Many future adventures await, and the mischief alone will be the stuff of legend. Alexandra, you are a princess and a brilliant mind. This book would not exist without your research and your ability to weave enjoyable stories from journal-bound science. I couldn't have done it without you. CureTogether.com rocks!

To Nate Green, the interviews (and therefore several chapters) quite simply wouldn't have been possible without your help. Thank you for the much-needed save and the deadlift kick-in-the-ass. I'll stick with sumo.

To Jack Canfield, you are an inspiration and have shown me that it is possible to make it huge and still be a wonderful, kind human being. *The 4-Hour Workweek,* which gave me permission to write this book, was just an idea until you encouraged me to take the leap. I cannot thank you enough for your wisdom, early support, and incredible friendship.

To Sifu Steve Goericke and Coach John Buxton, who taught me how to act in spite of fear and fight like hell for what I believe, this book—and my life—is a product of your influence. Bless you both. The world's problems would be far fewer if young men had more mentors like the two of you.

Last but not least, this book is dedicated to my parents, Donald and Frances Ferriss, who have guided me, encouraged me, loved me and consoled me through it all. I love you more than words can express.

PHOTO AND ILLUSTRATION CREDITS

Grateful acknowledgement is made to the following for permission to use their photographs, illustrations and graphics.

Page 33 © Philippe Halsman, The Halsman Archive
Page 43 © James Duncan Davidson
Page 44 © Marty Chobot, National Geographic Stock
Page 48 © Luiz Da Silva PhD
Page 49 © Body Composition Center, Redwood City, California
Page 56 © Trevor James Newell, Ray Cronise, Mike Wolfsbauer, Nathan Zaru
Page 57 © Anonymous, Erin Rhoades, Julee, Andrea Bell
Page 65 © Ramit Sethi
Page 68 © Phil Libin
Page 86 © Deborah Chud MD
Page 97 © Courtesy of author
Pages 108 and 109 © B. Jeffrey Madoff
Page 110 © Glenn McElhose
Pages 123, 126, and 131 © Ray Cronise
Page 135 © DexCom International
Pages 138, 140, and 141 © Courtesy of author
Page 154 © Wikipedia Commons: Harbin, Klaus Hoffmeier
Pages 159 and 160 © Mark Reifkind
Page 161 © Courtesy of author
Page 163 © Mark Reifkind
Pages 165 and 167 © B. Jeffrey Madoff
Page 172 © Courtesy of author
Page 175 © Mike Moran
Page 176 © B. Jeffrey Madoff
Pages 178 and 179 © B. Jeffrey Madoff
Pages 184 and 185 © Courtesy of author
Page 188 © Photos taken by Inge Cook, provided courtesy of Ellington Darden PhD
Pages 198, 199, 200, 201, 202, 211, and 212 © B. Jeffrey Madoff
Page 234 Used with Permission of the Author
Page 290 © Dustin Curtis

Pages 294, 295, and 296 © Courtesy of author
Page 301 © Phil Hoffmann Archive
Pages 306, 309, and 312 © Courtesy of author
Page 315 © Fotosearch
Pages 332–334 © Gray Cook
Page 333 © Courtesy of author
Page 341 © Gray Cook and Brett Jones
Pages 352 and 356 © B. Jeffrey Madoff
Page 358 © Courtesy of author
Page 363 © B. Jeffrey Madoff
Page 375 © Tertius A. Kohn PhD
Pages 376, 377, and 378 © Courtesy of author
Pages 381, 382, and 383 © Brian MacKenzie
Page 406 © Pavel Tsatsouline
Page 410 © Mike Lambert, *Powerlifting USA* Magazine
Page 415 © Barry Ross
Page 416 © Mike Lambert, *Powerlifting USA* Magazine
Page 421 © Pavel Tsatsouline
Pages 430 and 431 © Courtesy of author
Pages 437, 438, and 439 © Terry Laughlin
Pages 447 and 448 © Jaime Cevallos
Page 448 © Major League Baseball Photos
Pages 448–451 (besides MLB above) © Jaime Cevallos
Page 477 © Fotosearch
Page 485 © Universal Uclick
Pages 501 and 502 © Courtesy of author
Page 524 © Katie Hoehn

INDEX

B

C

D

L

M

Q

R

S

T

ABOUT THE AUTHOR

TIMOTHY FERRISS, nominated as one of *Fast Company*'s "Most Innovative Business People of 2007", is the author of the #1 *New York Times, Wall Street Journal* and *BusinessWeek* bestseller *The 4-Hour Workweek,* which has been published in 35 languages.

Wired magazine has called Tim "The Superman of Silicon Valley" for his manipulation of the human body. He is a tango world record holder, former national kickboxing champion (Sanshou), guest lecturer at Princeton University, and faculty member at Singularity University, based at NASA Ames Research Center.

He has been featured by more than 100 media outlets, including the *New York Times, The Economist, TIME, Forbes, Fortune,* CNN and CBS, and his blog is one of *Inc.* magazine's "19 Blogs You Should Bookmark Right Now". When not acting as a human guinea pig, Tim enjoys speaking to organizations ranging from Nike to the Harvard School of Public Health.

Find his latest case studies and experiments at
www.fourhourbody.com